Allergic Diseases: A Clinical Approach

Allergic Diseases:
A Clinical Approach

Edited by Trisha Coppola

hayle
medical

New York

Hayle Medical,
750 Third Avenue, 9ᵗʰ Floor,
New York, NY 10017, USA

Visit us on the World Wide Web at:
www.haylemedical.com

ISBN: 978-1-63241-643-8

Cataloging-in-Publication Data

Allergic diseases : a clinical approach / edited by Trisha Coppola.
   p. cm.
Includes bibliographical references and index.
ISBN 978-1-63241-643-8
1. Allergy. 2. Allergy--Immunological aspects. 3. Clinical immunology.
I. Coppola, Trisha.
QR188 .A44 2019
616.97--dc23

Table of Contents

Preface

The main aim of this book is to educate learners and enhance their research focus by presenting diverse topics covering this vast field. This is an advanced book which compiles significant studies by distinguished experts in the area of analysis. This book addresses successive solutions to the challenges arising in the area of application, along with it; the book provides scope for future developments.

Allergic diseases are the conditions of the human body that are induced due to a hypersensitivity of the immune system, usually in response to non-toxic substances in the environment. Some allergic diseases are anaphylaxis, atopic dermatitis, allergic asthma, food allergies and hay fever. Some symptoms of such allergic diseases are sneezing, an itchy rash, shortness of breath, red eyes or swelling. Allergens such as pollen, metals, medications and insect stings can also cause allergic reactions. The diagnosis of this is based on a review of the medical history of a person or through testing of the blood or skin. Allergic diseases are treated by the use of medications such as antihistamines and steroids, epinephrine, allergen immunotherapy, etc. This book covers in detail some existing theories and innovative concepts revolving around allergic diseases and their management. The objective of this book is to give a clinical view of the different aspects of allergic diseases. It will help the readers in keeping pace with the rapid changes in this field.

It was a great honour to edit this book, though there were challenges, as it involved a lot of communication and networking between me and the editorial team. However, the end result was this all-inclusive book covering diverse themes in the field.

Finally, it is important to acknowledge the efforts of the contributors for their excellent chapters, through which a wide variety of issues have been addressed. I would also like to thank my colleagues for their valuable feedback during the making of this book.

Editor

Genetic Aspects of Respiratory Allergy

Celso Pereira, Frederico S. Regateiro, Graça Loureiro, Beatriz Tavares and António Martinho

1. Introduction

Genetic and environmental factors contribute to the pathogenesis of asthma [44]. A clear familial incidence and genetic susceptibility was recognized in early XXth century and subsequent studies established high levels heritability [14, 42, 49, 67]. Analysis of genetic association to asthma susceptibility and disease traits has long been used to try and identify pathways involved in asthma pathogenesis and potential therapeutic targets.

In this chapter we review the recent advances in the understanding of the genetic factors contributing to asthma development. We also discuss some of our recent results on the association between allergic asthma and human leukocyte antigen (HLA) and cytokine loci. We present gene and protein expression analysis for some of these relevant disease markers in the context of allergen challenging of asthmatic patients.

1.1. Genetic studies

Asthma is a complex disease with heterogeneous presentations in different populations [44]. These variable presentations have been grouped into "endotypes" [41]. The high phenotypic diversity led others to propose that asthma is not a single disease but instead that the term "asthma" has been used to define a spectrum of related, overlapping syndromes [41].

At present, no single gene was found to be determinant for asthma susceptibility or, indeed, disease endotypes. Multiple molecular mechanisms seem to be involved in the pathogenesis of each disease feature and many genetic variations have been associated with risk and/or phenotypes. While some genes seem to contribute to asthma susceptibility, others might specifically influence disease features such as age of onset, atopy, progression (severity) or response to treatment. On the other hand, asthma is a multifactorial disease. In addition to genetic predisposition, there are well-established environmental or developmental factors that interact and influence gene expression [16, 52].

The knowledge in asthma genetics has evolved with the advances in biotechnology. Three major technical approaches have been used to search for associations between genes and disease (or phenotypes): genome-wide linkage studies, hypothesis-driven candidate gene association studies and genome-wide association studies (GWAS).

Genome-wide linkage studies using microsatellite markers performed in families identify chromosome segments associated with disease. Cloning of the "linked" alleles might then lead to the identification of genes and, potentially, to novel disease pathways, as it allows unbiased analysis of the genome. A downside of these linkage followed by positional candidate studies is the difficult study design and their poor resolution, as they often identify broad chromosome regions that might include hundreds of genes.

The sequencing of the whole human genome enabled the study of associations between disease/traits and single nucleotide polymorphisms (SNPs) in particular genes of interest. The candidate genes might be selected for their presumptive functional involvement in disease pathology or for their chromosomal position in a linkage region, or near a previous association signal (positional candidate). Association studies present some advantages over family linkage studies: use of independent case-controls and non-related populations, detect genes with modest effects, have a simpler study design and their results are easier to interpret. On the other hand, the candidate gene approaches require previous knowledge or assumptions about disease pathogenesis and, therefore, do not search for novel genes and pathways.

Linkage and candidate studies have contributed for pivotal discoveries in many monogenic diseases. However, genetic association studies provide limited information as only a small number of genes can be studied at a time. Furthermore, in complex diseases, such as asthma, the contribution of many genes is hard to encompass. Recently, the publication of the Human Genome Project in 2003 (www.genome.gov/) and the International HapMap Project (http:hapmap.ncbi.nlm.nih.gov) in 2005 (The International HapMap Consortium 2003) allowed the development of genome-wide association studies (GWAS), [26, 43]. GWAS analyse hundreds of thousands of genetic variants (such as SNPs) across the whole human genome and search for their association to a disease characteristic by comparing the frequency of a genetic variant among the afflicted population versus a control population. Powerful computational statistics are then required to analyse the data and find significant differences in frequency that support association and suggest involvement in disease pathogenesis. Case-control studies are useful to determine disease susceptibility. For particular disease characteristics, however, the associations might be better explored using case-only studies, comparing phenotypes, severity or response to treatment among subgroups of the diseased population.

GWAS brought significant improvement to previous genetic studies of disease because genetic variants are researched across the whole genome and a great number of patients and controls can be included. Importantly, the search is unbiased and does not require previous knowledge of the disease or the biological pathways involved, allowing the finding of unsuspected genes.

This advantage has, sometimes, proved thorny, as some identified genes have little biological plausibility. One important limitation in GWAS is the low detection of uncommon risk variants, as genotyping platforms mostly include common gene variants.

GWAS have now been used in many diseases with important results [26, 78]. The National Center for Biotechnology Information (part of the National Library of Medicine, USA) compiles data from GWAS performed in many diseases and conditions. Data can be accessed at the Database of Genotype and Phenotype at http://www.ncbi.nlm.nih.gov/gap and at the National Human Genome Research Institute, National Institutes of Health, USA: http://www.genome.gov/gwastudies/.

1.2. Linkage and candidate studies on the susceptibility and phenotypes of asthma

The first genome-wide linkage screening for asthma susceptibility loci was published in 1989 [9] and, in 2002, *ADAM33*, located in chromosome 20, was the first gene associated with asthma by positional cloning [75]. This association has then been replicated numerous times in different populations [27]. Ironically, the function of the encoded metallopeptidase in asthma pathogenesis is still unclear [72]. Only 9 genes were identified by positional candidate studies in linked regions [4, 12, 52]: *ADAM33, DPP10, PHF11, NPSR1, HLA-G, CYFIP2, IRAK3, COL6A5* and *OPN3 / CHML*.

Taking also into consideration the vast literature on candidate gene associations, more than 200 genes have been proposed as asthma related genes through human and murine studies [77]. In 2006, previous to the introduction of GWAS in asthma research, Ober and Hoffjan extensively reviewed the literature and identified a "top10" of genes more frequently associated to asthma [51]: *ADAM33, IL4, IL4RA, IL13, CD14, ADRB2, TNF, HLA-DRB1, HLA-DQB1* and *FCER1B*. Several of these genes are positioned on region 5q31-33, an early recognized and replicated association in linkage studies. This region includes genes for Th2 mediators [22, 51] thought to be involved in asthma development (e.g. IL4 or IL13), and also other genes that might contribute for asthma pathogenesis, such as environment interaction genes (e.g. *CD14*) and drug-response genes (e.g. *ADRB2*). *ADRB2* encodes the β2 adrenergic receptor expressed on bronchial smooth muscle cells and influences both the bronchial tonus and the response to adrenergic medications (e.g. albuterol). Further to asthma susceptibility, it has been associated also with several phenotypes, such as severity [8] or disease persistence into adulthood [24]. HLA genomic region (6p21) also has been repeatedly associated with asthma susceptibility, and in particular the *HLADRB1, HLA-DQB1* and *TNF* genes [45, 58, 60].

1.3. Genome-wide association studies in asthma

In 2007 the first GWAS on asthma susceptibility was published [46]. This study strongly associated gene *ORMDL3* in 17q21 with susceptibility to childhood asthma. This region includes also the gene *GSDBM*. Initially identified in populations of European ancestry [46, 61], many studies have now replicated the association of genes located in 17q21 with childhood-onset asthma and several asthma phenotypes [3, 4] also in Latin American [19, 69],

African American or African Caribbean [69, 19] European American [69], and Chinese [35] populations. *ORMDL3* gene encodes a transmembrane protein localized in the endoplasmic reticulum and may be involved in the endoplasmic reticulum response to stress and inflammation, increasing the unfolded-protein response [6]. The functional connections of *ORMDL3* and *GSDBM* to asthma development are not fully understood. Another GWAS on asthmatic children confirmed the relevance of 17q21 and found a novel association with the gene *DENND1B* (1q31) in children of European and African ancestry [62]. *DENND1B* is expressed by natural killer cells and dendritic cells and predicted to interact with TNF-alpha receptor [62].

So far, 43 GWAS were published on childhood and adult asthma using different populations – search at www.genome.gov, as of August 2014 – and a great deal of information is available about novel genes associations as well as confirmations of relevant genes previously described. This includes studies on asthma susceptibility as well as GWAS on several of asthma phenotypes, e.g., IgE [30], forced vital capacity [40], or response to glucocorticoid treatment [63]. Two important meta-analyses reviewed the published data.

In 2010, the **GABRIEL consortium** published a large-scale GWAS meta-analysis including European ancestry-matched 10365 asthmatic patients and 16110 controls [47]. Asthma was associated with *IL1RL1/IL18R1*, *HLA-DQB1*, *IL33*, *SMAD3*, *IL2R*, *GSDMB* and *GSDMA* genes, and using with a lower threshold to *SLC22A5*, IL13 and *RORA*. A stronger association was found between these genes and childhood-onset asthma than adult onset asthma, except for *HLA-DQ* which associates more with adult-onset. *ORMDL3* and *GSDMB* were associated only to childhood-onset asthma. No significant association was found for severe or occupational asthma. Notably, genes previously associated to asthma in other studies, such as *PDE4D*, *CHI3L1*, *DPP10*, *GPR154* [NPSR1], *ADAM33*, *PHF11*, *OPN3*, *IRAK3*, *PCDH1*, *HLA-G*, and *DENND1B*, were not found to be significantly associated with asthma in this study. High IgE serum levels were associated with previously described *FCER1A*, *IL13*, *STAT6* and *IL4R/IL21R* genes and to a new locus within MHC II – *HLA-DRB1*. Only *IL13* showed some association with asthma, whereas the others genes associated with serum high IgE levels were not associated with asthma. This is somewhat unexpected and suggests that asthma development is not related to the levels of IgE. Only *HLA-DR* was found to associate with high serum IgE levels [47].

The **EVE Consortium** meta-analysis searched for susceptibility genes across ethnic groups in North America: European American, African American or African Caribbean, and Latino ancestries [69]. Notably, four associations with asthma risk were found in all three ethnic groups: 17q21 region, *IL1RL1*, *TSLP* and *IL33*. Remarkably, some of these were associated in the two large published meta-analyses, GABRIEL and EVE [47, 69]. A novel asthma susceptibility locus was described by the EVE consortium at *PYHIN1* specifically in individuals of African ancestry [69].

It seems now clear that some genes are replicated across different populations whereas others seem to be ancestry specific. In another study, 6q14.1 was found to be related to asthma susceptibility in European and African patients [70].

1.4. Biological significance of genetic studies

It is reassuring that many of the genes identified were related to immunological physiopathology, e.g. several cytokines and antigen presentation genes. Particularly, genes coding for cytokines and pathways associated with Th2 cells (e.g. *IL13*, *IL2R*) and regulatory cells (e.g. SMAD, TGF-beta) were among them. This agrees with the vast literature showing roles for these cells in asthma, atopy and immune regulation. The role of epithelial cells in asthma pathogenesis is underlined by the associations with *TSLP*, *IL33* and *IL1RL1* (that encodes for the receptor of IL33, expressed on mast cells, Th2 cells, T-regulatory cells, and macrophages) [47, 69].

Some genes, however, do not immediately relate to immunological pathways. This was the case for *RAD50* [38]. In this study, Li and colleagues found that SNPs on *HLA-DQB1*, *HLA-DQA2* and *RAD50* region were associated with severe or difficult-to-treat asthma. *RAD 50* is a DNA repair gene and a connection with asthma pathogenesis is not obvious. Furthermore, the associated SNPs were found in an intron. Notably, previous research on Th2 cytokine expression in mice showed the presence of a locus control region (LCR) in this location that is an important regulator of the genes encoding the Th2 cytokines interleukins 4, 5 and 13 [33, 34]. Genetic ablation of this LCR did not affect the expression of a linked *RAD50* gene, but reduced long-range intrachromosomal interactions with the promoters of the Th2 cytokine genes. This example shows that some associations require further understanding of genetic or functional interactions of the genes. Nevertheless, some of the associated genes remain with no known immunological or genetic connection to asthma and more information is needed to understand their role in pathogenesis.

1.5. Limitations of GWAS results in asthma

The results obtained so far demonstrate the polygenic and multifactorial nature of asthma. Low levels of replication have been found between GWAS and individual study heritability estimates for the associated genes were found to be low [52] and, therefore, with little prognostic utility. These setbacks might be, at least in part, due to methodological or sampling differences between GWAS. A fundamental question is that some variants might increase risk only in specific individuals and not in others, for instance in the case of some genotype-environmental exposure interactions. Moreover, GWAS underestimate the role of rare genetic variants [65, 70] that might have an overall larger effect than common variants on the proportion of genetic risk for common diseases [15]. Epigenetic mechanisms [13] and epistatic effects might further difficult gene expression analysis [81].

The challenges with GWAS are discussed in further detail elsewhere [77]. Several methods have been proposed to improve the power of GWAS (De 2014). Utilizing a combination of approaches, in which GWAS-type studies are performed using selected SNPs of candidate genes, a strategy was devised and named "prioritized subset analysis" [37]. This strategy combines the strength of GWAS computational statistics with previous knowledge from the literature, allowing for power improvement [37]. Novel mathematical models have been proposed for data analysis in asthma [74].

In the future, the study of complex diseases might incorporate data from whole-genome sequencing [71] or exome sequencing to identify both common and rarer genetic variants in complex diseases [64]. These techniques and analysis are becoming more affordable and feasible on large numbers of individuals and therefore sufficient power will be possible for detecting associations with asthma. A recent study, for example, analysed the role of copy number variants asthma using whole genome sequencing [5].

Genetic approaches require replication and gene expression analysis. Ultimately, *in vitro/ex vivo/in vivo* studies are required to confirm the biological significance and to understand the precise functions of the associated genes in asthma pathogenesis. In this chapter, we analyse the expression of some candidate genes in the context of the allergen-specific response in allergy respiratory patients.

2. Experimental study

2.1. Cytokine single nucleotide polymorphism and HLA expression

2.1.1. Material and methods

2.1.1.1. Subjects

85 voluntary adult patients with respiratory allergy to *Dermatophagoides pteronyssinus* (Dp) under observation in outpatient Immunoallergy were enrolled for study (Group A). This group included patients of both sexes (female= 55; male=30; average age: 30.09±9.22 years), wherein 36 of them had the diagnosis of allergic rhinitis and the others 49 patients had simultaneously allergic asthma and rhinitis diagnosis, according criteria from ARIA and GINA guidelines [2, 20]. At the moment of the study all the patients were under clinical stability, and never were submitted to specific immunotherapy in the past.

Pregnancy, systemic inflammatory illness or other chronic disease, any exacerbation of allergic disease or a respiratory tract infection in the previous month to the study, as well as nasal polyposis or previous nasal surgery in the past were considered exclusion criteria.

2.1.1.2. Methods

DNA was extracted from polymorphonuclear blood cells (PMBC) using MagAttract DNA Blood Mini M48 Kit on the BioRobot *M48*. After extraction, the quality and quantification of DNA was evaluated and PCR -RSSO Cytokine SNP Typing kit from LIFECODES was used to investigate single cytokine polymorphism (SNP's) from 14 cytokines using bead array xMAP™ technology from Luminex™ .

The *HLA* genomic typing to class I (*locus* A and B) and class II (*locus* DR) were obtained from peripheral blood samples. The study of cytokine single nucleotide polymorphisms (SNP's) were also performed in the promoter region of IL-1 (α,β,R,RA), IL-2, IL-4, IL-6, IL-10, IL-12, IFN-γ, TGF-β and TNF-α.

2.1.1.3. Statistical analysis

Statistical analysis was performed using SPSS® Statistics 17.0 software. Were analyzed the frequency distribution for the different qualitative variables. For quantitative variables Average and Standard Deviation (SD) were calculated, according the two patients groups (A and C).

Differences between the two groups were analysed by means of χ^2 tests and Mann–Whitney test (two independent samples) for qualitative and quantitative variables respectively. A statistical significant difference was assumed with $p < 0.05$.

2.1.1.4. Results

In allergic group (A), it was observed a higher genotype frequency of *A*01* and *A*68* alleles, while *A*02* presented a lower frequency (Figure 1), compared to non-allergic healthy group (C). Concerning locus B (Figure 2), the most frequent allele was B*51, while B*35 was less frequent in the allergic population. With respect to HLA class II (Figure 3), the alleles DRB1*03 and DRB1*11 were more frequent in group A, while for DRB1*04 and DRB1*13 it was the opposite. None of these differences was statistically significant. The *A*01 B*08 DRB1*03* haplotype was the most frequent in both groups. Nevertheless in allergic patients the *A*02 B*51 DRB1*11* haplotype was the second most frequent, but the fifth one in healthy individuals (5.8% *vs* 1.4%, p=0.059).

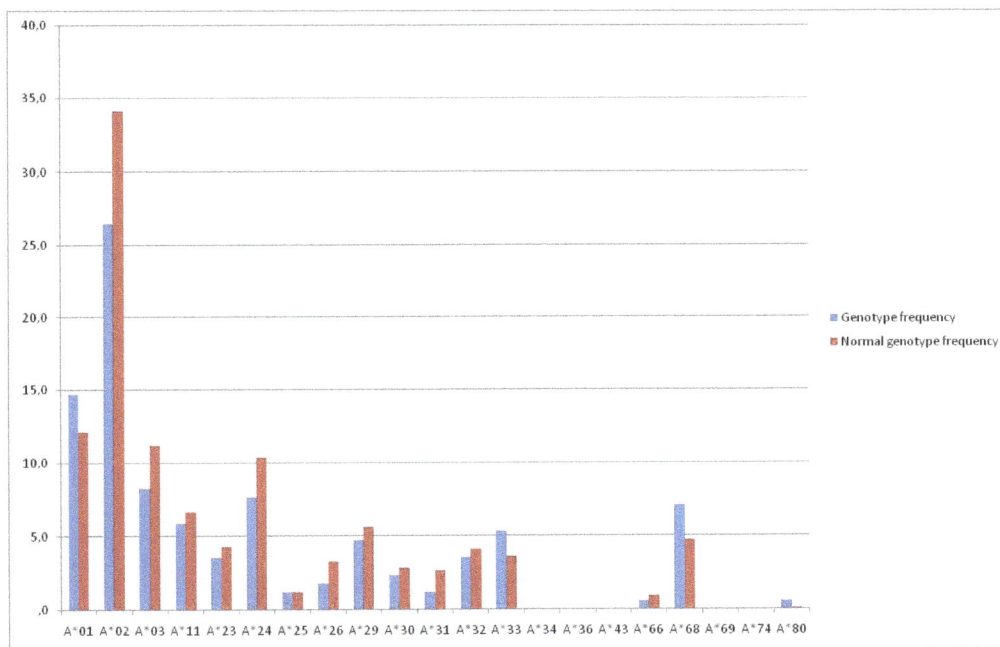

Figure 1. HLA class I, locus A. Frequency distribution of allergic patients (blue) compared to control group (red), not significant

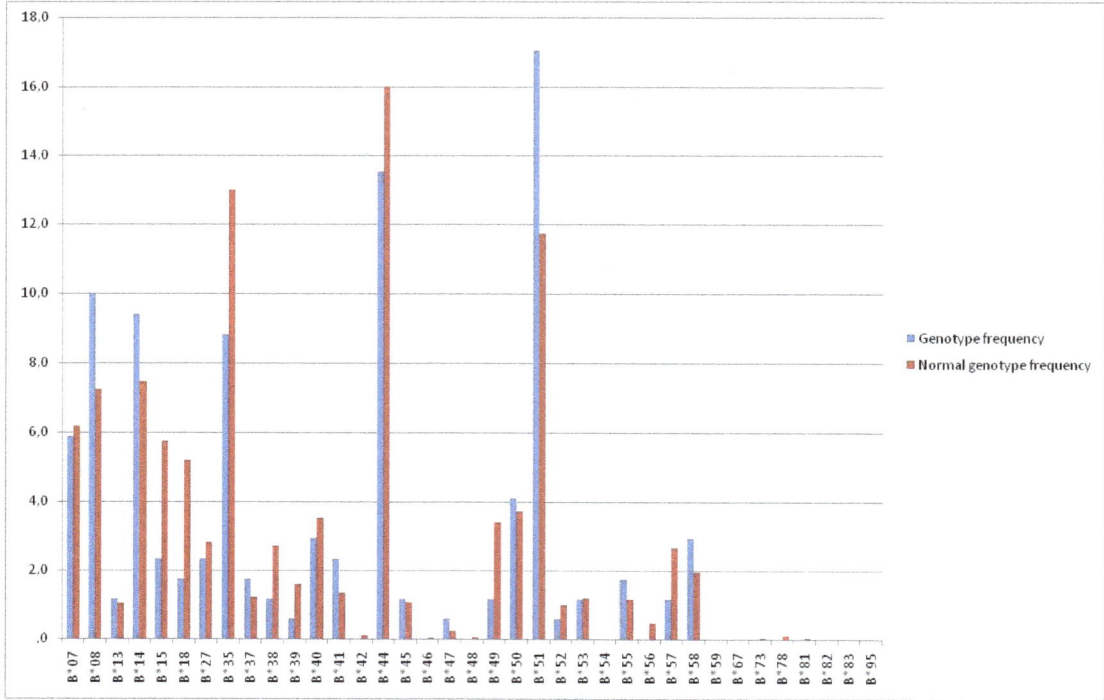

Figure 2. HLA class I, locus B. Frequency distribution of allergic patients (blue) compared to control group (red), not significant

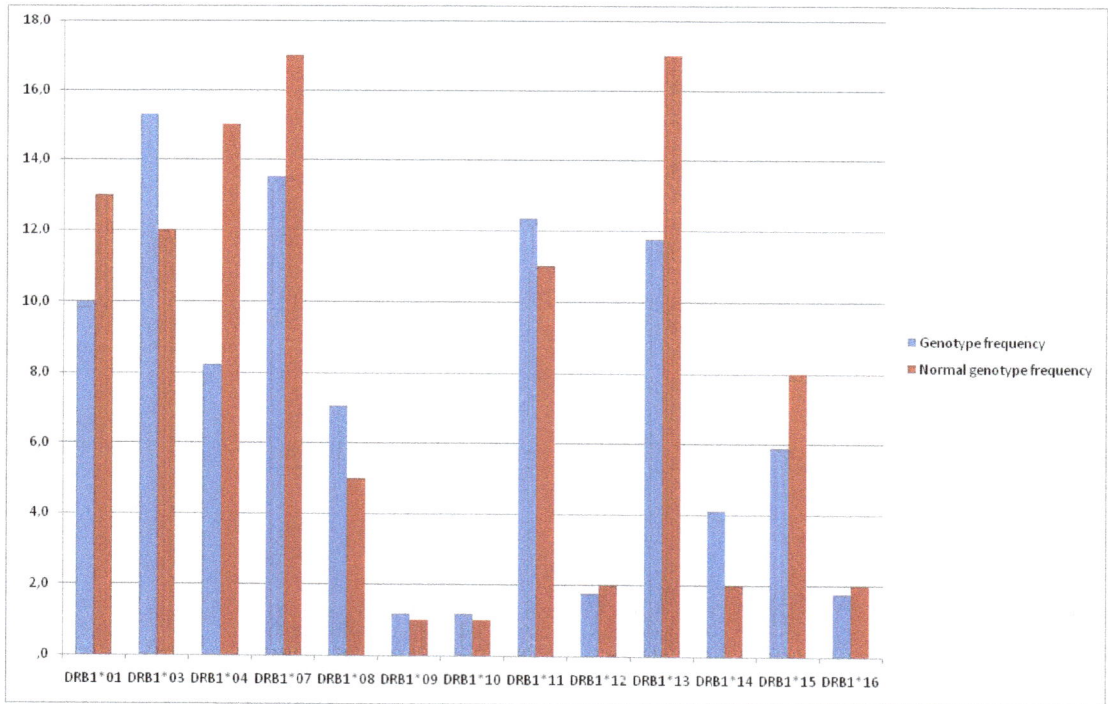

Figure 3. HLA class II, locus DR. Frequency distribution of allergic patients (blue) compared to control group (red), not significant

Results of phenotypic frequency of cytokine single nucleotide polymorphisms (SNP's) in the promoter region for subjects in the study the results are expressed in Figures 4 and 5.

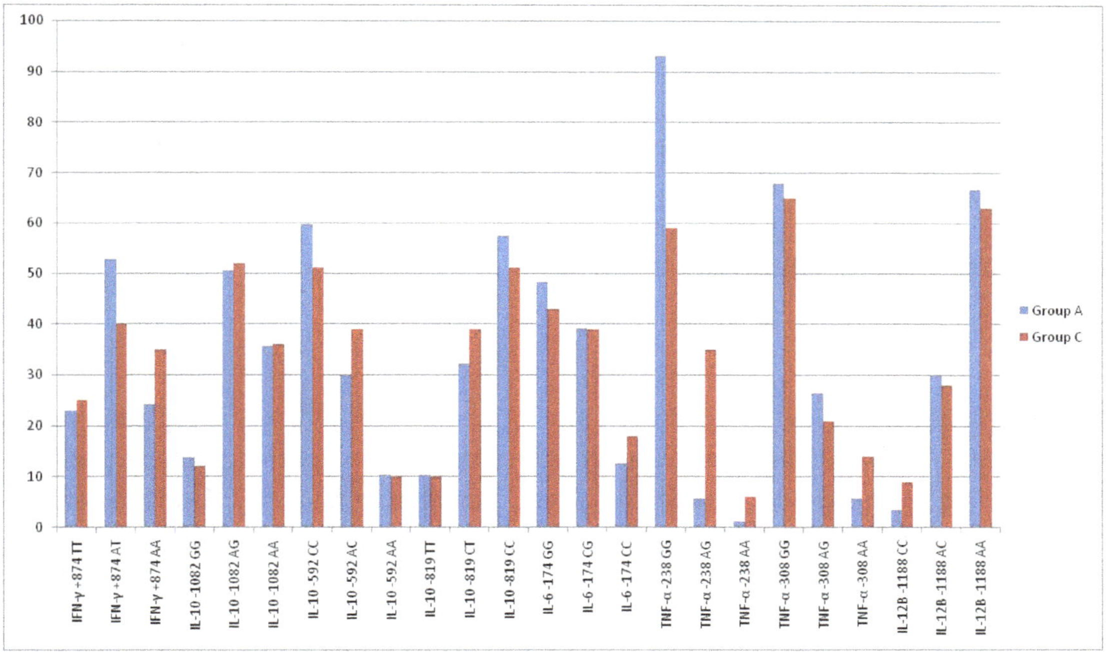

Figure 4. Cytokine single nucleotide polymorphisms (SNP's) : IFNg, IL-10, IL-6, TNFa, and IL-12b Frequency distribution of allergic patients (blue) compared to control group (red)

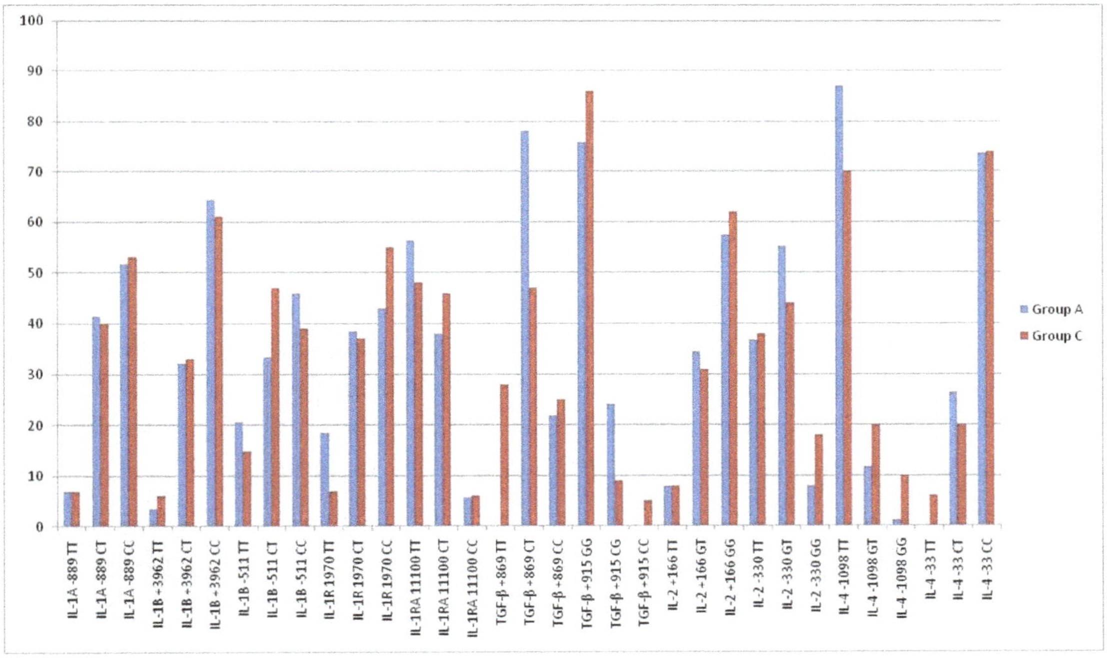

Figure 5. CCL4 gene expression in the patients submitted to CPT and NPT, before challenge (T0) and at 60 and 240 minutes after challenge (individual response values, average and SD).

It was found a higher phenotypic frequency for the following cytokine SNP's: TNFα-238GG (p<0.0001), TGFβ+869CT (p<0.0001) and IL4-1098TT (p=0.003). On the other hand, there were lower frequencies for TNFα-238AG (p<0.0001), TGFβ+915CC (p=0.024) and IL4-1098GG (p=0.005). In the allergic group it was not found any homozygous individual for TGFβ+869TT (p<0.0001), but conversely There was an increase of heterozygous individual compared with the control group (p=0.004).

No differences were observed between patients with concomitant asthma complaints and those with only rhinitis symptoms.

2.2. Gene expression and allergy challenge test

2.2.1. Subjects

From the previous mentioned 85 voluntary adult patients studied, with respiratory allergy to *Dermatophagoides pteronyssinus* (Dp) we selected a sample of 42 patients. These patients were enrolled to being submitted to an specific allergic challenge test, so H1-antihistamines and corticosteroids, either nasal or oral, were stopped 2 weeks and 4 weeks prior to the challenge test, respectively.

The specific allergic challenge test was performed using a standardized lyophilized *Dp* extract by nasal and ocular in 21 patients for each methodological procedure [21]. All patients were submitted to a previous respiratory function test (pletismography using *Master screen Body Jaeger®*) to assure the *standard* safe criteria ($FEV_1 \geq 80\%$ and $FEV_1/FVC \geq 80$).

Symptoms as dyspnoea, thoracic oppression, wheezing or cough were asked to being mentioned to all patients after challenge test.

The local ethics committee approved the study and all the participants gave written informed consent before entry.

2.2.2. Specific nasal and conjunctival challenge tests

All the patients performed skin prick tests with an aqueous extract of *Dp* with 5 mg/ml concentration (23 mg/ml of *Der p 1*, BialAristegui, Bilbao, Spain), with the dilutions of 1/1, 1/10, 1/100 and 1/1000 and negative and positive controls, according to standardized procedures [21, 54] (Dreborg 1993). The concentration used for specific provocation was the minimum that induced a prick test wheal at least equal to that induced by histamine.

All the specific challenge tests were performed after a period of adapting of room temperature for at least 30 minutes, and at the same period of the morning.

Nasal provocation test (NPT) were carry out by the administration of 160μl, corresponding a 2 consecutive puffs, of aerosolized spraying of *Dp* extract administered to the unilateral inferior nasal turbinate of the less congested nostril, and asking patients to perform apnea during the application of the allergen. Conjunctival provocation test (CPT) comprised on the unilateral administration of 50μl, one drop, of allergen extract in the inferior and external quadrant of the bulbar conjunctiva.

Both ocular and nasal symptoms were recorded after challenge test and registered filled at the 1st and the 5th minutes, according specific clinical score system [21, 39].

2.2.3. Clinical score scaling

For evaluation the clinical responses an adaptation of the previously used a nasal clinical score, NCS, [39] and ocular clinical score, OCS, [48] were applied at the 1st and the 5th minutes [21, 54] as well as the total clinical score (TCS), representing the sum of NCS (range: 0-15) and OCS (range: 0-13) ranging from 0 to 28 points.

Although the late record symptoms occurred 5 minutes later after the challenge test all patients remained under strictly clinical observation for at least 4 additional hours. Clinical evaluation scores was interrupted after the 5th minute, but all the patients maintained medical observation during the next 4 hours.

2.2.4. Patient groups

Blood samples were collect to PAXgene blood RNA tubes to all patients before the allergic challenge test (NPT or CPT) and at 60 or 240 minutes, according to the following subgroups.

T0 and T60 minutes	T0 and T240 minutes
CPT	**CPT**
n=11 [F=8+M=3]	n=11 [F=7+M=4]
Age: 28.36±5.0 years [20-36]	Age: 27.90±6.8 years [17-39]
NPT	**NPT**
n=12 [F=6+M=6]	n=10 [F=6+M=4]
Age: 32.5±8.7 years [19-43]	Age: 25.3±7.5 years [18-43]

2.2.5. Methods

Peripheral blood was collected in a PAXGene Blood RNA tube (Qiagen) and total RNA extraction performed with the PAXgene Blood RNA kit (Qiagen) according to the supplier's instructions in a QIAcube BioRobot [59]. Total RNA quantification and RNA integrity evaluation was analyzed using a 6000 Nano Chip kit, in an Agilent 2100 bioanalyzer (Agilent Technologies) and 2100 expert software.

RNA was reverse transcribed with SuperScript III First-Strand Synthesis SuperMix for qRT-PCR (Invitrogen), according to the manufacturer's instructions. Relative quantification of gene expression by real-time PCR was performed in the LightCycler 480 II (Roche Diagnostics).

Real-time PCR reactions were carried out using QuantiTect SYBR Green PCR Master Mix and QuantiTect Primer Assay (Qiagen) and 20 ng of cDNA sample, in a total volume of 10 µl. All samples were run in duplicate.

Real-time PCR results were analyzed with the LightCycler software (Roche Diagnostics). GeNorm Reference Gene Selection kit (PrimerDesign Ltd) in conjunction with the geNorm software (PrimerDesign Ltd.) were used to select the reference genes to normalize data. The normalized expression levels of the genes of interest were calculated by using the delta-Ct method.

2.2.6. Statistical analysis

Statistical analyses were performed using SPSS® Statistics 17.0 software. To determine the statistical significance of the differences observed, the non-parametric Mann–Whitney U-test and Wilcoxon paired-sample test were performed. A statistical significant difference was assumed with $p < 0.05$.

2.2.7. Results

All the patient groups demonstrated clinical positive response to a single dose of *Dp* extract [21], the symptoms were progressively decreasing, without need of therapeutic intervention. There were neither bronchial symptoms nor systemic reactions in any of the provocation tests.

It was observed in most of the patients, even at 60 minutes after challenge, differences in gene expression for cytokines, chemokines and nuclear transcription factors related to allergen exposure.

No differences were observed between patients with only nasal complaints compared to those that had associated clinical asthma.

We did not observe a similar pattern between the two routes of specific allergen challenge and in the two different periods of time in analysis.

Results of some chemokine gene expression after specific allergen challenge test are presented in figures 6 to 8.

The cytokine gene response to allergens did not show a homogeneous profile in the subgroups of patients studied, but it was evident that individually, there were changes in mRNA expression in many patients, as seen in Figures 9 and 12.

So we can distinguish two different groups of patients: one with very high values (also with high values of total serum IgE but without correlation with the clinical severity- data not shown) and the other with low expression of gene levels (Figures 13 and 14). However, this difference was not found for the cytokine receptor gene, IL-4R, Figure 15.

Figures 16-18 show the results of specific response to allergens in genes related to nuclear transcription factors on the four subgroups of patients.

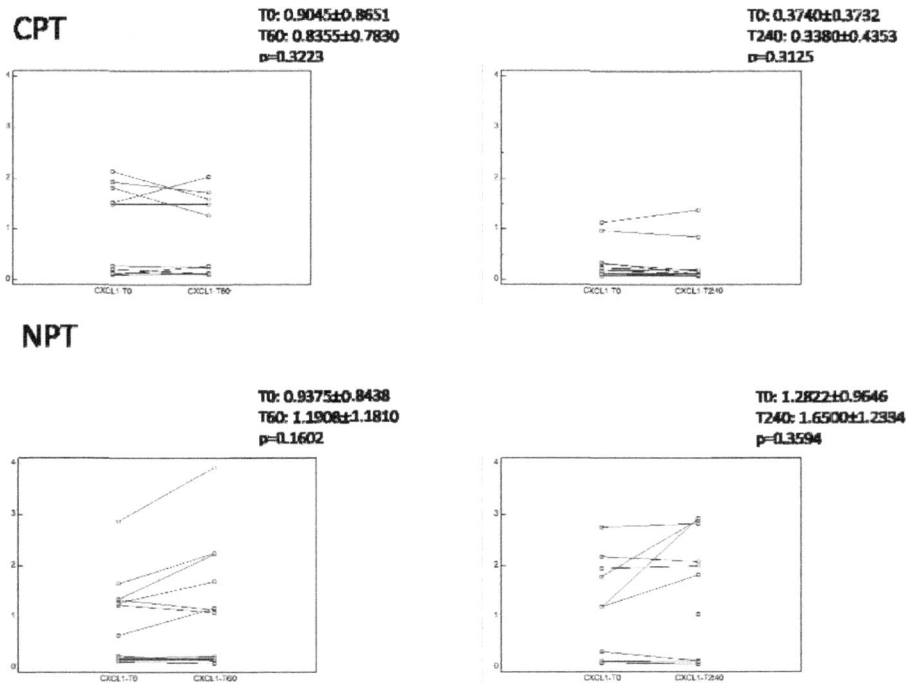

Figure 6. CXCL1 gene expression in the patients submitted to CPT and NPT, before challenge (T0) and at 60 and 240 minutes after challenge (individual response values, average and SD).

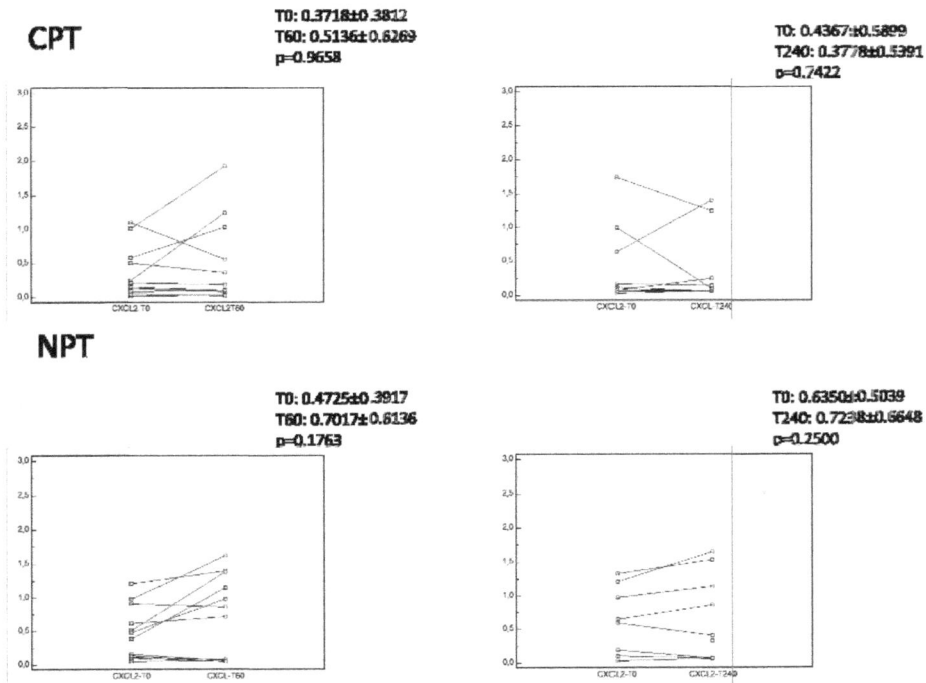

Figure 7. CXCL2 gene expression in the patients submitted to CPT and NPT, before challenge (T0) and at 60 and 240 minutes after challenge (individual response values, average and SD).

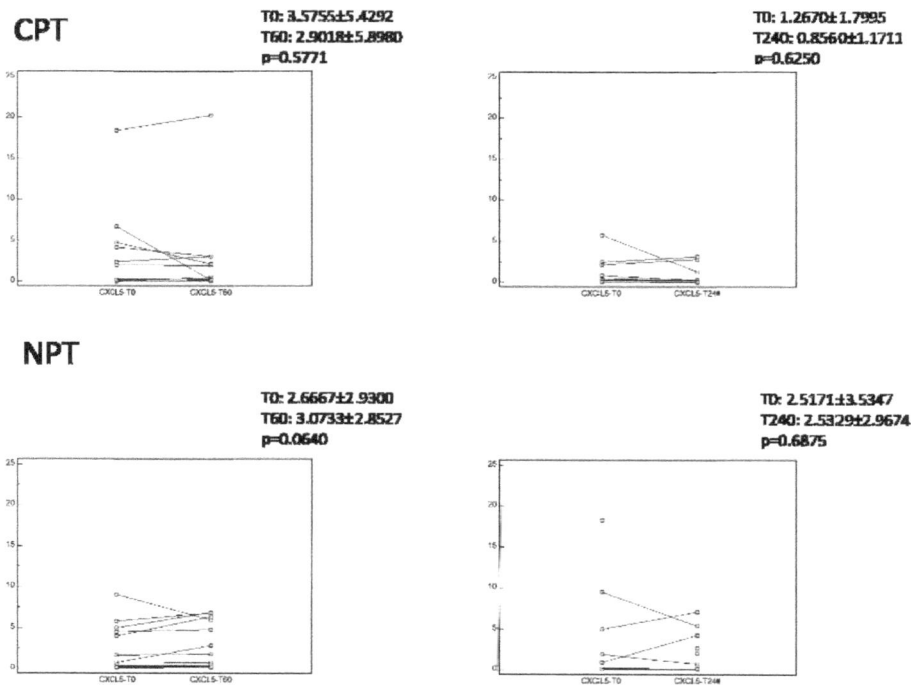

Figure 8. CXCL5 gene expression in the patients submitted to CPT and NPT, before challenge (T0) and at 60 and 240 minutes after challenge (individual response values, average and SD).

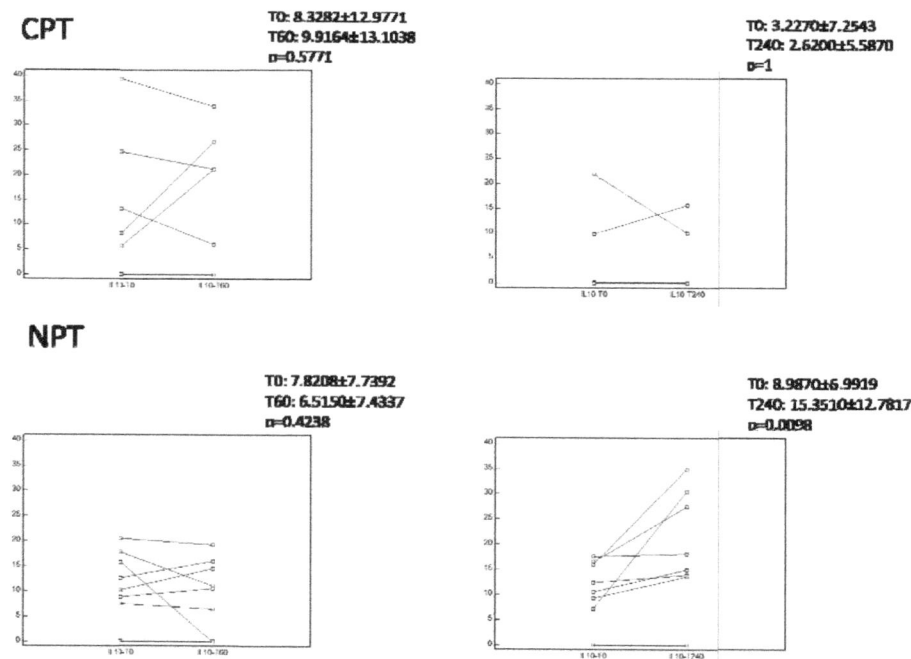

Figure 9. IL-10 gene expression in the patients submitted to CPT and NPT, before challenge (T0) and at 60 and 240 minutes after challenge (individual response values, average and SD).

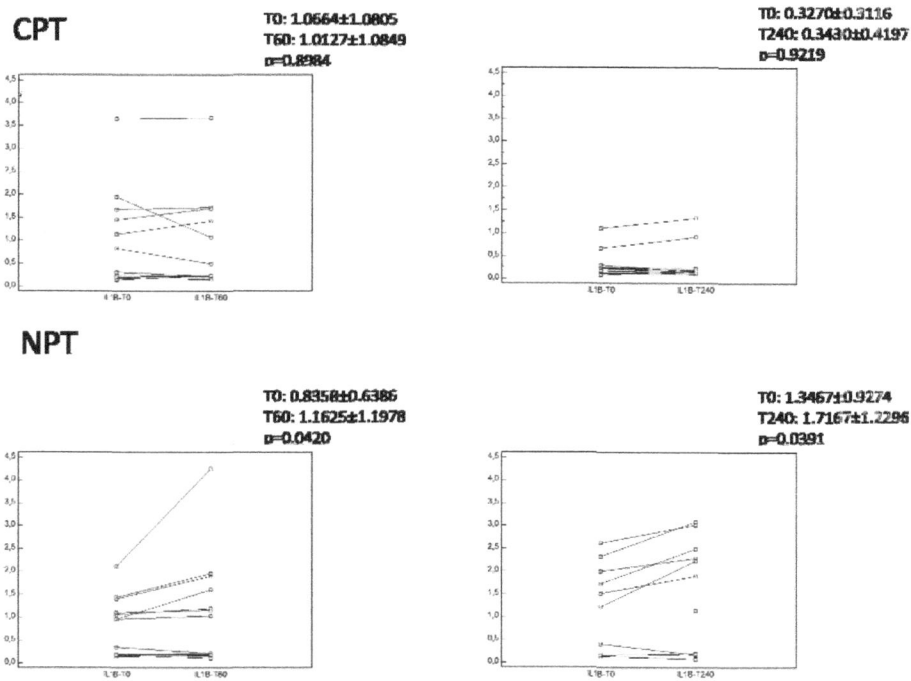

Figure 10. IL-1β gene expression in the patients submitted to CPT and NPT, before challenge (T0) and at 60 and 240 minutes after challenge (individual response values, average and SD).

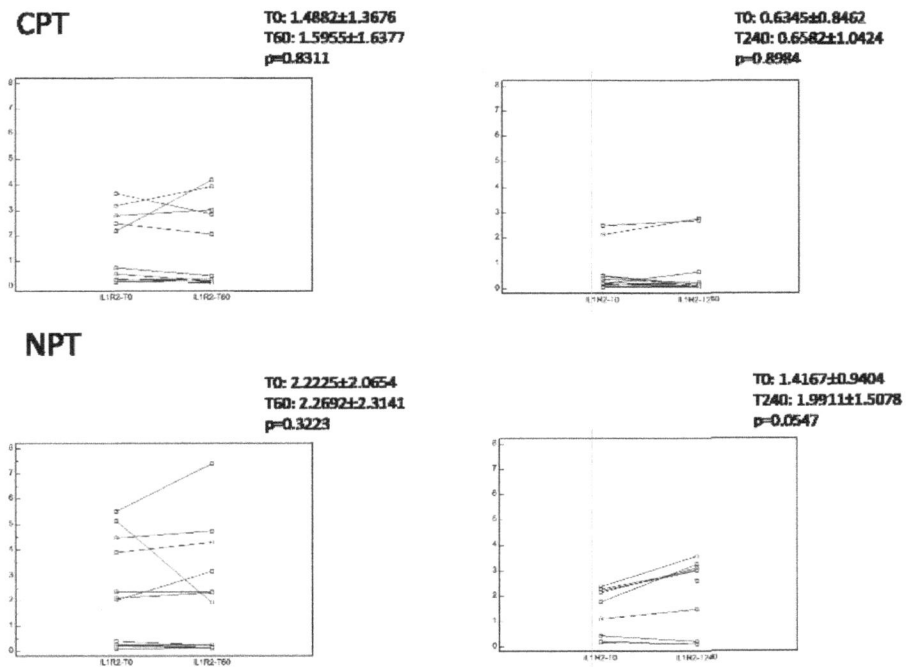

Figure 11. IL-1R2 gene expression in the patients submitted to CPT and NPT, before challenge (T0) and at 60 and 240 minutes after challenge (individual response values, average and SD).

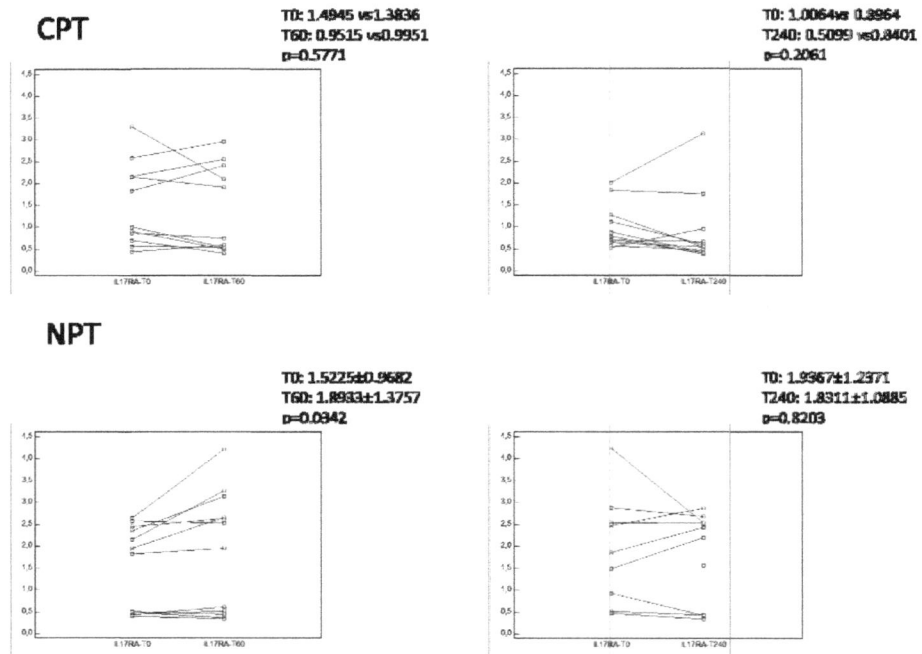

Figure 12. IL-17RA gene expression in the patients submitted to CPT and NPT, before challenge (T0) and at 60 and 240 minutes after challenge (individual response values, average and SD).

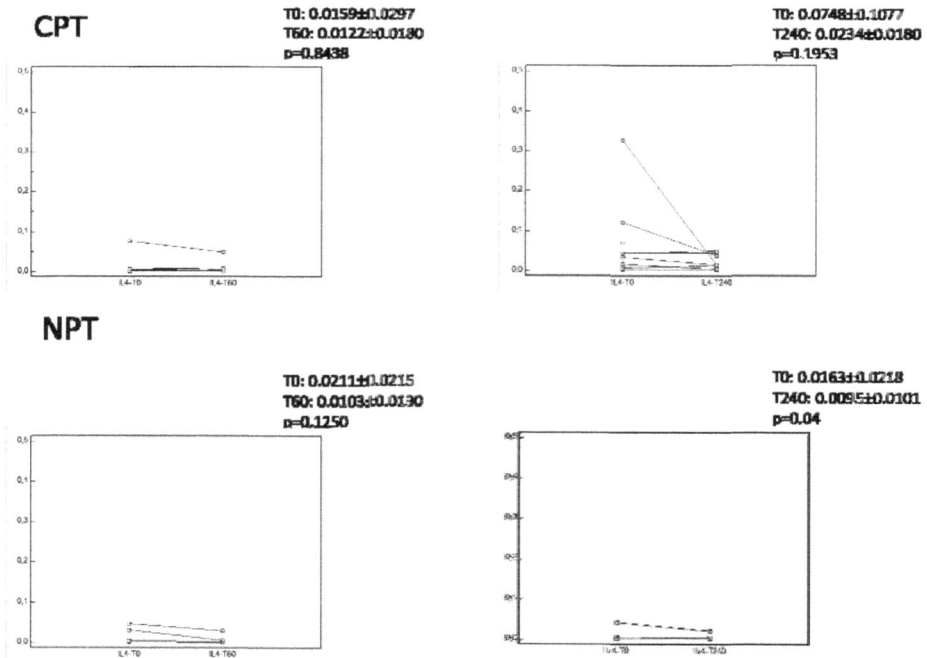

Figure 13. IL-4 (low levels) gene expression in the patients submitted to CPT and NPT before challenge (T0) and at 60 and 240 minutes after challenge (individual response values, average and SD).

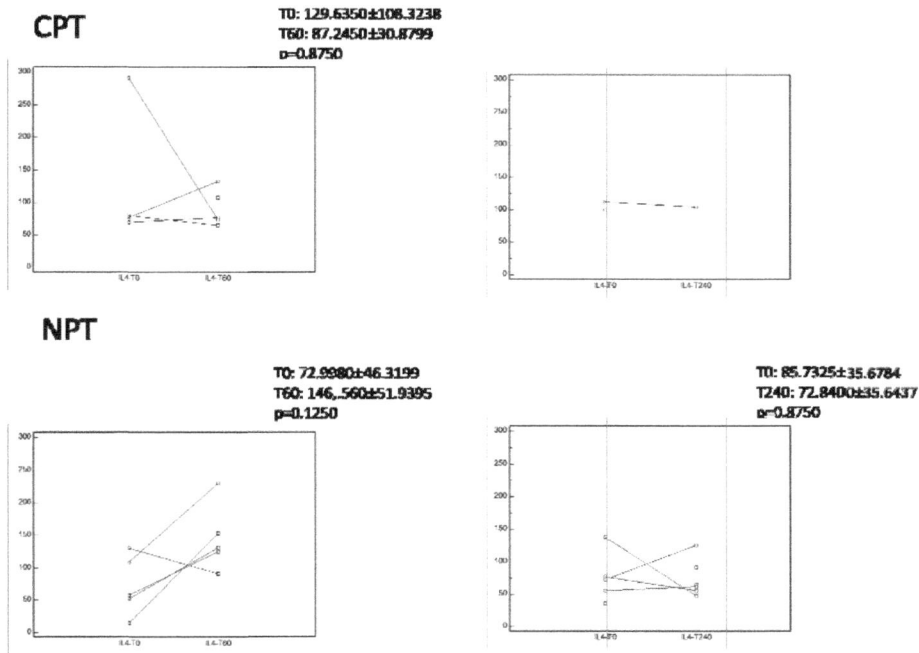

Figure 14. IL-4 (lhigh levels) gene expression in the patients submitted to CPT and NPT, before challenge (T0) and at 60 and 240 minutes after challenge (individual response values, average and SD).

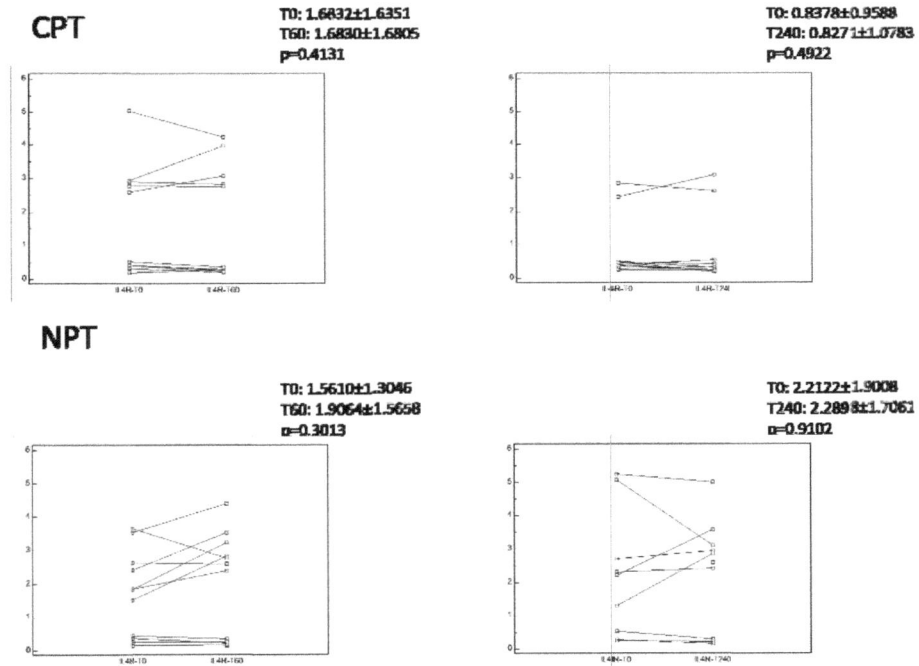

Figure 15. IL-4R gene expression in the patients submitted to CPT and NPT before challenge (T0) and at 60 and 240 minutes after challenge (individual response values, average and SD).

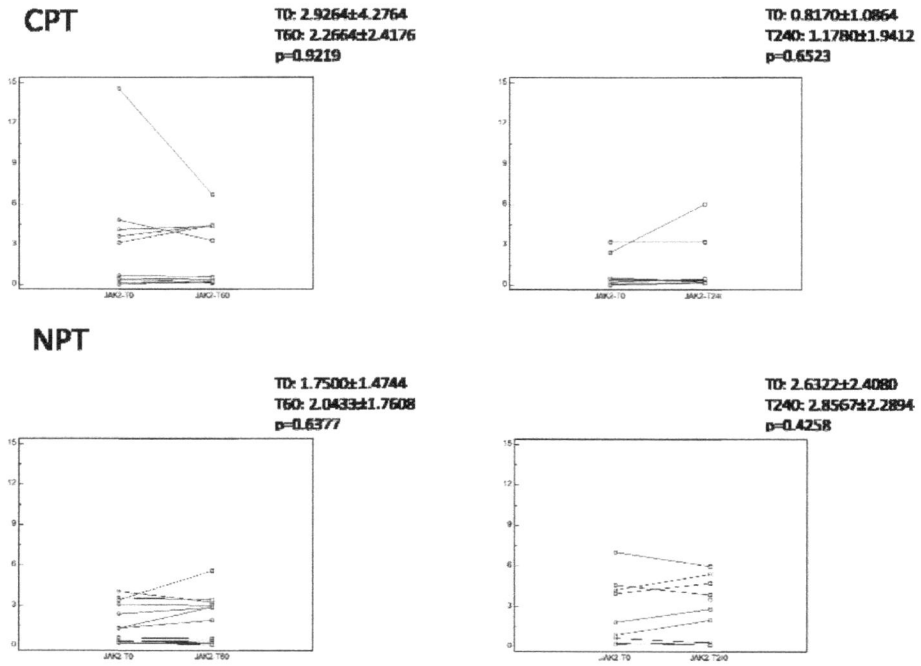

Figure 16. JAK2 gene expression in the patients submitted to CPT and NPT, before challenge (T0) and at 60 and 240 minutes after challenge (individual response values, average and SD).

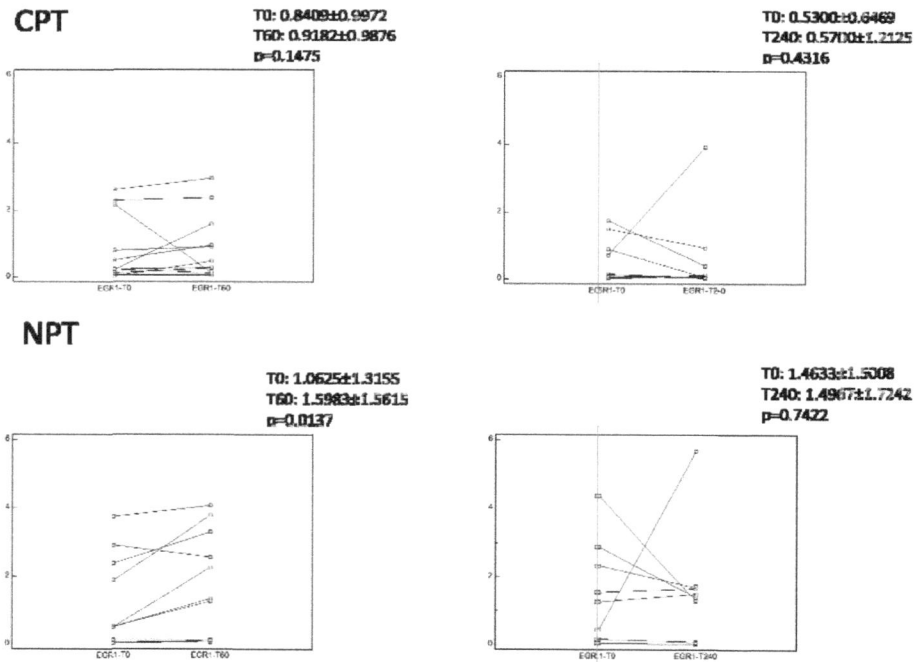

Figure 17. EGR1 gene expression in the patients submitted to CPT and NPT, before challenge (T0) and at 60 and 240 minutes after challenge (individual response values, average and SD).

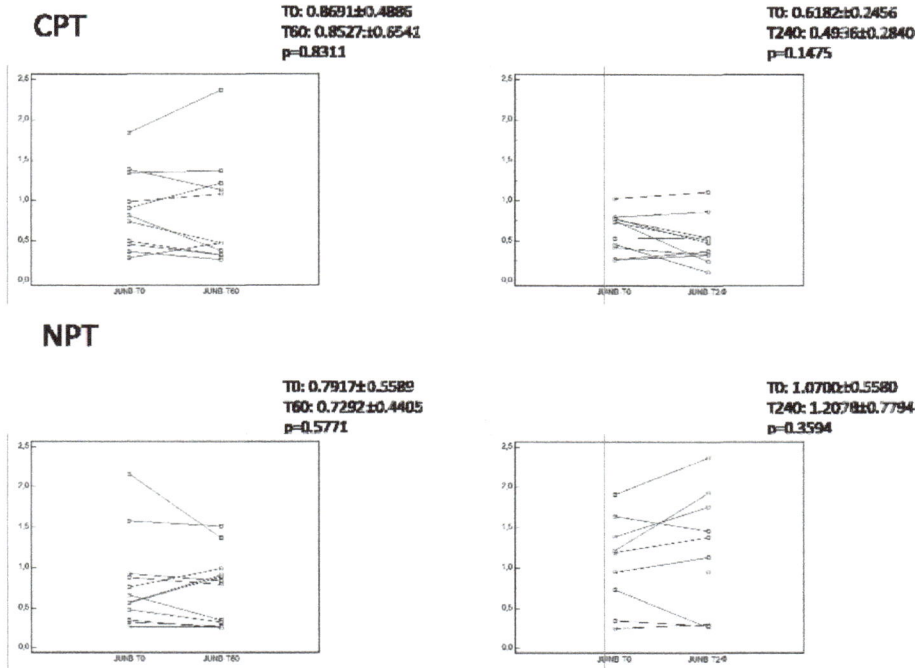

Figure 18. JUNB gene expression in the patients submitted to CPT and NPT, before challenge (T0) and at 60 and 240 minutes after challenge (individual response values, average and SD).

Overall, there seems that does not exist a specific profile of genes in response to cytokines, chemokines and nuclear transcription factors. However, even in first period of time after challenge (T60), many patients showed marked changes, since the beginning of the allergic reaction (Figures 19 to 21).

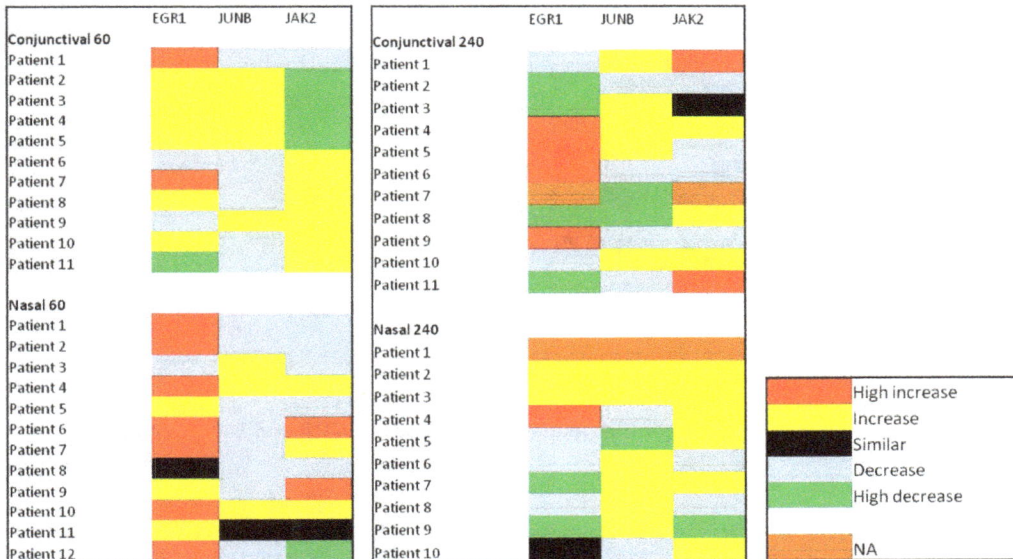

Figure 19. Global nuclear transcription factor gene responses in the patients submitted to CPT and NPT, according to the periods of time in study (A: 60 minutes; B: 240 minutes).

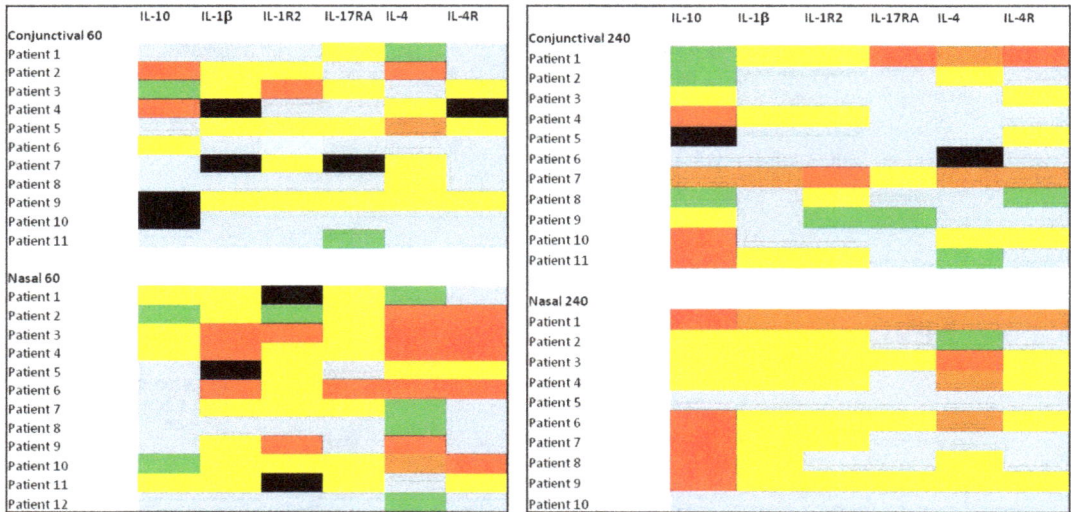

Figure 20. Global cytokine gene responses in the patients submitted to CPT and NPT, according to the periods of time in study (A: 60 minutes; B: 240 minutes).

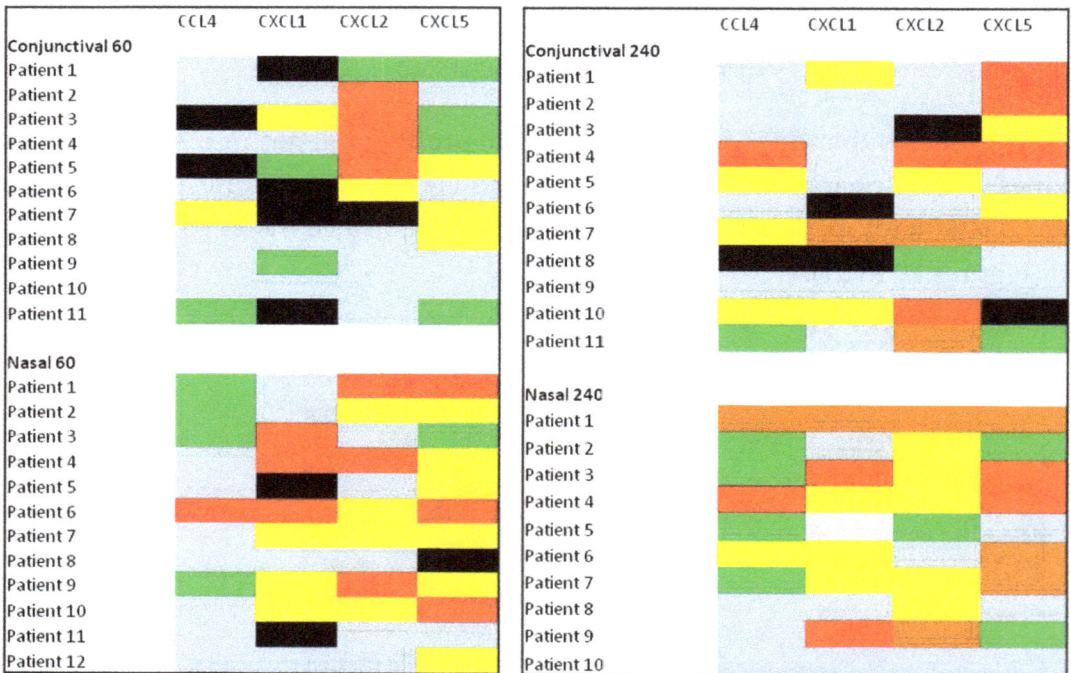

Figure 21. Global chemokine gene responses in the patients submitted to CPT and NPT, according to the periods of time in study (A: 60 minutes; B: 240 minutes).

2.2.8. Discussion

Allergic diseases and particularly respiratory allergy are complex disorders often present in the same family or closely related subjects. Genetic factors undoubtedly contribute to disease susceptibility but the expression of the disease can be modulated by environmental exposures and the interactions between the two. In this context it is emphasized the role of infection, allergens, pollutants, oxidative stress and cytokine dysregulation [50]. In the case of allergy and asthma in particular because they constitute a complex and multifactorial disease, each of the individual factors by itself can determine distinct phenotypes that result in the polarization of distinct cellular pathways, resulting into the final clinical expression.

The last decade has been marked by the publication of a lot of genome-wide association studies (GWAS) in asthma or allergy phenotypes. GWAS have reported novel and interesting genes but have also confirmed the role of some functionally relevant genes previously described. However, heritability of allergic diseases has not been elucidated completely so far [1].

Considering that respiratory allergy, like epigenetic mechanisms, is heritable, nevertheless exists a strongly familial condition (36% to 79% heritability) with a non-Mendelian pattern of inheritance and polymorphisms in more than 100 genes, but these associations have infrequently been replicated, scientifically supported, and so the genetic has explained only a small portion of the cause of this disease [80, 81].

In the selection of the sample of our patients we were intended to be homogenous, in particular to the type of allergen sensitivity, ethnicity and area of residence and similarly of environmental surrounding.

Although we found some more frequent haplotypes in allergic patients we could not identify significant differences compared to healthy subjects. However, the second most frequent haplotype was *A*02 B*51 DRB1*11*, corresponding to the fifth most frequent in control group.

Ours results are according to others studies, namely in Greek allergic children, that also failed to demonstrate a positive correlation between *HLA* haplotypes and allergy to *Dermatophagoides* species [53]. So, as previously reported by a European study, it seems reasonable to assume that specific sensitization is influenced by genetic variants leading to its initiation, as well as to its enhancement [32].

HLA super-locus is a genomic region in the chromosomal position 6p21 [31]. It is highly promising for future research particularly since it carries on the correlation of *HLA-DRB1* in allergic asthma, *HLA-DQB1* in occupational asthma and *HLA-DPB1* in aspirin-sensitive asthma. However, it is difficult to study the role of class II genes *in vivo* because of the tremendous heterogeneity of human population, the strong linkage disequilibrium among different class II genes, and also the highly complexity of MHC.

An interesting issue in this subject is the "epistasis", representing the action between 2-loci, in opposite side to Mendel's classical law of heredity. Epistasis designation applies when two or more loci interact to create a new phenotype, and when an allele at one locus masks or modifies the effects of alleles at one or more other loci. The phenotypic effect of a specific gene mutation entirely depends on the overall genetic background affected by many other gene mutations. Furthermore, the combined effects of more than 2 loci on phenotypes are not simply additive, but are either synergistic or antagonistic [81].

A wide range of studies has demonstrated the enormous variability of clinical phenotypes in allergic disease and respiratory allergy, representing the tremendous variability and gene diversity.

An interesting study, focused on single nucleotide polymorphisms (SNPs) from 17q21 locus, demonstrated scattering different frequencies of SNPs between distinct ethnic populations [36]. Therefore, comparisons of results between different populations are often hazardous as explained earlier.

Regarding the results of SNPs in our patients with respiratory allergy we stress relevant differences concerning IL-4, TNF-α and TGF-β genes.

TNF-α and IL-4 are relevant cytokines interested in the allergic reaction and also promotes the development of Th2 cell response to aeroallergens [7]. In the population that we studied we found strong increment of TNFα-238GG and IL4-1098TT phenotypes compared to healthy individuals. Conversely a decrease in phenotypic expression was found to TNFα-238AG and IL4-1098GG.

TGF-β is a master regulator of the immune response and exerts important anti-inflammatory functions [68] and is deeply involved in allergy. In our allergic patients TGFβ+869CT phenotype had a clearly increased frequency, and the genotype TGFβ+869TT was completely absent compared to healthy population.

So far, as our knowledge, this phenotype was not previously involved in allergy or asthma. A study in cystic fibrosis demonstrated that higher plasma levels of TGFβ1 were observed in patients carrying the TGFβ1 +869TT genotype, intermediate levels for +869CT genotype and low levels to +869CC genotype. Together with these results it was also observed that the +869CC genotype had a more severe phenotype, and the +869TT genotype had the higher rate of decline of lung function, compared to +869CT genotype [17].

The IgE-mediated allergic reaction dictates a premature systemic effect, which will develop simultaneously to immuno-inflammatory mechanisms at the local of allergen exposure. In previous studies we have demonstrated that in parallel to the immediate response that results from an IgE-dependent allergenic mechanism, the cellular response occurs early in the process, and the involvement of the central immune organs is crucial since the beginning of the reaction [54, 55].

In this study we provide evidence that mRNA gene expression take place earlier on peripheral T cells after allergen exposure, at least 60 minutes later. This fact occurs independently of the technique of allergen provocation, in spite of the differences on the mechanisms and cell traffic ways involved, because they are distinct mucosae. Obviously, this modification in the production of mRNA does not imply that all of it will be completed in an efficient manner, particularly since there are strictly necessary requirements in cell regulation and biological skill conditions that allows the synthesis of the protein or its biological mediator.

Naturally, this modification in the production of mRNA does not imply that all of it will be completed in an efficient manner, particularly since in cell regulation there are specific requirements and biological conditions allowing the synthesis of the corresponding protein or its biological mediator.

In this context, it is very important to analyse the individual results in the different subgroups, since the high individual variation does not allow an unequivocal evaluation of the average values of the sample. For this study we did not considered to be relevant the existence of a separate control group of allergic patients, since the time point T0 would be a better internal control [54]. It was also evident that the individual response of each patient is highly variable, most likely depending on the genetic endowment of each patient, although the clinical pattern and the allergic sensitization (Dp) was the same.

During the inflammatory mechanism a set of different cytokine and chemokine molecules are able to promote not only the appropriate regulation of leukocytes and other cells recruitment but also the efficient network that permitting an accurate intracellular signaling control [73].

The existence of 23 chemokine receptors and 48 chemokine ligands guarantees a tight control and fine-tuning of the immune system [83]. Conceptually, it is considered that these biological mediators require long periods of cell maturation and synthesis, as described in several papers using culture cells [25; 29].

However, our results support the involvement of genic cytokines and chemokines are earlier events, indeed consistent with the early cell trafficking between places of allergenic aggression and those dependent on the central and secondary immune system, as noted in previous work

However, our results support that the involvement of genic cytokines and chemokines are earlier events, indeed consistent with the quickly cell trafficking between the local site of allergenic aggression and those sites dependents on the central and secondary immune system, as noted in previous research from our group [55].

More than a common standard for the same respiratory allergic disease and for the same the most important allergic sensitization is the observation of the individual profile of each patient. Indeed, IgE-mediated allergy in spite of a pathogenic mechanism conductor has at clinical level, is extremely heterogeneous. The results shown in Figures 18 to 20 also showed a tremendous heterogeneity in gene expression after allergen provocation, between our patients.

The gene expression levels of IL-4 results are extremely interesting, because unquestionably two distinct profiles are observed (high and low levels), but without correspondence with those achieved for IL-4R. Also, the level of gene expression of IL-4 was correlated with total serum IgE levels, but without correlation with the clinical severity profile, as supported by clinical practice [18].

Unlike other diseases, allergy and asthma appear to be arguably multifactorial and multigenic disorders, and therefore it has not been possible identify till now one or a set of specific genes that may be genetic markers [57, 81], although recent paper identifies the involvement of *GSTO2 loci* in asthma, and *GSTA1* as risk factor for asthma and allergies in Italian patients [56], while Genome-wide association studies (GWAS) represent the most powerful approach for asthma, have identified several distinct others genotypes from IL-18R1, IL-33, *SMAD3*, *ORMDL3*, *HLA-DQ* and IL-2RB loci [31].

As mentioned before, allergy and asthma are chronic inflammatory and polygenic disorders, and so any isolated specific gene could claim be an asthma gene. Therefore, recently in order to best understanding the intricate heterogeneity of this disease the designation of phenotype and endotype have been used to stress the complexity of the mechanisms and clinical patterns [10, 31].

In the pathogenesis of chronic inflammatory diseases such as asthma several transcription (signal transducer and activator) factors are known to play a crucial role, acting as agonists or antagonists [79]. A transcription factor is formed by a sequence-specific DNA-binding factor. It is a protein that specific binds to specific DNA sequences, so it is able to controlling the rate of transcription of genetic information from DNA to messenger RNA.

These factors perform this purpose alone or with other proteins in a complex, by promoting (activator), or blocking (repressor) the recruitment of RNA polymerase. These enzymes permit the efficient genetic transcription from DNA to RNA to a specific gene.

A defining feature of transcription factors is that they contain one or more DNA-binding domains, which linked to specific sequences of DNA adjacent to the genes that they regulate.

For an efficient transcription are needed additional proteins (not classified as transcription factors) such as coactivators, chromatin remodelers, histone acetylases, deacetylases, kinases, and methylases, having crucial roles in gene regulation, but lack DNA-binding domains.

So these factors are very important and therefore we also studied three of them.

EGR1, also knew as early growth response protein 1, have engaged in multi functions such as transcriptional regulator, mitogenesis, cell proliferation and differentiation regulation, apoptosis and tumor suppressor gene [28]. Previous report had highlighted the potential stimulatory and inhibitory effects on *EGR1* by *STAT6* (Th2 differentiation enhancer) and *STAT1* (Th1 differentiation enhancer), respectively.

Overall our patients, we have observed at 60 minutes later the allergen exposure an increase of expression of *EGR1*, favoring the allergic reaction, but at 240 minutes after provocation levels had decreased, possibly due to mechanisms of self-control of allergic reaction.

In opposite, the *JUNB* expression decreased at least after 60 minutes of the beginning of the allergic reaction, and going increasing later at 240 minutes. This factor is mainly a Th2 cell related transcription factor (Il-4), but also have role favoring other cytokines: IL-1, IL-2, and IL-10 [79]. So, we hypothesize that the earlier involvement could favouring the beginning of the allergic reaction, but also could be later a down-regulator factor.

JAK2 belongs to a tyrosine kinase family, and its activation engages the transcription factor *STAT3* to initiate *JAK-STAT* pathway [82]. It signalizes the interferon receptors, and GM-CSF receptor family (IL3R, IL5R, GM-CSF-R). In our patients we did not observed. In our patients, we did not observe relevant performance for this transcription factor.

Allergic diseases are complex and multifaceted, and asthma in particular was widely recognized as condition in which both genes and the environment play critical roles.

Currently, GWAS try to identifying a number of candidate genes evocative of biological relevance, but have failed to report for more than a reduced amount of phenotypic variance – a situation that has come to be known as the problem of the missing or hidden heritability [13, 76].

In our patients we could verify that the allergen challenge determines a very early cellular response with gene and protein expression.

At present, the environmental influence with direct effects on epigenetic plan offers an explanation for this extreme individual variability, one clinical disease but different phenotypes and endotypes, not yet fully characterized.

So, in spite of the same genetic heritage, each individual and each patient, with an equal number of chromosomes and genes, have a specificity and uniqueness: all equals but all different from one to each other.

In Figure 22 we present the results of 4 allergic patients with asthma and rhinitis.

		IL10	IL1B	IL1R2	IL17RA	IL4	IL4R
Severe	Conjunctival 240	↓↓	↓	↓↓	↓	↓	↓
Moderate	Nasal 240	↑	↑	↑	↓	↓↓↓	=
Mild	Nasal 60	↓↓↓	↑	↓↓	↑	↑↑↑	↑↑
Moderate	Conjunctival 60	↓	↓	↓↓	↓	↓	↓↓

		EGR1	JUNB	JAK2
Severe	Conjunctival 240	↓	↑	=
Moderate	Nasal 240	↑	↑↑	↓
Mild	Nasal 60	↑↑	↓	↓↓
Moderate	Conjunctival 60	↑	↓↓	↓

		CCL4	CXCL1	CXCL2	CXCL5
Severe	Conjunctival 240	↓	↓	↓	↓
Moderate	Nasal 240	↓	↓	↑	↓↓
Mild	Nasal 60	↓↓	↓	↑	↑
Moderate	Conjunctival 60	↓	↓	↓	↓

Figure 22. Overall results of 4 patients with allergic asthma and rhinitis

Gene expression of cytokines and chemokines seem to have a strictly correlation with the results obtained in the study of nuclear transcription factors, *ERG1* and *JUNB*, as discussed before.

The susceptibility to elicit an allergic response or in opposite side its own inhibition is under liability of a time-dependent dynamic response since the allergen exposure. It might be more appropriate to view genes as a frame surrounding a complex network of biological processes. The frame delimits and supports the network, but the connections within the network determine its functions.

Besides the identification of novel pathological mechanisms and therapeutics, the wealth of information leads to the vision of genes forecasting asthma risk and phenotypes, with genetic scores and eventual personalized medicine with more effective treatments. Gene-environment interactions might difficult the achievement of such knowledge. Thus, even after the completed sequence of the human genome, the scientific community maintains expectations that genetics may be a decisive tool in the allergic risk prediction and personalized tailor-made treatments. At present asthma epigenetics is still in its infancy and a promise to keep [13].

Author details

Celso Pereira*, Frederico S. Regateiro, Graça Loureiro, Beatriz Tavares and António Martinho

*Address all correspondence to: celsopereira.pt@gmail.com

Clinic Immunology, Medicine Faculty, Coimbra University. Immunoallergology Department, Coimbra University Center Hospital. Blood and Transplantation Center of Coimbra / Portuguese Institute of Blood and Transplantation., Portugal

References

[1] Binia A, Kabesch M (2012). Respiratory medicine - genetic base for allergy and asthma. Swiss Med Wkly, Vol 142, (August 2012), pp. w13612, ISSN 1424-3997.

[2] Bousquet J.; et al, (2012). Allergic Rhinitis and its Impact on Asthma (ARIA): achievements in 10 years and future needs. J Allergy Clin Immunol, Vol 131, nº 2, (November 2012), pp. 1049-62, ISSN 0091-6749.

[3] Bouzigon E, Corda E, Aschard H, et al (2008). Effect of 17q21 variants and smoking exposure in early-onset asthma. N Engl J Med, Vol. 359, nº 19, (November 2008), pp. 1985-94, ISSN 1533-4406.

[4] Bouzigon E, Forabosco P, Koppelman GH, et al (2010). Meta-analysis of 20 genome-wide linkage studies evidenced new regions linked to asthma and atopy. Eur J Hum Genet, Vol. 18, nº 6, (June 2010), pp. 700-6, ISSN 1018-4813.

[5]   Campbell CD, Mohajeri K, Malig M, et al. (2014) Whole-Genome Sequencing of Individuals from a Founder Population Identifies Candidate Genes for Asthma. PLoS ONE, Vol. 9, nº 8, (August 2014), pp. e104396, ISSN 1932-6203.

[6]   Cantero-Recasens G, Fandos C, Rubio-Moscardo F, Valverde MA, Vicente R (2010). The asthma-associated ORMDL3 gene product regulates endoplasmic reticulum-mediated calcium signaling and cellular stress. Hum Mol Genet, Vol. 19, nº 1, (January 2010), pp. 111-21, ISSN 1460-2083.

[7]   Choi JP, Kim YS, Kim OY, et al (2012). TNF-alpha is a key mediator in the development of Th2 cell response to inhaled allergens induced by a viral PAMP double-stranded RNA. Allergy, Vol 67, nº 9, (September 2012), pp. 1138-48, ISSN 1398-9995.

[8]   Contopoulos-Ioannidis DG, Manoli EN, Ioannidis JP (2005). Meta-analysis of the association of beta2-adrenergic receptor polymorphisms with asthma phenotypes. J Allergy Clin Immunol, Vol. 115, nº 5, (May 2005), pp. 963-72, ISSN 0838-1925.

[9]   Cookson WO, Sharp PA, Faux JA, Hopkin JM (1989). Linkage between immunoglobulin E responses underlying asthma and rhinitis and chromosome 11q. Lancet, Vol. 1, nº 8650, (June 1989), pp. 1292-5, ISSN 0140-6736.

[10] Corren J (2013). Asthma phenotypes and endotypes: an evolving paradigm for classification. Discov Med, Vol 15, nº 83, (April 2013), pp. 243-9, ISSN 1539-6509.

[11] De R, Bush WS, Moore JH (2014). Bioinformatics challenges in genome-wide association studies (GWAS). Methods Mol Biol, Vol. 1168, pp. 63-81, ISSN 1064-3745.

[12] Denham S, Koppelman GH, Blakey J, et al (2008). Meta-analysis of genomewide linkage studies of asthma and related traits. Respir Res, Vol. 9, nº 1, (April 2008), pp. 38, ISSN. 1465-9921.

[13] Devries A, Vercelli D (2013). Epigenetics of human asthma and allergy: promises to keep. Asian Pac J Allergy Immunol, Vol 31, nº 3, (September 2013), pp. 183-9, ISSN 2228-869.

[14] Duffy DL, Martin NG, Battistutta D, Hopper LL, Mathews JD (1990). Genetics of asthma and hay fever in Australian twins. Am Rev Respir Dis (1990), Vol, nº 6, December 1990), pp. 142, 1351-8, ISSN 0003-0805.

[15] Eichler EE, Flint J, Gibson G, et al (2010). Missing heritability and strategies for finding the underlying causes of complex disease. Nat Rev Genet, Vol. 11, nº 6, (June 2010), pp. 446-50, ISSN 1471-0056.

[16] Ege MJ, Mayer M, Normand AC, et al (2011). Exposure to environmental microorganisms and childhood asthma. N Engl J Med, Vol. 364, nº 8, (February 2011), pp. 701-9, ISSN 1533-4406.

[17] Eickmeier O, Boom Lv, Schreiner F, et al (2013). Transforming growth factor β1 genotypes in relation to TGFβ1, interleukin-8, and tumor necrosis factor alpha in induced

sputum and blood in cystic fibrosis. Mediators Inflamm, (August 2013), pp. 913135, ISSN 0962-9351.

[18] Gadermaier E, Levin M, Flicker S, Ohlin M (2014). The human IgE repertoire. Int Arch Allergy Immunol, Vol 163, nº 2, (November 2014), pp. 77-91, ISSN 1018-2438.

[19] Galanter J, Choudhry S, Eng C. et al (2008). ORMDL3 gene is associated with asthma in three ethnically diverse populations. Am J Respir Crit Care Med, Vol. 177, nº 11, (June 2009), pp. 1194-200, ISSN 0003-0805.

[20] Global Strategy for Asthma Management and Prevention, May 2014. www.ginasthma.org. (28/07/2014).

[21] Graça Loureiro, Beatriz Tavares, Daniel Machado and Celso Pereira (2012). Nasal Provocation Test in the Diagnosis of Allergic Rhinitis, Allergic Rhinitis, Prof. Marek Kowalski (Ed.), ISBN: 978-953-51-0288-5, InTech, DOI: 10.5772/39069.

[22] Guerra S, Martinez FD (2008). Asthma genetics: from linear to multifactorial approaches. Annu Rev Med, Vol. 59, pp. 327-41, ISSN 0066-4219.

[23] Halapi E, Gudbjartsson DF, Jonsdottir GM, et al (2010). A sequence variant on 17q21 is associated with age at onset and severity of asthma. Eur J Hum Genet, Vol. 18, nº 8, (August 2010), pp. 902-8, ISSN 1018-4813.

[24] Hall IP, Blakey JD, Al Balushi KA, et al (2006). Beta2-adrenoceptor polymorphisms and asthma from childhood to middle age in the British 1958 birth cohort: a genetic association study. Lancet, Vol. 368, nº 9537, (August 2006), pp. 771-79, ISSN 0140-6736.

[25] Hamid Q (2012). Pathogenesis of small airways in asthma. Respiration, Vol 84, nº 1, (June 2012), pp. 4-11, ISSN 0025-7931.

[26] Hirschhorn JN, Daly M J (2005). Genome-wide association studies for common diseases and complex traits. Nature Rev Genet, Vol. 6, nº 2, (February 2005), pp. 95-108, ISSN 1471-0064.

[27] Holgate ST (2013). Mechanisms of asthma and implications for its prevention and treatment: a personal journey. Allergy, Asthma Immunol Res, Vol. 5, nº 6, (November 2013), pp. 343-7, ISSN 2092-7355.

[28] Ingram JL, Antao-Menezes A, Mangum JB, et al (2006). Opposing actions of Stat1 and Stat6 on IL-13-induced up-regulation of early growth response-1 and platelet-derived growth factor ligands in pulmonary fibroblasts. J Immunol, Vol 177, nº 6, (September 2006), pp. 4141-8, ISSN 0022-1767.

[29] Islam SA, Luster AD (2012). T cell homing to epithelial barriers in allergic disease. Nat Med, Vol 18, nº 5, (May 2012), pp. 705-15, ISSN 1078-8956.

[30] Kim JH, Cheong HS, Park JS, et al (2013). A genome-wide association study of total serum and mite-specific IgEs in asthma patients. PLoS One, Vol. 8, nº 8, (August 2013), pp. 71958, ISSN 1932-6203.

[31] Kontakioti E, Domvri K, Papakosta D, Daniilidis M (2014). HLA and asthma phenotypes/endotypes: A review. Hum Immunol, Vol 75, nº 8, (August 2014), pp. 930-9, ISSN 0198-8859.

[32] Kurz T, Strauch K, Heinzmann A, et al (2000). A European study on the genetics of mite sensitization. J Allergy Clin Immunol, Vol 106, nº 5, (November 2000), pp. 925-32. ISSN0091-6749.

[33] Lee G, Fields P, Griffin T, Flavell R (2003). Regulation of the Th2 cytokine locus by a locus control region. Immunity, Vol. 19, nº 1, (July 2003), pp. 145-53, ISSN 1074-7613.

[34] Lee GR, Spilianakis CG, Flavell RA (2005). Hypersensitive site 7 of the TH2 locus control region is essential for expressing TH2 cytokine genes and for long-range intrachromosomal interactions. Nat Immunol, Vol. 6, nº 1, (December 2005), pp. 42-8, ISSN 1529-2908.

[35] Leung TF, Sy HY, Ng MC, et al (2009). Asthma and atopy are associated with chromosome 17q21 markers in Chinese children. Allergy, Vol. 64, nº 4, (April 2009), pp. 621-8, ISSN 1398-9995.

[36] Leung TF, Ko FW, Sy HY, Tsui SK, Wong GW (2014). Differences in asthma genetics between Chinese and other populations. J Allergy Clin Immunol, Vol 133, nº 1, (January 2014), pp. 42-8, ISSN 0091-6749.

[37] Li C, Li M, Lange EM, Watanabe RM (2008). Prioritized subset analysis: improving power in genome-wide association studies. Hum Hered, Vol. 65, nº 3, (Octuber 2008), pp. 129-41, ISSN 1423-0062.

[38] Li X, Howard TD, Zheng SL, et al (2010). Genome-wide association study of asthma identifies RAD50-IL13 and HLA-DR/DQ regions. J Allergy Clin Immunol, Vol. 125, nº 2, (February 2010), pp. 328-335.e11, ISSN 0838-1925.

[39] Linder, A. (1988). Symptom scores as measures of the severity of rhinitis. Clin Allergy, Vol.18, No.1 (January 1988), pp 29-37, ISSN 0009-9090.

[40] Loth DW, Artigas MS, Gharib SA, et al (2014). Genome-wide association analysis identifies six new loci associated with forced vital capacity. Nat Genet, Vol. 46, nº 7, (July 2014), pp. 669-77, ISSN 1061-4036.

[41] Lötvall J, Akdis CA, Bacharier LB et al (2011). Asthma endotypes: a new approach to classification of disease entities within the asthma syndrome. J Allergy Clin Immunol, Vol. 127, nº 2, (Bebruary 2011), pp. 355-60, ISSN 0091-6749.

[42] Los H, Postmus PE, Boomsma DI (2001). Asthma genetics and intermediate phenotypes: a review from twin studies. Twin Res, Vol. 4, nº 2, (April 2001), pp. 81-93, ISSN 1832-4274.

[43] Manolio TA, Collins FS (2009). The HapMap and genome-wide association studies in diagnosis and therapy. Annu Rev Med, Vol. 60, pp. 443-56, ISSN 0066-4219.

[44] Martinez FD, Vercelli D (2013). Asthma. Lancet, Vol. 382, nº 9901; (Octuber 2013), pp. 1360-72, ISSN 0140-6736.

[45] Moffatt MF, James A, Ryan G, et al. (1999). Extended tumour necrosis factor/HLA-DR haplotypes and asthma in an Australian population sample. Thorax, Vol. 54, nº 9, (September 1999), pp. 757-61, ISSN 1468-3296.

[46] Moffatt MF, Kabesch M, Liang L, et al (2007). Genetic variants regulating ORMDL3 expression are determinants of susceptibility to childhood asthma. Nature, Vol. 448, nº 7152, (June 2007), pp. 470-3, ISSN 0028-0836.

[47] Moffatt MF, Gut IG, Demenais F, et al (2010). A large-scale, consortium-based genomewide association study of asthma. N Engl J Med, Vol. 363, nº 13, (September 2010), pp. 1211-21, ISSN 1533-4406.

[48] Mortemousque, B. (2007). Les tests de provocation conjonctivaux. *J Fr Ophtalmol,* Vol. 30, No. 3 (March 2007), pp. 300-305, ISSN 0181-5512.

[49] Nieminen, MM, Kaprio J, Koskenvuo M (1991). A population-based study of bronchial asthma in adult twin pairs. Chest, Vol. 100, nº 1, (July 1991), pp. 70-5, ISSN 1931-3543.

[50] Novershtern N, Itzhaki Z, Manor O, Friedman N, Kaminski N (2008). A functional and regulatory map of asthma. Am J Respir Cell Mol Biol, Vol 38, nº 3 (March 2008), pp. 324-36, ISSN 1535-4989.

[51] Ober C, Hoffjan S, (2006). Asthma genetics 2006: the long and winding road to gene discovery. Genes Immun, Vol. 7, nº 2, (March 2006), pp. 95-100, ISSN 1466-4879.

[52] Ober C, Yao TC (2011). The genetics of asthma and allergic disease: a 21st century perspective. Immunol Rev, Vol. 242, nº 1, (June 2011), pp. 10-30, ISSN 1600-065X.

[53] Parapanissiou E, Papastavrou T, Deligiannidis A, et al (2005). HLA antigens in Greek children with allergic bronchial asthma. Tissue Antigens, Vol 65, nº 5, (May 2005), pp. 481-4, ISSN 1399-0039.

[54] Pereira C, Loureiro G, Martinho A, et al. (2012a). T cell receptor excision circles (TREC) and recent thymic migrant cells in specific immunotherapy and respiratory allergy to Dermatophagoides pteronyssinus. Eur Ann Allergy Clin Immunol, Vol 44, nº 2, (April 2012), pp. 61-72, ISSN 1764-1489.

[79] Yamashita M, Onodera A, Nakayama T (2007). Immune mechanisms of allergic airway disease: regulation by transcription factors. Crit Rev Immunol, Vol 27, nº 6, pp. 539-46, ISSN 1040-8401.

[80] Yang IV, Schwartz DA (2012). Epigenetic mechanisms and the development of asthma. J Allergy Clin Immunol, Vol. 130, nº 6, (December 2012), pp. 1243-55, ISSN 0838-1925.

[81] Yoshikawa T, Kanazawa H, Fujimoto S, Hirata K (2014). Epistatic effects of multiple receptor genes on pathophysiology of asthma - its limits and potential for clinical application. Med Sci Monit, Vol 17, nº 20, (January 2014) pp. 64-71, ISSN 1234-1010.

[82] Zouein FA, Duhé RJ, Booz GW (2011). JAKs go nuclear: emerging role of nuclear JAK1 and JAK2 in gene expression and cell growth. Growth Factors, Vol 29, nº 6, (December 2011), pp. 245-52, ISSN 0897-7194.

[83] Zweemer AJ, Toraskar J, Heitman LH, IJzerman AP (2014). Bias in chemokine receptor signalling. Trends Immunol, Vol 35, nº 6, (June 2014), pp. 243-52, ISSN 1471-4906.

2

Eosinophilic Esophagitis

Rebecca Scherr and Mary Beth Hogan

1. Introduction

Eosinophilic gastrointestinal diseases (EGIDS) are immune mediated diseases with varying clinical presentations but are characterized pathologically by eosinophilic infiltrate of the epithelium of the gastrointestinal tract. Eosinophilic esophagitis has become the most recognized entity over the last twenty years and great strides have been made to understand it. In the 1970s and 1980s, case reports of patients with esophageal eosinophilia were reported but the significance of these findings was not known or were attributed to GERD. In the 1990s the field of Pediatric Gastroenterology was emerging and endoscopy of children became more common. In addition, pediatric gastroenterologists knew that inflammation could occur despite macroscopically "normal" appearing tissue and therefore routine biopsies during endoscopy have been standard of care. This led to wider understanding of the clinical presentation and outcomes of children with prominent eosinophilia of the esophagus. These children did not respond to the typical antacid regimen. They had a wide range of clinical symptoms including vomiting, regurgitation, and abdominal pain and feeding refusal. It was also noted that many had concurrent atopic diseases including food allergies, eczema and asthma.[1-4] The fields of allergy and gastroenterology were beginning to converge on a disease process that would prove more complex to manage than many other food allergies. Today gastroenterologists and allergists have come to depend on one other in the management of these patients.

Eosinophilic esophagitis is becoming a recognized common cause of esophagitis in children and adults. The most current definition comes from the consensus statement published in 2011 in The Journal of Allergy and Clinical Immunology. The new criteria is less restrictive then definitions put forth in the past. In addition, the authors changed the abbreviation from EE to EoE because across disciplines EE can have different meanings (e.g. erosive esophagitis). This expert panel wanted to conceptualize the definition so that it could represent the wide range of patients and clinical scenarios. The expert panel agreed upon the definition that "eosinophilic esophagitis represents a chronic, immune/antigen-mediated esophageal disease characterized clinically by symptoms related to esophageal dysfunction and histologically by eosinophil-predominant inflammation".[5]

Histologic criteria include the presence of ≥15 eosinophils per high power field on esophageal biopsy. This requirement should make diagnosis more standardized; however, the definition of "high power" field can vary and therefore change the number of eosinophils reported. They did allow for exceptions to the 15 per high power field in the case of other histologic features including microabscess, superficial layering or extracellular eosinophilic granules. [5]

2. Epidemiology

The epidemiology of eosinophilic esophagitis is becoming better understood. From multiple studies it has become apparent that EoE effects males at least 3 times more frequently than females.[6-11] EoE patients are more likely to have atopic disease than the general population. [12-17] Whites appear to have a higher incidence than other races. All age groups are effected including infants and there is a report of a 98 year old with EoE.[11] However, most patients are children, adolescents and adults younger than 50 years old. In a large epidemiological study the prevalence was highest in men age 35-39 years old.[18]

The prevalence and incidence has been hard to determine. Data suggests that the incidence and prevalence is increasing. While it could be hypothesized that this was due to increased awareness, retrospective studies of esophageal biopsy specimens have indicated that the incidence and prevalence are truly increasing. This increase in incidence and prevalence remains when adjusted for the increased use of endoscopy.[19, 20] The incidence has been reported to be 6 to 13 cases per 100,000 in studies from the United States, Canada, and Switzerland.[13, 21-23] Denmark and Netherlands report lower incidence at less than 2 cases per 100,000.[24] The prevalence has been estimated anywhere between 10-80 cases per 100,000, depending on the population being studied.[18] A recent study using a large US database of health insurance claims of over 35 million patients showed a period prevalence of 56.7 per 100,000 through the years 2009-2011.[18]

3. Differential diagnosis

The differential diagnosis for esophageal eosinophilia includes celiac disease, Crohn's disease, esophageal achalasia, connective tissue disorders, drug reactions, hypereosinophilic syndromes and graft versus host disease and these disorders need to be ruled out prior to making the diagnosis of EoE. The most problematic differential diagnosis is gastroesophageal reflux (GERD). In the past, eosinophilia was attributed to GERD. During the treatment of patients with prominent eosinophilic infiltrate it was noted that they were less responsive to antacids, both clinically and histologically. Trying to understand the relationship between GERD, eosinophilia of the esophagus and EoE is one of the most important and difficult tasks facing clinicians who diagnose and treat EoE. Food allergy is also a major component of EoE and dietary therapy can be first line therapy in many cases. The relationship between food allergy and EoE is also only partially realized.

4. Eosinophils

An understanding of EoE requires a review of the primary effector cell in the pathology, the eosinophil. New developments in our understanding of eosinophil responses reveal that their role in immunology goes beyond attacking helminthes. Eosinophils are highly complex hematopoietic cells which participate actively in the immune response. First, eosinophil released granule products such as eosinophil cationic protein (ECP) are capable of chemoattracting antigen presenting cells such as macrophages.[25] This granule is believed to have direct antimicrobial action as well as directing macrophage recruitment to the site of ECP release. Recruitment of myeloid dendritic cells to draining lymph nodes, a critical step to specific immune responses, is influenced by eosinophils.[26] Further downstream, in the immunologic response, eosinophils are capable of regulating B cell numbers via influencing B cell proliferation.[27]Further evidence that eosinophils can participate in the immune response to pathogens is the presence of pattern recognition receptors on the eosinophil receptor. These toll-like receptors, NOD, dectin-1 and RAGE receptors are innate, non-specific responses to various elements of the microbial cell wall which result in initiating and amplifying the host immune response.[28] Studies have demonstrated toll-like receptor expression on eosinophils occurs in EoE.[29] The immunobiology of the eosinophil is intimately related to the allergic response. The understanding that eosinophils and allergies are related in the experimental research in EoE is new. Due to the recent gains in the knowledge of the pathophysiology of EoE there are gaps in the clinical applications. Therefore other atopic diseases, such as asthma, will be utilized as a model to demonstrate the eosinophil's complex capabilities. Particular emphasis will be placed on those components of the allergic response which likely contribute to EoE.

Eosinophils are hematopoietic cells, derived from the bone marrow. Normal hematopoiesis involves tight control on eosinophil differentiation from a common progenitor cell. New data suggests that eosinophils and basophils share a common lineage with the erythrocytes and megakaryocytes.[30] However, commitment from the common progenitor cell into an eosinophil progenitor (CD 34+IL5R+) requires the presence of IL-5 predominately, but GM-CSF and IL-3 also affect eosinophilopoiesis.[31] Sources of IL-5 in the bone marrow include the bone marrow stromal cell, hematopoietic cells, T lymphocytes and bone marrow endothelial cells.[32] Data suggests that a newly discovered hematopoietic cell ILC2, an innate lymphoid cell present locally in peripheral tissues, may be capable of controlling eosinophilopoiesis. [33] These ILC2 cells produce profound amounts of IL-5 which is released into the systemic circulation directing the bone marrow to increase eosinophil production. IL-5's role in EoE is under investigation, as it has been found in the blood vessels of esophageal biopsies of pediatric EoE patients.[34]

Increases of eosinophil progenitor cells and mature eosinophils in the bone marrow are described in both human and murine studies of allergen sensitization and occurs independent of T lymphocytes or specific IgE activation of the bone marrow.[35-37] This model of accelerated response of eosinophilopoiesis is linked to an acute response to allergens in multiple strains of mice. However, the eosinophilic potential to have ongoing bone marrow eosinophilia linked to chronic disease and fibrosis development in the asthmatic airway may not be a universal response in the disease and may require a specific genetic background. [38] This may have implications for disease severity in both asthma and EoE in determining which individuals have disease progression due to eosinophil influenced severe fibrosis.

Eosinophil progenitor cells may be able to finish differentiation to mature eosinophils locally in the effected peripheral tissue, like the esophagus, stomach and intestines. Eosinophil progenitors are released into the peripheral blood stream in asthmatic individuals and are attracted to peripheral tissues that are involved in the asthmatic response.[39] Interestingly, topical glucocorticoid therapy in asthma decreases eosinophil progenitors circulating in the peripheral blood. [37] In addition, interfering with chemotactic signaling of eosinophil progenitors early in the asthmatic response to allergen challenge to the lung decreases lung eosinophil progenitor and mature eosinophil numbers.[39] This demonstrates that control of eosinophilopoiesis may be an important component to controlling eosinophil derived diseases. Investigations into the potential for eosinophilic mucosa to support eosinophilopoiesis could provide a key understanding of the pathophysiology of EoE.

Progenitor cells are attracted to peripheral tissue and so are mature eosinophils. The primary chemokines responsible for recruiting mature eosinophils to their targets are IL-5, eotaxin, MCP and RANTES.[40] These cytokines are produced by inflammatory cells present in the tissue during allergic responses. Other cytokines released by tissue cells in the allergic response such as IL-4 and IL-13 may play an indirect role in eosinophil trafficking role by increasing eotaxin expression. Epithelial cell production of IL-5, IL-13 and eotaxin has been found in biopsies obtained from pediatric EoE patient.[34, 41] and are decreased with glucocorticoid therapy in EoE. Blockade of these chemotactic signals results in reduction of the eosinophilic response peripherally.

Once recruited to peripheral tissues, eosinophils are activated by multiple extracellular proteins and cytokines. Eosinophils have integrins on their surface that interact with the extracellular matrix. This interaction can increase survival of eosinophils and also increase recruitment of more eosinophils through several pathways. For instance, platelet-activating factor primes eosinophil adherence to tissue through both beta-1 and beta-2 integrins.[40] Periostin, an extracellular matrix protein, is a strong chemotactic agent.[42] Periostin production has been shown to be inducible by transforming growth factor-beta and IL-13 after allergen exposure in a corresponding murine model of EoE.[43] Periostin exists in both the human lung and esophagus. Levels of periostin have been found to be higher in EoE patients than controls. Increased accumulation of eosinophils was correlated to increased levels of periostin in these studies.[44] Therefore it may be that periostin recruits and retains eosinophils at the peripheral tissue in eosinophilic disease. Fibronectin is another extracellular matrix protein that binds with Beta-1 integrin (VL-4) on the surface of eosinophils. This interaction has shown to enhance eosinophil survival.[45]

Therapeutic approaches that target the adhesion and interactions of eosinophils with tissue and plasma elements will be difficult due to multiple interactions and pathways involved once eosinophils are activated. Highly activated integrin molecules on eosinophils are associated with survival independent of exogenous IL-5 signaling.[42, 46] Eosinophils activated by endothelial fibronectin will also autologously produce survival factors including IL-5, IL-3 and GM-CSF.[47] Dexamethasone reduces the endothelial production of these survival factors.[48] However, this autologous production of survival factors from adherent stimulated eosinophils will make development of a novel single agent anti-cytokine therapy to treat EoE more difficult. The capability of the eosinophil to survive without exogenous IL-5 will also limit the use of anti-IL-5 therapies as sole pharmacotherapy in the armentarium of EoE treatment.

Negative regulators of chemotaxis and survival of eosinophils include, IL-12 which reduces platelet activating effects on eosinophils and reduces eotaxin dependent tissue migration. [49] Activation of the Siglec-F receptor on eosinophils induces eosinophil apoptosis. IL-5 and GM-CSF failed to rescue eosinophils from this fate, suggesting that this may be one viable way to eliminate eosinophils once they have migrated to peripheral tissues.[50] A proof of concept study has been performed in a murine model of allergic EoE in which Siglec-F activation resulted in decreased eosinophil numbers in the esophagus.[51] Other inhibitory mechanisms which the immune system uses, such as FOXP3, CD25+and TH17 may play a role in this process.[52] While TGF-beta has been linked to fibrotic activity it also has an apoptotic effect on eosinophils as a negative feedback regulatory mechanism. [50-52] The only currently used therapeutic agent which prevents eosinophil priming in eosinophilia is glucocorticoids.[53] Glucocorticoid effect is thought to be from altering eosinophil and other immune mediated cell cytokine production. Glucocorticoids also bias hematopoiesis towards neutrophil production.

5. IgE mediated allergic mechanisms

Allergy is the immune pathway mediated by IgE binding to allergen and subsequently activating mast cell release of prototypic cytokines. These preformed mediators include histamine, tryptase, IL-5, cysteinyl leukotrienes amongst other cytokines. This is known as the immediate phase reaction. It is responsible for the wheal and flare during functional skin prick testing to allergens, and immediate airway contraction in asthma. These agents also cause vomiting, diarrhea, and abdominal cramping after an IgE mediated food allergy. Release of these agents subsequently causes an inflammatory recruitment of eosinophils and lymphocytes, known as the late phase reaction.

Some EoE patients appear to have this basic immediate phase response. IL-5 and IL-13 correlate with eotxin-3 and eosinophil levels.[44] In addition some EoE patients have both eosinophils and mast cells in esophageal biopsies.[54] In fact, the presence of IgE bearing intraepithelial mast cells in EoE patients distinguished allergic EoE patients from non-allergic EoE patients. [17] Mastocytosis and degranulated mast cells have been found in the biopsies of EoE patient. [55] In asthma, contact of eosinophils with mast cells was the most potent driver of eosinophil survival.[56] The presence of IL-13 in EoE would also increase IL-4 and IL-13 and cause B cell isotype switching to IgE production.

In addition, TH2 cell production of cytokines such as IL-4, 5, 13 is a hallmark feature of allergy. The importance of IL-13 in immediate phase reactions is demonstrated by inhibition of IL-13 by an anti-IL-13 Fab fragment resulting in decreased eosinophilia, inflammatory infiltrate and airway hyper-reactivity in a murine model of asthma.[57] Anti-IL5 therapy is being investigated in eosinophilic diseases such as asthma and Churg Strauss disease. Anti-IL4 therapeutic targets are being investigated in atopic dermatitis. These Th2 driven processes are also amplified by innate lymphoid cells (ILC2) at the mucosal surface. [58] These cytokines along with TGF-beta encourages eosinophil induced fibrosis and motility disorders in EoE patients.[43]

Some allergens will also actively participate in the subsequent immediate phase reactions. Allergens which are proteases (insect derived or fungal) have been found to deceitfully act in an innate fashion with initial exposure. These allergic proteases activate IL-25, IL-33 and TSLP mucosal production resulting in ILC2 activation in the lung tissue.[59] In this study ILC2 expressed IL-5 and ILl-13. Eosinophil recruitment has been identified in the lung with fungal chitinase exposure.[60] Interestingly a murine model of EoE induced by cockroach and dust mite has been described.[61] This model was characterized by esophageal eosinophilia, mastocytosis, increased IgE, IL-5 and eotaxin after cockroach and dust mite exposure but not cat or dog exposure. Protease inhibition in a murine asthma model with cockroach extract reduced eosinophil counts in BALF.[62]

6. GERD and eosinophils

In 1982 Winter, et al. described esophageal eosinophils in series of pediatric patients and concluded that increased eosinophils was a marker for more severe GERD.[63] Four theories have been proposed for the association between esophageal eosinophilia and GERD. First, EoE and GERD can both be present but they are unrelated. The 2011 consensus statement has chosen not to exclude the diagnosis of EoE even in the setting of abnormal pH probe. This recognizes the hypothesis that GERD and EoE can coexist. The basis of this hypothesis from an epidemiologic view, is that approximately 20% of adults have GERD so a certain percentage of adult EoE patients will also have GERD. [64, 65] In addition, pathologic GERD is rare in children with EoE.[66] This latter claim could be disputed since pH monitoring is not always done in children and there are no standardized norms. However, other research has found higher incidences of GERD among adult patients with EoE.[67, 68]

Another proposed mechanism is that GERD causes esophageal eosinophilia but it is not eosinophilic esophagitis. The criteria for the number of esophageal eosinophils to be greater than 20 was suggested after it was noted that patients with more than 15 eos/hpf were less likely to respond to anti-reflux medication.[69, 70] In lab models it has been shown that acid stimulates the release of many substances that could potentially attract and activate eosinophils. These substances include platelet activating factor, interleukin-8, eotaxin-1, eotaxin-2, exotoxin-3, macrophage inflammatory protein and RANTES (regulated upon activation of normal T cell expressed and secreted).[71-76] These factors have also been isolated from biopsy specimens from patients with GERD.[76] However, it is still not known if the eosinophilia associated with GERD is a separate entity from eosinophilic esophagitis.

Another hypothesis is that EoE contributes to or causes GERD. Eosinophils produce substances that are cytotoxic and other factors that may alter esophageal motility. For example, eosinophils produce vasoactive intestinal peptide and PAF which can lower esophageal pressure, inducing GERD.[77, 78] Secretion of IL-6 can weaken esophageal muscle contraction and peristalsis.[79] In asthma, cytotoxic substances can damage tight junctions.[80] In the esophagus this could lead to increased permeability to acid and induce pain receptors and the clinical symptoms of GERD.[81, 82]

Finally, one hypothesis blames GERD for EoE. GERD can cause inflammation and increase the permeability of the esophageal epithelium; thereby allowing large molecules to enter. This influx of gastric contents could include potential allergens that induce EoE.[72, 74, 83-85] In addition, refluxed gastric contents can activate many eosinophil chemoattractants including IL-8, PAF, eotaxin-1-3 and MIP-1α.[74, 85] Other non-eosinophil immune cells and inflammatory mediators can also be attracted to the esophagus after exposure to gastric material.[86] Proving any of these is a complex task involving multiple pathways in the systemic and gastrointestinal immune systems.

7. Proton pump inhibitors

Due to the complexity of the relationship between GERD and EoE, proton pump inhibitors have been at the center of much therapeutic research. When esophageal eosinophils were first described they were attributed to GERD. Therefore patients were treated with anti-acid medications. As mentioned earlier, only some of these patients responded to this therapy. These patients are now considered to have "proton pump inhibitor responsive eosinophilic esophagitis" (PPI-REE) according to the 2011 consensus recommendations.[5] The consensus statement does not recommend PPI as a sole treatment for patients with esophageal eosinophils that are not responsive to PPI therapy. However, they state that even these patients could be treated with a PPI in addition to other treatment for their EoE. The use of PPI in patients with EoE is multifactorial. First, GERD may be a comorbid disease in these patients. These patients may have additional symptomatic relief with PPI therapy. PPI are used in acid suppression because of their inhibitory effect on the H+K+ATPase of the gastric parietal proton pump cell.[87] According to some hypotheses the suppression of acid in the gastric reflux contents could decrease the production of acid stimulated eosinophilic chemoattractants and other inflammatory cytokines. Also, decreasing esophageal acid damage would decrease esophageal permeability and exposure to allergens which can induce eosinophilia. However, PPI's may affect esophageal eosinophilia through other mechanisms outside of acid suppression. They have been found to have anti-inflammatory effects on epithelial and endothelial cells. They have demonstrated inhibitory effects against eotaxin-3 production and decrease the expression of adhesion molecules and other inflammatory cytokines.[88, 89] PPI's also display anti-oxidant properties, including scavenging hydroxyl radicals, preventing oxidative damage, and increasing levels of other anti-oxidants.[90-94] Proton pumps are found on cell types other than parietal cells including neutrophils and monocytes. In vitro studies have demonstrated PPI's inhibit the oxidative burst, impair phagocytosis, impair neutrophil migration, and decrease expression of adhesion molecules on monocytes and neutrophils. [95-98] Despite these added effects of PPI's, they cannot be used alone to treat EoE.[5]

8. Food allergy and dietary therapy

The link between allergens and EoE has now been accepted; however, the best way to determine which allergens are most responsible and in which patients is still an area undergoing intense research. Food elimination was first described by Kelly, et al. in 1995 with positive results.[99] Currently there are three frequently prescribed dietary therapies. First, complete elimination diet using amino acid-based formula. Second, six food elimination diet (SFED), which restricts milk, soy, eggs, wheat, tree nuts/peanuts, and fish/shellfish. Last, targeted elimination diet (TED) based off of skin prick and atopy patch testing. This last therapy sometimes includes combination of empiric six food elimination and targeted food elimination.

In a study of EoE patients by Spergel, et al. they determined food allergen prevalence through biopsy results and symptom reports. They found the most common food allergen, diagnosed by both symptoms and biopsy findings, in these patients was milk. Most common food allergens diagnosed with biopsy were milk, egg, wheat, followed by beef, soy and chicken. The most common foods diagnosed by symptoms were milk, egg and soy.[3] This has been substantiated in the EoE literature where many of the studies have also used skin prick testing and atopy patch testing to determine contributing food allergens.[9, 10, 100-103] The most common food allergies reported in the EoE literature are milk, eggs, soy, wheat, nuts (peanuts and tree nuts), and fish/shellfish.[100, 104, 105]

Henderson et al., in a retrospective study compared complete food elimination, targeted elimination diet based from skin prick and atopy testing and six food elimination diet to determine the effectiveness of each therapy.[6] They identified ninety eight patients that were proton pump resistant and non-steroid treated who went on dietary therapy. They rated remission as complete (<1 eos/hpf), partial (1-15 eos/hpf) and non-remission (>15 eos/hpf). Patients on complete elimination diet had significantly higher complete remission rate (<1 eos/ hpf) and lower non-remission rate than the targeted elimination diet. They concluded that the complete elimination diet was superior to targeted elimination or the six food elimination diet and there was no difference between SFED and TED.[6] Other studies have shown similar results with a histologic remission rate for compete elimination diet to be over 90%.[106] Studies of SFED in adults and children have shown that majority of patients have complete histologic response with rates varying from 64-85%. A greater proportion have significant response even if it is not complete resolution.[102, 105, 107]

Gonsalves' study of adults with EoE all patients had skin prick testing for aeroallergens and food allergens.[107] In all patients food allergens tested included the food items in the SFED; eggs, milk, peanuts, tree nuts, fish, shellfish, wheat, and soy, in addition to other foods self-reported as exacerbating symptoms. They found the skin prick test was predictive of only 13% of inciting agents. Also, 67% of the patients who had positive biopsy findings after reintroduction of one of the foods in the SFED had tested negative for that food on SPT. In addition, a recent meta-analysis found that allergy test result-directed food elimination remission rate (<15 eos/hpf) was only 45.5%, with high variability of remission rate between studies.[108, 109] The finding that elemental diet is superior to targeted elimination diet indicates that other pathways are involved.

Aeroallergens/ pollen have also been studied as contributors of eosinophilic esophagitis. Determining if aeroallergens are directly responsible for EoE via ingestion/inhalation or their potential to cross react with sensitized foods is under research. Interestingly, common immune epitopes (pan-allergens) exist between fruits, vegetables and pollen, and shellfish and insects such as cockroach and dust mite. Some of the broad based allergy response may be linked such as ragweed and melon or profiling in birch with celery and apple. In a mouse model, eosinophlic esophagitis could be induced by intranasal aeroallergen exposure.[110] In addition, in both children and adults there is higher incidence of EoE diagnosis in seasons with high aeroallergen counts.[111-113] Some have proposed that esophageal accumulation of eosinophilia in the background of aeroallergens is eotaxin and IL-5 dependent and others propose it is through the TH2/IL-13 response.[114-116] Rayapudi, et al. tested the aeroallergen trigger hypothesis via intranasal cockroach and dust mite allergen exposure on IL-5 and eotaxin levels in CCR-3 deficient mice and wild-type mice. The deficient mice had a dampened esophageal response to the allergens and they concluded indoor insect allergens induce IL-5 and eotaxin mediated EoE.[61] In addition, it has been reported that patients with allergies treated with sublingual pollen immunotherapy may have the unintended side effect of inducing EoE. A recent meta-analysis concluded that 2.7% of patients undergoing oral immune therapy for IgE mediated allergies develop EoE.[117]

Children and adults placed on an elemental diet show resolution of EoE in nearly all patients. Elemental diet may be effective as they could also eliminate pollen pan-allergens and food cross reactivity Issues. Elemental diets may also have effects unrelated to hypersensitivity reactions. This has been investigated by Erwin,et al.[7] Patients with EoE were tested for IgE sensitization using skin prick testing and a screening panel of specific IgE tests. They also tested patients for non-IgE mediated food sensitivities with atopy patch testing. In order to determine overall sensitization they included aeroallergens, common food allergens, cross-reactive carbohydrate determinants, and common commensal elements of the GI tract (Candida albicans and Helicobacter pylori) in the serum, skin prick testing and atopy patch testing. They found that 20-30% of patients with EoE had no detectable immune sensitivity.[7] This suggests an intrinsic defect not relatable to allergic immune responses may be responsible. In some patients non-IgE mediated responses are found in asthma, hay fever, and atopic dermatitis at approximately 30% of each patient population. Investigators in these three diseases hypothesize that it is possible to induce pure IL-5 response to stimuli without activating allergic antibody (IgE) responses via IL-4 and IL-13.

9. Steroids

Although corticosteroids are not currently approved for use in EoE, they are frequently used off-label in the treatment of PPI non-responsive esophageal eosinophilia. Dietary management has shown to be effective however, due to compliance difficulties, topical steroids have been used and have been found to be effective in majority of cases of EoE. The two most commonly used preparations are swallowed aerosolized fluticasone propionate and oral viscous budesonide. Systemic corticosteroids can be used if topical steroids are not effective or the patient needs rapid improvement in symptoms, like a food impaction. [118]

Four open-label trials have been conducted using fluticasone propionate.[68, 118-120] Two trials were pediatric patients and two were in adult patients. All four studies reported a significant symptom response rate. Complete symptom response ranged from 90-100% in patients. In addition, all patients on fluticasone had significant decreases in the number of esophageal eosinophils. Complete histologic response rates varied from 21-74% between the studies.[68, 120]

In pediatric and adult placebo controlled trials using fluticasone or oral viscous budesonide, patients on topical steroids had significant histologic response compared to placebo.[121-125] Symptom response was variable in the studies. One study found no significant difference in symptom response between the treatment and placebo groups. However, majority of the patients in the topical steroid group had decrease in dysphagia symptoms, as opposed to less than half in the placebo group.[121]

Four controlled trials have compared a proton pump inhibitor to topical steroids in the adult population. Peterson, et al. compared fluticasone 440 µg twice daily to omeprazole 40 mg once daily for 8 weeks. The histologic response between the two groups was not statistically significant.[67] They also found no difference in dysphagia scores. Moaward, et al studied the same drugs and doses.[126] They also had no statistical difference in histologic response between the two groups at eight weeks. They did have a statistically significant difference in dysphagia scores. The proton pump inhibitor had greater symptom response. The patients with abnormal pH probes were stratified to both groups and these patients had response to omeprazole but not to fluticasone.

Francis, et al. in a prospective trial, compared patients with esophageal eosinophilia who had positive pH probe results compared to patients with negative pH probe results.[127] The positive pH probe patients were prescribed omeprazole 40 mg twice daily and the patients with negative pH probe results were treated with oral viscous budesonide 1 mg twice daily.

The symptom and histologic response rates between the omeprazole and steroid groups was not statistically significant.

Dellon, et al. compared two topical steroid treatments; oral viscous budesonide 1 mg twice daily to nebulized then swallowed budesonide 1 mg twice daily in a randomized trial.[128] They performed scintigraphy to measure esophageal mucosal contact time with the drug. The oral viscous budesonide had statistically significant more mucosal contact time than the nebulized then swallowed budesonide. This correlated with a significant decrease in eosinophil counts in the oral viscous budesonide group. Both groups showed improvement in symptoms and symptom response was not correlated with histologic response.

One randomized, comparator controlled study has been done in pediatrics. This study compared prednisone 1 mg/kg/day (40 mg maximum) to fluticasone propionate 220 µg QID or 440 µg QID (depending on weight) for 4 weeks.[129] The study also had an 8 week weaning protocol. Decrease in esophageal eosinophil counts at 4 weeks were significant in both groups but the prednisone group had a greater degree of histologic response. Those in the prednisone group had 100% symptom resolution at 4 weeks and 97% of fluticasone patients had symptom resolution. Symptom relapse occurred at 12 weeks in approximately 50% of patients, regardless of the treatment received. In addition, systemic adverse effects were reported in 40% of the prednisone group; while the only adverse effect in the fluticasone group was esophageal *Candida* occurrence in 15% of the patients. The incidence of esophageal candidiasis as a result of topical steroid treatment for EoE has been reported in studies of adults and pediatrics at rates ranging from 5-26%. Most report that the infection was found incidentally on endoscopy, was not not symptomatic and was the only adverse effect.[68, 120, 121, 123, 125, 126, 128]

Topical steroids have been shown to be effective at inducing histologic and symptom response. However, length of therapy and role of maintenance therapy is still debated. Eosinophilic esophagitis over time, can create fibrosis and subsequent strictures of the esophagus. Whether or not this should be avoided even in asymptomatic patients is the basis of the maintenance therapy debate. Straumann, et al. conducted a placebo controlled maintenance trial comparing those with continued medication therapy versus placebo after steroid induced remission.[122] They reported symptomatic recurrence rate of 64% and histologic relapse of 100% at 1 year in the placebo group. However, others have found that more than half of patients were symptom free after 3-11 years even if they had persistent esophageal eosinophilia.[130, 131] It is not known which patients will develop fibrosis or if long-term topical steroid treatment will prevent it.

The path of eosinophilic esophagitis to fibrosis is being investigated to help distinguish which patients should receive long-term therapy to avoid esophageal fibrosis. Eosinophilic fibrosis occurs as a consequence of tissue remodeling. As discussed earlier in the chapter, asthma has been used as a model to understand EoE. These principles are used to understand the mediators responsible for remodeling in EoE. For example, IL-5 and IL-13 have shown to increase collagen in animal models.[43, 51, 132, 133] In addition, other mediators including periostin, TGF-B1, TSLP, Smad 3, and Siglec-F that have been studied in EoE pathogenesis are involved in tissue remodeling through multiple mechanisms.[43, 51, 134, 135] The mast cell-eosinophil interaction has also shown to be important in the disease process. Mast cells are also producers of the mediators and cytokines responsible for pathogenesis of EoE, includingTGFB1. Eosinophils produce factors such as IL-9 that work in mast cell survival and recruitment. Mast cells and eosinophils are both found in esophageal biopsies of EoE models. Murine models with mast cell deficient mice show decrease in smooth muscle hypertrophy and proliferation. Therefore indicating that mast cells may play a role in fibrosis and also esophageal dysmotility in EoE.[55, 134, 136]

10. Future therapies

Treatment research is focused on understanding the mechanism behind the effectiveness of dietary and steroid therapy. In addition, therapy directed at specific mediators in the pathogenesis of EoE are also of great interest. Currently clinical trials are being conducted to find effective non-steroidal therapy. Anti-IL-5, anti-IL-13, and a CRTH2 receptor antagonist therapies are being studied in placebo controlled trials in adult and pediatric EoE patients and they have all shown that they can induce significant decreases in number of esophageal eosinophils compared to placebo.[137-141] However, their ability to resolve symptoms has not been repeatedly demonstrated. An IL-4 α-subunit antagonist is showing promise in asthma patients and may be a potential therapy for EoE.[142-144] As our knowledge of the immune pathways associated with EoE increase then other receptors could also be targets for therapies.

Eosinophilic esophagitis is a chronic immune mediated disease of the gastrointestinal tract. The diagnosis of the disease and its' subsequent treatment requires the expertise of the allergist/immunologist and the gastroenterologist. Allergists have a unique understanding of the pathophysiology of atopic diseases. The diagnosis of EoE is likely to occur at the time of atopic evaluation at an allergy clinic. The allergist can be of great assistance to the gastroenterologist in assessing food allergic individuals. In addition, allergists are in a position to identify and treat, with immunotherapy or biologics, pollen associated EoE. In our center a multi-disciplinary approach with GI and A/I has produced better outcomes for symptom response and overall improvement of disease compared to a fragmented approach to care (abstract accepted). The allergist needs to be able identify atopic patients who have risk for eosinophilic esophagitis. Likewise, the gastroenterologist who encounters a patient with food impaction and discovers esophageal eosinophilia should consult an allergist for potential triggers and possible joint treatment approaches. A cooperative multi-disciplinary clinic allows for coordinated food introductions with endoscopic follow-up evaluation. In addition, allergists routinely educate patients regarding food avoidance, sources of contamination and cross-reactivity. This type of detailed education has been a proven asset to dietary compliance. Allergists will also have the experience with biologics, such as anti-IL5 and anti-IL-4 monoclonal antibodies, which may not be currently used in gastroenterology practices.

Author details

Rebecca Scherr[1*] and Mary Beth Hogan[2]

*Address all correspondence to: rscherr@medicine.nevada.edu

1 Division of Gastroenterology, Hepatology, and Nutrition, University of Nevada School of Medicine, Department of Pediatrics, USA

2 Division of Allergy and Immunology, University of Nevada School of Medicine, Department of Pediatrics, USA

References

[1] Attwood, S.E. and G.T. Furuta, *Eosinophilic esophagitis: historical perspective on an evolving disease.* Gastroenterol Clin North Am, 2014. 43(2): p. 185-99.

[2] Dalby, K., et al., *Eosinophilic oesophagitis in infants and children in the region of southern Denmark: a prospective study of prevalence and clinical presentation.* J Pediatr Gastroenterol Nutr, 2010. 51(3): p. 280-2.

[3] Spergel, J.M., et al., *Identification of causative foods in children with eosinophilic esophagitis treated with an elimination diet.* J Allergy Clin Immunol, 2012. 130(2): p. 461-7 e5.

[4] Spergel, J.M., et al., *14 years of eosinophilic esophagitis: clinical features and prognosis.* J Pediatr Gastroenterol Nutr, 2009. 48(1): p. 30-6.

[5] Liacouras, C.A., et al., *Eosinophilic esophagitis: updated consensus recommendations for children and adults.* J Allergy Clin Immunol, 2011. 128(1): p. 3-20 e6; quiz 21-2.

[6] Henderson, C.J., et al., *Comparative dietary therapy effectiveness in remission of pediatric eosinophilic esophagitis.* J Allergy Clin Immunol, 2012. 129(6): p. 1570-8.

[7] Erwin, E.A., et al., *Serum IgE measurement and detection of food allergy in pediatric patients with eosinophilic esophagitis.* Ann Allergy Asthma Immunol, 2010. 104(6): p. 496-502.

[8] Liacouras, C.A., et al., *Eosinophilic esophagitis: a 10-year experience in 381 children.* Clin Gastroenterol Hepatol, 2005. 3(12): p. 1198-206.

[9] Kagalwalla, A.F., et al., *Identification of specific foods responsible for inflammation in children with eosinophilic esophagitis successfully treated with empiric elimination diet.* J Pediatr Gastroenterol Nutr, 2011. 53(2): p. 145-9.

[10] Spergel, J.M., et al., *Treatment of eosinophilic esophagitis with specific food elimination diet directed by a combination of skin prick and patch tests.* Ann Allergy Asthma Immunol, 2005. 95(4): p. 336-43.

[11] Kapel, R.C., et al., *Eosinophilic esophagitis: a prevalent disease in the United States that affects all age groups.* Gastroenterology, 2008. 134(5): p. 1316-21.

[12] Spergel, J.M. and M. Shuker, *Nutritional management of eosinophilic esophagitis.* Gastrointest Endosc Clin N Am, 2008. 18(1): p. 179-94; xi.

[13] Noel, R.J., et al., *Clinical and immunopathologic effects of swallowed fluticasone for eosinophilic esophagitis.* Clin Gastroenterol Hepatol, 2004. 2(7): p. 568-75.

[14] Assa'ad, A.H., et al., *Pediatric patients with eosinophilic esophagitis: an 8-year follow-up.* J Allergy Clin Immunol, 2007. 119(3): p. 731-8.

[15] Sugnanam, K.K., et al., *Dichotomy of food and inhalant allergen sensitization in eosinophilic esophagitis.* Allergy, 2007. 62(11): p. 1257-60.

[16] Guajardo, J.R., et al., *Eosinophil-associated gastrointestinal disorders: a world-wide-web based registry.* J Pediatr, 2002. 141(4): p. 576-81.

[17] Mulder, D.J., et al., *Atopic and non-atopic eosinophilic oesophagitis are distinguished by immunoglobulin E-bearing intraepithelial mast cells.* Histopathology, 2012. 61(5): p. 810-22.

[18] Dellon, E.S., et al., *Prevalence of eosinophilic esophagitis in the United States.* Clin Gastroenterol Hepatol, 2014. 12(4): p. 589-96 e1.

[19] DeBrosse, C.W., et al., *Identification, epidemiology, and chronicity of pediatric esophageal eosinophilia, 1982-1999.* J Allergy Clin Immunol, 2010. 126(1): p. 112-9.

[20] Vanderheyden, A.D., et al., *Emerging eosinophilic (allergic) esophagitis: increased incidence or increased recognition?* Arch Pathol Lab Med, 2007. 131(5): p. 777-9.

[21] Hruz, P., et al., *Escalating incidence of eosinophilic esophagitis: a 20-year prospective, population-based study in Olten County, Switzerland.* J Allergy Clin Immunol, 2011. 128(6): p. 1349-1350 e5.

[22] Prasad, G.A., et al., *Epidemiology of eosinophilic esophagitis over three decades in Olmsted County, Minnesota.* Clin Gastroenterol Hepatol, 2009. 7(10): p. 1055-61.

[23] Arias, A. and A.J. Lucendo, *Prevalence of eosinophilic oesophagitis in adult patients in a central region of Spain.* Eur J Gastroenterol Hepatol, 2013. 25(2): p. 208-12.

[24] van Rhijn, B.D., et al., *Rapidly increasing incidence of eosinophilic esophagitis in a large cohort.* Neurogastroenterol Motil, 2013. 25(1): p. 47-52 e5.

[25] Liu, Y.S., et al., *Chemoattraction of macrophages by secretory molecules derived from cells expressing the signal peptide of eosinophil cationic protein.* BMC Syst Biol, 2012. 6: p. 105.

[26] Jacobsen, E.A., et al., *Eosinophils regulate dendritic cells and Th2 pulmonary immune responses following allergen provocation.* J Immunol, 2011. 187(11): p. 6059-68.

[27] Wong, T.W., et al., *Eosinophils regulate peripheral B cell numbers in both mice and humans.* J Immunol, 2014. 192(8): p. 3548-58.

[28] Kvarnhammar, A.M. and L.O. Cardell, *Pattern-recognition receptors in human eosinophils.* Immunology, 2012. 136(1): p. 11-20.

[29] Mulder, D.J., et al., *Expression of tcll-like receptors 2 and 3 on esophageal epithelial cell lines and on eosinophils during esophagitis.* Dig Dis Sci, 2012. 57(3): p. 630-42.

[30] Gorgens, A., et al., *Revision of the human hematopoietic tree: granulocyte subtypes derive from distinct hematopoietic lineages.* Cell Rep, 2013. 3(5): p. 1539-52.

[31] Yamaguchi, Y., et al., *Purified interleukin 5 supports the terminal differentiation and proliferation of murine eosinophilic precursors.* J Exp Med, 1988. 167(1): p. 43-56.

[32] Hogan, M.B., D. Piktel, and K.S. Landreth, *IL-5 production by bone marrow stromal cells: implications for eosinophilia associated with asthma.* J Allergy Clin Immunol, 2000. 106(2): p. 329-36.

[33] Nussbaum, J.C., et al., *Type 2 innate lymphoid cells control eosinophil homeostasis.* Nature, 2013. 502(7470): p. 245-8.

[34] Tantibhaedhyangkul, U., et al., *Increased esophageal regulatory T cells and eosinophil characteristics in children with eosinophilic esophagitis and gastroesophageal reflux disease.* Ann Clin Lab Sci, 2009. 39(2): p. 99-107.

[35] Hogan, M.B., et al., *Regulation of eosinophilopoiesis in a murine model of asthma.* J Immunol, 2003. 171(5): p. 2644-51.

[36] Wood, L.J., et al., *Changes in bone marrow inflammatory cell progenitors after inhaled allergen in asthmatic subjects.* Am J Respir Crit Care Med, 1998. 157(1): p. 99-105.

[37] Gauvreau, G.M., et al., *Effects of an anti-TSLP antibody on allergen-induced asthmatic responses.* N Engl J Med, 2014. 370(22): p. 2102-10.

[38] Hogan, M.B., et al., *Asthma progression to airway remodeling and bone marrow eosinophil responses in genetically distinct strains of mice.* Ann Allergy Asthma Immunol, 2008. 101(6): p. 619-25.

[39] Neighbour, H., et al., *Safety and efficacy of an oral CCR3 antagonist in patients with asthma and eosinophilic bronchitis: a randomized, placebo-controlled clinical trial.* Clin Exp Allergy, 2014. 44(4): p. 508-16.

[40] Blanchard, C. and M.E. Rothenberg, *Biology of the eosinophil.* Adv Immunol, 2009. 101: p. 81-121.

[41] Romano, C., et al., *Mucosal cytokine profiles in paediatric eosinophilic oesophagitis: a case-control study.* Dig Liver Dis, 2014. 46(7): p. 590-5.

[42] Johansson, M.W. and D.F. Mosher, *Integrin activation States and eosinophil recruitment in asthma.* Front Pharmacol, 2013. 4: p. 33.

[43] Blanchard, C., et al., *Periostin facilitates eosinophil tissue infiltration in allergic lung and esophageal responses.* Mucosal Immunol, 2008. 1(4): p. 289-96.

[44] Blanchard, C., et al., *A striking local esophageal cytokine expression profile in eosinophilic esophagitis.* J Allergy Clin Immunol, 2011. 127(1): p. 208-17, 217 e1-7.

[45] Higashimoto, I., et al., *Regulation of eosinophil cell death by adhesion to fibronectin.* Int Arch Allergy Immunol, 1996. 111 Suppl 1: p. 66-9.

[46] Johansson, M.W., D.S. Annis, and D.F. Mosher, *alpha(M)beta(2) integrin-mediated adhesion and motility of IL-5-stimulated eosinophils on periostin.* Am J Respir Cell Mol Biol, 2013. 48(4): p. 503-10.

[47] Walsh, G.M., F.A. Symon, and A.J. Wardlaw, *Human eosinophils preferentially survive on tissue fibronectin compared with plasma fibronectin.* Clin Exp Allergy, 1995. 25(11): p. 1128-36.

[48] Lamas, A.M., G.V. Marcotte, and R.P. Schleimer, *Human endothelial cells prolong eosinophil survival. Regulation by cytokines and glucocorticoids.* J Immunol, 1989. 142(11): p. 3978-84.

[49] Davoine, C., et al., *Adducts of oxylipin electrophiles to glutathione reflect a 13 specificity of the downstream lipoxygenase pathway in the tobacco hypersensitive response.* Plant Physiol, 2006. 140(4): p. 1484-93.

[50] Nutku, E., et al., *Ligation of Siglec-8: a selective mechanism for induction of human eosinophil apoptosis.* Blood, 2003. 101(12): p. 5014-20.

[51] Rubinstein, E., et al., *Siglec-F inhibition reduces esophageal eosinophilia and angiogenesis in a mouse model of eosinophilic esophagitis.* J Pediatr Gastroenterol Nutr, 2011. 53(4): p. 409-16.

[52] Fuentebella, J., et al., *Increased number of regulatory T cells in children with eosinophilic esophagitis.* J Pediatr Gastroenterol Nutr, 2010. 51(3): p. 283-9.

[53] Lamas, A.M., O.G. Leon, and R.P. Schleimer, *Glucocorticoids inhibit eosinophil responses to granulocyte-macrophage colony-stimulating factor.* J Immunol, 1991. 147(1): p. 254-9.

[54] Dellon, E.S., et al., *Markers of Eosinophilic Inflammation for Diagnosis of Eosinophilic Esophagitis and Proton Pump Inhibitor-Responsive Esophageal Eosinophilia: A Prospective Study.* Clin Gastroenterol Hepatol, 2014.

[55] Abonia, J.P., et al., *Involvement of mast cells in eosinophilic esophagitis.* J Allergy Clin Immunol, 2010. 126(1): p. 140-9.

[56] Elishmereni, M., et al., *Physical interactions between mast cells and eosinophils: a novel mechanism enhancing eosinophil survival in vitro.* Allergy, 2011. 66(3): p. 376-85.

[57] Hacha, J., et al., *Nebulized anti-IL-13 monoclonal antibody Fab' fragment reduces allergen-induced asthma.* Am J Respir Cell Mol Biol, 2012. 47(5): p. 709-17.

[58] Saenz, S.A., et al., *IL-25 simultaneously elicits distinct populations of innate lymphoid cells and multipotent progenitor type 2 (MPPtype2) cells.* J Exp Med, 2013. 210(9): p. 1823-37.

[59] Van Dyken, S.J., et al., *Chitin activates parallel immune modules that direct distinct inflammatory responses via innate lymphoid type 2 and gammadelta T cells.* Immunity, 2014. 40(3): p. 414-24.

[60] O'Dea, E.M., et al., *Eosinophils Are Recruited in Response to Chitin Exposure and Enhance Th2-Mediated Immune Pathology in Aspergillus fumigatus Infection.* Infect Immun, 2014. 82(8): p. 3199-205.

[61] Rayapudi, M., et al., *Indoor insect allergens are potent inducers of experimental eosinophilic esophagitis in mice.* J Leukoc Biol, 2010. 88(2): p. 337-46.

[62] Saw, S. and N. Arora, *Protease Inhibitor Reduces Airway Response and Underlying Inflammation in Cockroach Allergen-Induced Murine Model.* Inflammation, 2014.

[63] Winter, H.S., et al., *Intraepithelial eosinophils: a new diagnostic criterion for reflux esophagitis.* Gastroenterology, 1982. 83(4): p. 818-23.

[64] Locke, G.R., 3rd, et al., *Prevalence and clinical spectrum of gastroesophageal reflux: a population-based study in Olmsted County, Minnesota.* Gastroenterology, 1997. 112(5): p. 1448-56.

[65] Shaheen, N. and D. Provenzale, *The epidemiology of gastroesophageal reflux disease.* Am J Med Sci, 2003. 326(5): p. 264-73.

[66] Sant'Anna, A.M., et al., *Eosinophilic esophagitis in children: symptoms, histology and pH probe results.* J Pediatr Gastroenterol Nutr, 2004. 39(4): p. 373-7.

[67] Peterson, K.A., et al., *Comparison of esomeprazole to aerosolized, swallowed fluticasone for eosinophilic esophagitis.* Dig Dis Sci, 2010. 55(5): p. 1313-9.

[68] Remedios, M., et al., *Eosinophilic esophagitis in adults: clinical, endoscopic, histologic findings, and response to treatment with fluticasone propionate.* Gastrointest Endosc, 2006. 63(1): p. 3-12.

[69] Liacouras, C.A., et al., *Primary eosinophilic esophagitis in children: successful treatment with oral corticosteroids.* J Pediatr Gastroenterol Nutr, 1998. 26(4): p. 380-5.

[70] Ruchelli, E., et al., *Severity of esophageal eosinophilia predicts response to conventional gastroesophageal reflux therapy.* Pediatr Dev Pathol, 1999. 2(1): p. 15-8.

[71] Cheng, L., et al., *Acid-induced release of platelet-activating factor by human esophageal mucosa induces inflammatory mediators in circular smooth muscle.* J Pharmacol Exp Ther, 2006. 319(1): p. 117-26.

[72] Souza, R.F., et al., *Gastroesophageal reflux might cause esophagitis through a cytokine-mediated mechanism rather than caustic acid injury.* Gastroenterology, 2009. 137(5): p. 1776-84.

[73] Lampinen, M., S. Rak, and P. Venge, *The role of interleukin-5, interleukin-8 and RANTES in the chemotactic attraction of eosinophils to the allergic lung.* Clin Exp Allergy, 1999. 29(3): p. 314-22.

[74] Ma, J., et al., *HCl-induced and ATP-dependent upregulation of TRPV1 receptor expression and cytokine production by human esophageal epithelial cells.* Am J Physiol Gastrointest Liver Physiol, 2012. 303(5): p. G635-45.

[75] Luster, A.D. and M.E. Rothenberg, *Role of the monocyte chemoattractant protein and eotaxin subfamily of chemokines in allergic inflammation.* J Leukoc Biol, 1997. 62(5): p. 620-33.

[76] Isomoto, H., et al., *Elevated levels of chemokines in esophageal mucosa of patients with reflux esophagitis.* Am J Gastroenterol, 2003. 98(3): p. 551-6.

[77] Cheng, L., et al., *Hydrogen peroxide reduces lower esophageal sphincter tone in human esophagitis.* Gastroenterology, 2005. 129(5): p. 1675-85.

[78] Farre, R., et al., *Pharmacologic characterization of intrinsic mechanisms controlling tone and relaxation of porcine lower esophageal sphincter.* J Pharmacol Exp Ther, 2006. 316(3): p. 1238-48.

[79] Cao, W., et al., *Proinflammatory cytokines alter/reduce esophageal circular muscle contraction in experimental cat esophagitis.* Am J Physiol Gastrointest Liver Physiol, 2004. 287(6): p. G1131-9.

[80] Ohashi, Y., et al., *[Relationship between bronchial reactivity to inhaled acetylcholine, eosinophil infiltration and a widening of the intercellular space in patients with asthma].* Arerugi, 1990. 39(11): p. 1541-5.

[81] Orlando, R.C., *Pathophysiology of gastroesophageal reflux disease.* J Clin Gastroenterol, 2008. 42(5): p. 584-8.

[82] Krarup, A.L., et al., *Acid hypersensitivity in patients with eosinophilic oesophagitis.* Scand J Gastroenterol, 2010. 45(3): p. 273-81.

[83] Untersmayr, E. and E. Jensen-Jarolim, *The effect of gastric digestion on food allergy.* Curr Opin Allergy Clin Immunol, 2006. 6(3): p. 214-9.

[84] Tobey, N.A., et al., *Dilated intercellular spaces and shunt permeability in nonerosive acid-damaged esophageal epithelium.* Am J Gastroenterol, 2004. 99(1): p. 13-22.

[85] Cheng, E., R.F. Souza, and S.J. Spechler, *Eosinophilic esophagitis: interactions with gastroesophageal reflux disease.* Gastroenterol Clin North Am, 2014. 43(2): p. 243-56.

[86] Hirano, I. and S.S. Aceves, *Clinical implications and pathogenesis of esophageal remodeling in eosinophilic esophagitis.* Gastroenterol Clin North Am, 2014. 43(2): p. 297-316.

[87] Shin, J.M. and G. Sachs, *Pharmacology of proton pump inhibitors.* Curr Gastroenterol Rep, 2008. 10(6): p. 528-34.

[88] Cheng, E., et al., *Omeprazole blocks eotaxin-3 expression by oesophageal squamous cells from patients with eosinophilic oesophagitis and GORD.* Gut, 2013. 62(6): p. 824-32.

[89] Zhang, X., et al., *Omeprazole blocks STAT6 binding to the eotaxin-3 promoter in eosinophilic esophagitis cells.* PLoS One, 2012. 7(11): p. e50037.

[90] Biswas, K., et al., *A novel antioxidant and antiapoptotic role of omeprazole to block gastric ulcer through scavenging of hydroxyl radical.* J Biol Chem, 2003. 278(13): p. 10993-1001.

[91] Blandizzi, C., et al., *Lansoprazole prevents experimental gastric injury induced by non-steroidal anti-inflammatory drugs through a reduction of mucosal oxidative damage.* World J Gastroenterol, 2005. 11(26): p. 4052-60.

[92] Takagi, T., Y. Naito, and T. Yoshikawa, *The expression of heme oxygenase-1 induced by lansoprazole.* J Clin Biochem Nutr, 2009. 45(1): p. 9-13.

[93] Lapenna, D., et al., *Antioxidant properties of omeprazole.* FEBS Lett, 1996. 382(1-2): p. 189-92.

[94] Simon, W.A., et al., *Hydroxyl radical scavenging reactivity of proton pump inhibitors.* Biochem Pharmacol, 2006. 71(9): p. 1337-41.

[95] Martins de Oliveira, R., et al., *The inhibitory effects of H+K+ATPase inhibitors on human neutrophils in vitro: restoration by a K+ionophore.* Inflamm Res, 2007. 56(3): p. 105-11.

[96] Ohara, T. and T. Arakawa, *Lansoprazole decreases peripheral blood monocytes and intercellular adhesion molecule-1-positive mononuclear cells.* Dig Dis Sci, 1999. 44(8): p. 1710-5.

[97] Wandall, J.H., *Effects of omeprazole on neutrophil chemotaxis, super oxide production, degranulation, and translocation of cytochrome b-245.* Gut, 1992. 33(5): p. 617-21.

[98] Agastya, G., B.C. West, and J.M. Callahan, *Omeprazole inhibits phagocytosis and acidification of phagolysosomes of normal human neutrophils in vitro.* Immunopharmacol Immunotoxicol, 2000. 22(2): p. 357-72.

[99] Kelly, K.J., et al., *Eosinophilic esophagitis attributed to gastroesophageal reflux: improvement with an amino acid-based formula.* Gastroenterology, 1995. 109(5): p. 1503-12.

[100] Spergel, J.M., et al., *The use of skin prick tests and patch tests to identify causative foods in eosinophilic esophagitis.* J Allergy Clin Immunol, 2002. 109(2): p. 363-8.

[101] Al-Hussaini, A., E. Al-Idressi, and M. Al-Zahrani, *The role of allergy evaluation in children with eosinophilic esophagitis.* J Gastroenterol, 2013. 48(11): p. 1205-12.

[102] Spergel, J.M., *Eosinophilic esophagitis in adults and children: evidence for a food allergy component in many patients.* Curr Opin Allergy Clin Immunol, 2007. 7(3): p. 274-8.

[103] Wen, T., et al., *Molecular diagnosis of eosinophilic esophagitis by gene expression profiling.* Gastroenterology, 2013. 145(6): p. 1289-99.

[104] Rona, R.J., et al., *The prevalence of food allergy: a meta-analysis.* J Allergy Clin Immunol, 2007. 120(3): p. 638-46.

[105] Kagalwalla, A.F., et al., *Effect of six-food elimination diet on clinical and histologic outcomes in eosinophilic esophagitis.* Clin Gastroenterol Hepatol, 2006. 4(9): p. 1097-102.

[106] Markowitz, J.E., et al., *Elemental diet is an effective treatment for eosinophilic esophagitis in children and adolescents.* Am J Gastroenterol, 2003. 98(4): p. 777-82.

[107] Gonsalves, N., et al., *Elimination diet effectively treats eosinophilic esophagitis in adults; food reintroduction identifies causative factors.* Gastroenterology, 2012. 142(7): p. 1451-9 e1; quiz e14-5.

[108] Arias, A., et al., *Efficacy of dietary interventions for inducing histologic remission in patients with eosinophilic esophagitis: a systematic review and meta-analysis.* Gastroenterology, 2014. 146(7): p. 1639-48.

[109] Liacouras, C.A., J. Spergel, and L.M. Gober, *Eosinophilic esophagitis: clinical presentation in children.* Gastroenterol Clin North Am, 2014. 43(2): p. 219-29.

[110] Mishra, A., et al., *An etiological role for aeroallergens and eosinophils in experimental esophagitis.* J Clin Invest, 2001. 107(1): p. 83-90.

[111] Almansa, C., et al., *Seasonal distribution in newly diagnosed cases of eosinophilic esophagitis in adults.* Am J Gastroenterol, 2009. 104(4): p. 828-33.

[112] Fogg, M.I., E. Ruchelli, and J.M. Spergel, *Pollen and eosinophilic esophagitis.* J Allergy Clin Immunol, 2003. 112(4): p. 796-7.

[113] Wang, F.Y., S.K. Gupta, and J.F. Fitzgerald, *Is there a seasonal variation in the incidence or intensity of allergic eosinophilic esophagitis in newly diagnosed children?* J Clin Gastroenterol, 2007. 41(5): p. 451-3.

[114] Yamazaki, K., et al., *Allergen-specific in vitro cytokine production in adult patients with eosinophilic esophagitis.* Dig Dis Sci, 2006. 51(11): p. 1934-41.

[115] Mishra, A., et al., *IL-5 promotes eosinophil trafficking to the esophagus.* J Immunol, 2002. 168(5): p. 2464-9.

[116] Mishra, A. and M.E. Rothenberg, *Intratracheal IL-13 induces eosinophilic esophagitis by an IL-5, eotaxin-1, and STAT6-dependent mechanism.* Gastroenterology, 2003. 125(5): p. 1419-27.

[117] Lucendo, A.J., A. Arias, and J.M. Tenias, *Relation between eosinophilic esophagitis and oral immunotherapy for food allergy: a systematic review with meta-analysis.* Ann Allergy Asthma Immunol, 2014.

[118] Boldorini, R., F. Mercalli, and G. Oderda, *Eosinophilic oesophagitis in children: responders and non-responders to swallowed fluticasone.* J Clin Pathol, 2013. 66(5): p. 399-402.

[119] Arora, A.S., J. Perrault, and T.C. Smyrk, *Topical corticosteroid treatment of dysphagia due to eosinophilic esophagitis in adults.* Mayo Clin Proc, 2003. 78(7): p. 830-5.

[120] Teitelbaum, J.E., et al., *Eosinophilic esophagitis in children: immunopathological analysis and response to fluticasone propionate.* Gastroenterology, 2002. 122(5): p. 1216-25.

[121] Alexander, J.A., et al., *Swallowed fluticasone improves histologic but not symptomatic response of adults with eosinophilic esophagitis.* Clin Gastroenterol Hepatol, 2012. 10(7): p. 742-749 e1.

[122] Straumann, A., et al., *Long-term budesonide maintenance treatment is partially effective for patients with eosinophilic esophagitis.* Clin Gastroenterol Hepatol, 2011. 9(5): p. 400-9 e1.

[123] Konikoff, M.R., et al., *A randomized, double-blind, placebo-controlled trial of fluticasone propionate for pediatric eosinophilic esophagitis.* Gastroenterology, 2006. 131(5): p. 1381-91.

[124] Dohil, R., et al., *Oral viscous budesonide is effective in children with eosinophilic esophagitis in a randomized, placebo-controlled trial.* Gastroenterology, 2010. 139(2): p. 418-29.

[125] Straumann, A., et al., *Budesonide is effective in adolescent and adult patients with active eosinophilic esophagitis.* Gastroenterology, 2010. 139(5): p. 1526-37, 1537 e1.

[126] Moawad, F.J., et al., *Randomized controlled trial comparing aerosolized swallowed fluticasone to esomeprazole for esophageal eosinophilia.* Am J Gastroenterol, 2013. 108(3): p. 366-72.

[127] Francis, D.L., et al., *Results of ambulatory pH monitoring do not reliably predict response to therapy in patients with eosinophilic oesophagitis.* Aliment Pharmacol Ther, 2012. 35(2): p. 300-7.

[128] Dellon, E.S., et al., *Viscous topical is more effective than nebulized steroid therapy for patients with eosinophilic esophagitis.* Gastroenterology, 2012. 143(2): p. 321-4 e1.

[129] Schaefer, E.T., et al., *Comparison of oral prednisone and topical fluticasone in the treatment of eosinophilic esophagitis: a randomized trial in children.* Clin Gastroenterol Hepatol, 2008. 6(2): p. 165-73.

[130] Levine, J., et al., *Conservative long-term treatment of children with eosinophilic esophagitis.* Ann Allergy Asthma Immunol, 2012. 108(5): p. 363-6.

[131] Khanna, s., Kujath, C., Katzka, D., *The natural history of symptomatic esophageal eosinophilia: a longitudinal follow-up over 5 years..* American Journal of Gastroenterology, 2011. 106(S19): p. 45.

[132] Mishra, A., et al., *Esophageal remodeling develops as a consequence of tissue specific IL-5-induced eosinophilia.* Gastroenterology, 2008. 134(1): p. 204-14.

[133] Zuo, L., et al., *IL-13 induces esophageal remodeling and gene expression by an eosinophil-independent, IL-13R alpha 2-inhibited pathway.* J Immunol, 2010. 185(1): p. 660-9.

[134] Aceves, S.S., et al., *Mast cells infiltrate the esophageal smooth muscle in patients with eosinophilic esophagitis, express TGF-beta1, and increase esophageal smooth muscle contraction.* J Allergy Clin Immunol, 2010. 126(6): p. 1198-204 e4.

[135] Rieder, F., et al., *T-helper 2 cytokines, transforming growth factor beta1, and eosinophil products induce fibrogenesis and alter muscle motility in patients with eosinophilic esophagitis.* Gastroenterology, 2014. 146(5): p. 1266-77 e1-9.

[136] Niranjan, R., et al., *Pathogenic role of mast cells in experimental eosinophilic esophagitis.* Am J Physiol Gastrointest Liver Physiol, 2013. 304(12): p. G1087-94.

[137] Straumann, A., et al., *Anti-interleukin-5 antibody treatment (mepolizumab) in active eosinophilic oesophagitis: a randomised, placebo-controlled, double-blind trial.* Gut, 2010. 59(1): p. 21-30.

[138] Straumann, A., et al., *Anti-eosinophil activity and clinical efficacy of the CRTH2 antagonist OC000459 in eosinophilic esophagitis.* Allergy, 2013. 68(3): p. 375-85.

[139] Otani, I.M., et al., *Anti-IL-5 therapy reduces mast cell and IL-9 cell numbers in pediatric patients with eosinophilic esophagitis.* J Allergy Clin Immunol, 2013. 131(6): p. 1576-82.

[140] Assa'ad, A.H., et al., *An antibody against IL-5 reduces numbers of esophageal intraepithelial eosinophils in children with eosinophilic esophagitis.* Gastroenterology, 2011. 141(5): p. 1593-604.

[141] Spergel, J.M., et al., *Reslizumab in children and adolescents with eosinophilic esophagitis: results of a double-blind, randomized, placebo-controlled trial.* J Allergy Clin Immunol, 2012. 129(2): p. 456-63, 463 e1-3.

[142] Wenzel, S., et al., *Dupilumab in persistent asthma with elevated eosinophil levels.* N Engl J Med, 2013. 368(26): p. 2455-66.

[143] Wills-Karp, M. and F.D. Finkelman, *Untangling the complex web of IL-4-and IL-13-mediated signaling pathways.* Sci Signal, 2008. 1(51): p. pe55.

[144] Izuhara, K., K. Arima, and S. Yasunaga, IL-4 and IL-13: their pathological roles in allergic diseases and their potential in developing new therapies. Curr Drug Targets Inflamm Allergy, 2002. 1(3): p. 263-9.

3

Therapeutic and Immunologic Effects of *Zingiber officiale* in Allergic Rhinitis

Abdulghani Mohamed Alsamarai,
Mohamed Abdulsatar Hamid and
Amina Hamed Ahmed Alobaidi

1. Introduction

Allergic diseases are the most common problem in our community an d globally [1]. Allergic rhinitis is one of the most common allergic diseases in Iraq and probably in the world and nowadays it is increasing. It is with a chronic natural history and may appear at any age of life and subsequently converted into asthma [2] Up to now, there is no curative treatment for allergic rhinitis and most of the drugs that are used can only induce symptomatic relief and some of them have serious side effects and can cause withdrawal symptoms which lead the patients to continue treatment ending in more side effects [1]. There are marked increase in allergic diseases in developing countries as reported recently [3,4].

Allergic rhinitis with possibility of either under diagnosis in a ccuntries with lower prevalence or difference in risk factors in these areas of the world [5]. In Iraq, the allergic diseases were increased with time including AR [6]. To date there were no curative treatment for AR, however, many pharmacotherapeutic treatment evaluated in different studies and suggested a variable clinical response [3]. Recently an interest was launched which is the evaluation of plant products in the treatment of allergic rhinitis [7].

Environmental control measures and allergen avoidance, pharmacological management, and immunotherapy are the main three approaches for treatment of allergic rhinitis [8-10]. However, most of these approaches are palliative and not curative and may be not cost effective due to the chronicity of the disease [11,12]. Although allergic rhinitis is not a life-threatening condition, various complications can occur and result in significant impairment in quality of life [11,12], eventually leading to increase medical cost and may be converted into asthma [1]. Immunotherapy another option of treatment is reserved for patients with a less than adequate response to usual treatments and reported to be effective [13,14]. Although the effectiveness of SIT in the treatment of allergic rhinitis and allergic asthma has been proven, however its delayed time of action and adverse local and systemic side effects have limited its use as a treatment modality by majority of the patients [15-19].

Ginger is the rhizome of the plant *Zingiber officinal*, belong to Zingiberaceae plant family and it used as therapy in ancient medicine, spice or a tea [20]. Reported studies [21-26] suggest that ginger extract may exert its benefit as medicine through blocking of serotonin receptors, antioxidant activity, antiglycating mechanisms. In addition, ginger extract may be effective in treating nausea, vomiting and heart burn [27-31] and demonstrate antibacterial activity [32]. However, the extract should be not used during pregnancy because of it is mutagenic [28]. Furthermore, ginger may have analgesic, antipyretic, and antitumor activity [33-39].

Ginger adverse reactions that include some drugs interaction, increase of bile secretion, and induction of allergic reaction, may restrict its usage as medicine [40,41]. Since reported studies suggested the anti-inflammatory, suppressive effects on production of cytokines and reduction of IgE serum level [42-44], we conduct this study to evaluate the therapeutic effect of ginger in allergic rhinitis.

Aim of the study:

The aim of this study is to study the clinical and immunological efficacy of Zingiber officinale (Z.O) on the treatment of allergic rhinitis.

2. Materials and methods

2.1. Patients

A total of 79 patients allergic rhinitis were included in the study. Those patients were recruited from patients attending Aljumhory Teaching Hospital in Mosul and were selected on the basis that was with high total IgE serum levels. The study done during the period from November 2010 to October 2012. The patients were with age of > 10 years old. The patients divided into active and control group. The active group includes 42 patient and 37 patients were in control group. Each patients in active group received Zingiber officinale (Z.O) capsules, twice daily after meal. While each patient in control group received the same dose of sucrose powder capsules for 2 months, through which clinical follow up occurred completely in each monthly visit with recording the notes.

2.2. Diagnosis of asthma and allergic rhinitis

Allergic rhinitis diagnosis was performed according to previously reported guidelines [45].

2.3. Skin prick test

The skin prick tests were performed for all patients and control and evaluated in accordance with European Academy of Allergy and Clinical [1]. Immunology subcommittee on allergy standardization and skin tests using standards allergen panel (Stallergen, France). The panel for skin test include: dust mite (Dermatophagoides farina, Dermatophagoides peteronyssinus), Aleternaria, Cladosprium, Penicillum mixture, Aspergillus mixture, Grasses mixture, Feather mixture, Dog hair, Horse hair, Cat fur, Fagacae, Oleaceae, Betulaceae, Plantain, Bermuda grass, Chenopodium and Mugworth. All tests were performed in the outpatient Asthma and Allergy Centre, Mosul by a physician using a commercial allergen extracts (Stallergen, France) and a lancet skin prick test device. A wheal diameter of 3 mm or more in excess of the negative control was considered as positive test result.

2.4. Determination of total serum IgE

ELISA was performed to estimate the total serum IgE level as a serological marker for treatment response monitoring [1]. Total serum IgE was determined by enzyme linked immunosorbant assay kit (Biomaghreb). Results were interpreted as allergy not probable if serum IgE was lower than 20 IU/ml, allergy is possible if IgE value is between 20 and 120 IU/ml and allergy is very probable if IgE is more than 120 IU/ml.

2.5. Treatment schedule and assessment

Z. officinale was given as capsules, one capsule twice daily after each meal. Each capsule contained about 0.5 gm (500 mg) of Z.O powder.

The control group received the same capsules but they were contained sucrose sugar powder, the treatment was given for 2 months. The results were recorded on the patient's questionnaire in each visit. The same routine physical examination & laboratory investigations as mentioned earlier were done in each visit & recorded with clinical evaluation which was done according to the following criteria and as reported previously[6]:

1. Clinical assessment (symptoms score); during each visit, the patients was examined clinically for vital signs & questioned about the improvement in his day & night symptoms (rhinorrhoea, nasal obstruction, paroxysm of sneezing, night snoring, chest tightness, wheezes, cough, shortness of breath, work & school attendance, skin wheals, itchy skin, swelling & the lip or eye lid, shortness on exertion.....etc).

2. Tolerability to the exacerbating factors: Many precipitating factors such as aeroallergens exposure, cold exposure, infection (sinusitis), drugs, exertion....etc. may precipitate the condition, so the response to the exacerbating factors were assessed in each visit.

2.6. Side effects

Side effects that were shown by the patients were recorded in all patients & for all allergies type.

2.7. Statistical analysis

SPSS version 19 analytic system: Paired Samples test; Independent Samples test & Descriptive Statistics were used to compare between active & placebo groups. Chi square also was used in this statistics of the research.

3. Results

3.1. Baseline estimation

A total of 79 patients were included, 51.9 % (41patients) male and 48.1% (38 patients) female. Those patients were classified according to their disease pattern into seasonal 39.2 % (31 patients) and perennial 60.7 % (48 patients), of the total 49.3 % (39 patients) had positive family history of atopic diseases while 50.6 % (40 patients) were with negative family history of atopic disease. They were subdivided into active (42 patients) and control group (37 patients) as show in Table 1.

Total number	79	
Gender	Male	41
	Female	38
Type	Seasonal	31
	Perennial	48
Family history	Positive	39
	Negative	40
Smoking	Positive	27
	Negative	52
Subgroups	Active	42
	Control	37

Table 1. Allergic rhinitis patients baseline information.

3.2. Frequency distribution of the patients according to the age

Table 2 shows the frequency distribution of patients according to their ages. It shows that the peak incidence age occurred within the age of 10-19 years which account for 30.3% (24 patients).

Age/year	Number of patients
10-19 years	24 (30.3%)
20-29 years	19 (24%)
30-39 years	16 (20.2%)
40- above	20 (25.3%)

Table 2. Frequency distribution of the patients according to the age

3.3. Frequency distribution of the patients according to the duration of the disease

Table 3 shows the frequency distribution of the patients according to their duration of the disease. It shows that the peak incidence duration of the disease range between 1-5 years and this account for 64.5% (51patients).

Duration/ years	Number of patients
1-5 years	51 (64.5%)
6-10 years	14 (17.7%)
11-15 years	8 (10.1%)
16-20 years	1 (1.2%)
21- above years	5 (6.3%)

Table 3. Frequency distribution of the patients according to the duration of the disease

3.4. Relationship between family history of atopic disease and total IgE level in allergic rhinitis patients

The relationship between family history of atopic disease and total IgE level in allergic rhinitis patients is shown in Table 4. There was a significant relationship (p= 0.001) between family history of atopy and total IgE serum level.

Family history of atopy	Patients number	mean	Standard deviation	P value
Negative history	40	206.8	54.9	0.001
Positive history	39	335.2	223.2	

Independent Samples test

Table 4. Relationship between family history of atopic disease and total IgE level in allergic rhinitis patients

3.5. Relationship between smoking and total IgE level in allergic rhinitis patients

There was a non-significant relationship (p=0.124) between smoking and total IgE serum level in allergic rhinitis as shown in (Table 5).

Smoking	Patients number	Mean	Standard deviation	P value
Negative history	52	248.5	146.8	0.124
Positive history	27	311.9	211.6	

Independent Samples test

Table 5. Relationship between smoking and total IgE level in allergic rhinitis patients

3.6. Subgroups of allergic rhinitis patients

Table 6 shows the subgroups of allergic rhinitis patients: active group of allergic rhinitis included 42 patients (22 male, 20 female), (19 seasonal, 23 perennial), (21 positive family history of atopy while 21 with negative family history),(28 smoking cigarette while 14 not smoking cigarette). On the other hand, control group included 37(19 male,18 female), (12 seasonal,25 perennial), (18 had positive family history of atopy while 19 had not),(25 smoke cigarette, 12 not).

Group		Active	Control
Number		42	37
Sex	Male	22	19
	Female	20	18
Type	Seasonal	19	12
	Perennial	23	25
Family history	Positive	21	18
	negative	21	19
Smoke	Positive	28	25
	negative	14	12

Table 6. Subgroups of allergic rhinitis patients

3.7. Immunological effect (on total IgE level) after 2 months treatment

The effect of treatment on total IgE level is shown in Table 7 : It shows that the effect of *Z. officinale* is highly significant after the first month of treatment (p = 0.027) which also stayed significant after the second month treatment (p =0.002). While in case of placebo capsules, there is no significant decrease in the level of total IgE after first month (p= 0.112) nor after second month (p= 0.64).

Group	Month	Number of patients	Mean	Standard deviation	P value
Active	0	42	258.4	170.5	-------
	1	42	229.3	133.7	**0.027**
	2	42	175.7	85.5	**0.002**
Control	0	37	383.6	177.2	------
	1	37	256.1	157.8	0.112
	2	37	239.2	108.5	0.64

Table 7. Immunological Effect of treatment on Total IgE level in AR patients

3.8. Clinical effect after 2 months treatment

Clinical improvement after 2 months of treatment for both groups is seen in Table 8, from total, 78.5 %(33 patients) were improved in the active group after first month of treatment while 21.4

%(9 patients) were improved from placebo treating group. There was a significant difference (p=0.010) between active and placebo treated groups. At the end of 2nd month, the result stayed significant (p=0.011) with 92.8 %(39 patients) were improved from active group corresponding to 35.1 %(13 patients) were improved from placebo treating group.

Months of Treatment	Subgroups	Improved patients Number	Not improved Patients Number	P value
Month 1	Active	33 (78.5%)	9 (21.4%)	0.010
	Control	10 (27 %)	27 (72.9 %)	
Month 2	Active	39 (92.8%)	3 (7.1%)	0.011
	Control	13 (35.1 %)	24 (64.8 %)	

Table 8. Clinical improvement in general condition in A.R patients after treatment

3.9. Effect on specific clinical features

The comparison between the improvement in specific nasal allergic symptoms in both subgroups(experimental and placebo) after 2 months of treatment is shown in Table 9. It shows that sinusitis had improved in 83.3% (35 patient) of experimental group while only 21.6% (8 patients) in control group demonstrate improvement and this difference was significant(p=0.002). Nasal itching had improved in 78.5% (33 patients) in experimental patients while it improved in 32.4 % (12 patients) in control group (p=0.027). While rhinorrhoea had improved in 69.0% (29 patients) in active group corresponding to 37.8 % (14 patients) in control group which is insignificant (p=0.126). Sneezing had decreased in 61.9% (26 patients) in experimental group while in control group it had improved in 24.3%(9 patients) with significant difference (p=0.033).

Clinical features	Active group improved patients	Control group patients improved	P value
Sinusitis	35 (83.3%)	8 (21.6%)	**0.002**
Nasal itching	33 (78.5%)	12 (32.4%)	**0.027**
Rhinorrhoea	29 (69.0%)	14 (37.8%)	0.126
Sneezing	26 (61.9%)	9 (24.3%)	**0.033**
Post nasal drainage	17 (40.4%)	5 (13.5%)	**0.042**
Conjunctivitis	11 (26.1%)	6 (16.2%)	0.385
Others	8 (19.0%)	4 (10.8%)	0.381

Chi square test

Table 9. Effect on specific clinical features after 2 months treatment

Post nasal drainage had decreased significantly (p=0.042) in 40.4% (17 patients) of active group while it had decreased in 13.5 % (5 patients) of control group. Conjunctivitis had decreased in 26.1% (11 patients) in experimental group but it had decreased in 16.2% (6 patients) in control group, but not with significant difference (p=0.381) result.

3.10. Medication score

Medication score of conventional therapy had been decreased in 71.4 % (30 patients) in active group and in 27.4 % (10 patients) in control in 1st month of treatment and the difference was significant (p=0.021). The significance degree became larger in the second month (p=0.004), which statistically measured the results of decreased conventional therapy use in active group which account for 88 % (37 patients) corresponding to 27 %(10 patients) in the placebo treating group.

Months of treatment	Subgroups	Patients with decreased medication	Patients not with decreased medications	P value
Month 1	Active	30 (71.4%)	12 (28.5%)	0.021
	Control	10 (27%)	27 (72.9%)	
Month 2	Active	37 (88%)	5 (11.9%)	0.004
	Control	10 (27%)	27 (72.9%)	

Chi square test

Table 10. Medication score

4. Discussion

Pharmacotherapy is still the corner stone in the management of allergic disease followed by immunotherapy. All therapeutic strategies have many side effects. Some of them may prove dangerous or even lethal, in addition, mostly there is no curative therapy [3,4]. One of the good substitutions is the use of herbal medicine and one of the ancient herb that was used medically for many diseases was *Zingiber officinale* [21,22]. This herb has been used for many diseases since no signs of serious adverse effects were known in antiquity.

Male were affected slightly more with AR than female. This result accords with other studies that showed no sex difference or slight male predominance [46] About 54% of patients were less than 30 years old which means that the onset mainly started at the days of childhood adolescence. This goes in line with other studies [47] because allergy is a less common cause of rhinitis in elderly as compared with form of rhinitis like atrophic rhinitis [48].

Concerning duration of the disease, 64.5% of patients had duration less than 5 years. That means the allergic state in Iraq increased progressively in the last years especially after the last war in 2003 due to increased air pollutions. Our study demonstrated a significant association between family history and IgE serum level in allergic rhinitis patients. This finding is in accordance with well documented fact in allergic diseases [49-51].

The present study not shows a significant relationship between smoking and IgE serum level and this result is not agreed with that reported for Canada [52]. Z.O treatment showed a significant effect on total IgE level. This is not strange for Z.O because it has potent immunological effect in different studies [42-44]. Ginger extract seems to be with a wide range of therapeutic effects that include multiorgan [53] such as the immune response, metabolism, and gastrointestinal.

In the present study the patients showed excellent improvement in clinical symptoms and clinical response after 2 months treatment duration especially in patients as compared with control group. This may be due to the anti-mucous effect mainly, in addition to anti allergic effect that present in its contents. Ginger demonstrate effective therapeutic effects in the treatment of asthma and other respiratory diseases through its ability to loosen and expel phlegm from the sinuses and lungs [42].

In Japanese cedar pollinosis patients, and in the most sever cedar pollen scattering period, allergy symptoms (blowing the nose, itching eyes....etc) were significantly relieved in experimental group taking tea containing ginger extract for 13 weeks as compared with placebo group. Stuffy nose, sore throat medication score were significantly relieved. [54].

Medication score showed good decrease in conventional treatment of allergic rhinitis after 2 months uses of Z.O therapy as compared with control group. These results were a reflection and explanation of the improvement in clinical symptoms and augment the idea that says herbal treatment is benefit in medical fields.

In conclusion, *Zingiber officinale* is effective treatment for allergic rhinitis and significantly reduced serum total IgE after 4 weeks of treatment course.

Author details

Abdulghani Mohamed Alsamarai[*], Mohamed Abdulsatar Hamid and Amina Hamed Ahmed Alobaidi

*Address all correspondence to: galsamarrai@yahoo.com

Tikrit University College of Medicine, Tikrit, Iraq

References

[1] Alhalwani M, Alobaidi AH, Alsamarai AGM. Evaluation of the Therapeutic Effect of Combined Conventional Asthma Drugs with Tianeptine in Treatment of Asthma: Double-Blind Controlled Trial. Pharmacothewrapy 2014, IN Tech, in press.

[2] Alsamarai AM, Alwan AM, Ahmed AH. The relationship between asthma and allergic rhinitis in Iraqi population. Allergology International 2009;58:549-555.

[3] Sur DK, Scandale S. Treatment of allergic rhinitis. Am Fami Physician 2010;81:1440-1446.

[4] Alsamarai AGM, Amina Hamed Ahmad Alobaidi, Sami Mezher Alrefaiei and Amar Mohamed Alwan. House Dust Mite Immunotherapy in Iraqi Patients with Allergic Rhinitis and Asthma, Pharmacotherapy 2012, Dr. Farid Badria (Ed.), ISBN: 978-953-51-0532-9, InTech, Available from: http://www.intechopen.com/ books/ pharmacotherapy /house-dust-mite-immunotherapy-in-iraqi-patients-withallergic-rhinitis-and-asthma.

[5] Worldwide variation in prevalence of symptoms of asthma, allergic rhinoconjunctivitis & a topic eczema: ISAAC. The International study of Asthma & Allergies in childhood (ISAAC) Steering committee. Lancet 1998; 351: 1225- 1232.

[6] Alsamarai AGM, Abdul Satar M, Alobaidi AHA. Evaluation of Therapeutic Efficacy of Nigella sativa (Black Seed) for Treatment of Allergic Rhinitis", Allergic Rhinitis, 2012, Prof. Marek Kowalski (Ed.), ISBN: 978-953-51-0288-5, InTech, Available from: http://www.intechopen.com /books/allergic-rhinitis/evaluation-of-therapeutic-efficacy-of-nigella-sativa-blackseed-for-treatment-of-allergic-rhinitis].

[7] Alsamarai AGM, Abdulsatar M, Alobaidi AHA. Evaluation of topical black seed in the treatment of allergic rhinitis. AIAAMC 2014.

[8] Platts-Mills TA. Allergen avoidance. *J. Allergy Clin. Immunol.* Mar 2004,113(3),388-91.

[9] Denisek, S.; Stephanie, S. Treatment of Allergic Rhinitis. *Am. Fam. Physician.* 2010, 81(12), 1440-1446.

[10] Alzakar, E.; Alsamarai, A. Efficacy of immunotherapy for treatment of asthma in children. *Asthma Allergy Proceeding*, 2010, 31,324-330.

[11] Blaiss MS. Quality of life in allergic rhinitis. *Ann. Allergy Asthma Immunol.*, Nov 1999,83(5),449-54..

[12] Thompson, A.K.; Juniper, E.; Meltzer, E.O. Quality of life in patients with allergic rhinitis. *Ann. Allergy Asthma Immunol.* Nov 2000,85(5),338-47.

[13] Passalacqua, G.; Durham, S.R. Allergic rhinitis and its impact on asthma update: allergen immunotherapy. *J. Allergy Clin. Immunol.* 2007, 119,881-891.

[14] Jacobsen, L.; Niggemann, B.; Dreborg, S.; et al. Specific immunotherapy has long term preventive effect of seasonal and perennial asthma: 10 year follow up on the PAT study. *Allergy*, 2007, 62,943-948.

[15] Cohn, J.R.; Pizzi, A. Determinants of patient's compliance with allergen immunotherapy. *J. Allergy Clin. Immunol.*, 1993, 91,734-737.

[16] Tinkelman, D.G.; Cole, W.Q.; Tunno, J. Immunotherapy: a one year prospective study to evaluate risk factors of systemic reactions. *J. Allergy Clin. Immunol.*, 1995, 95,8-14.

[17] Taubi, E.; Kessel, A.; Blant, A.; Golan, T.D. Follow-up after systemic adverse reactions of immunotherapy. *Allergy*, 1999, 54,617-620.

[18] Tamir, R.; Levy, I.; Duer, S.; et al. Immediate adverse reactions to immunotherapy in allergy. *Allergy*, 1992, 47, 260-263.

[19] Zeldin, Y.; Weiler, Z.; Magen, E.; Tiosano, L.; Kidon, M.I. Safety and efficacy of allergen immunotherapy in the treatment of allergic rhinitis and asthma in real life. *IMAJ*, 2008, 10,869-872.

[20] http://acawo.com/ginger091824.htm.

[21] Nievergelt A, Huonker P, Schoop R, Altmann KH, Gertsch J. Identification of serotonin 5-HTIA receptor partial agonists in ginger. Bioorganic & Medicinal Chemistry. 2010;18(9): 3345-51.

[22] http://www.aseanbiodiversity.info/Abstract/51006851. pdf

[23] http://www.scienedaily.com/releases/2010/05/100519131130.htm

[24] Saraswat M, Suryanarayana P, Reddy PY, Patil M, ABalakrishna N, Reddy GB. Antiglycating potential of Zingiber officinalis and delay of diabetic cataract in rats. Molecular Vision. 2010; 16: 1525-37.

[25] Al-Amin ZM, Thomson M, Al-Qattan KK, Peltonen- Shalaby R, Ali M. Anti- diabetic and hypolipidaemic properties of ginger (Zingiber officinale) in streptozotocin- induced diabetic rats. British Journal of Nutrition (Cambridge University Press) 2006;96 (4): 660-666. doi: 10.1079/BJN20061849. PMID 17010224.

[26] Afshari, Ali taghizadeh et al.; Shirpoor, A; Farshid, A; Saadation, R; Rasmi, Y; Saboory, E; Ilkhanizadeh, B; Allameh, A. The effect of ginger on diabetic nephropathy, plasma antioxidant capacity and lipid peroxidation in rate. Food Chemistry (Elsevier) 2007;101 (1): 148-153. doi: 10.1016/j.foodchem.2006.01.013.

[27] http://medind.nic.in/ibi/t03/i1/ibit03i1p32.pdf.

[28] Ernst, E, Pittler, M.H. Efficacy of ginger for nausea and vomiting: a systematic review of randomized clinical trials. British Journal of Anesthesia 200;84 (3): 367-371. PMID 10793599.

[29] Wood C, Pittler MH. Comparison of ginger with various anti motion sickness drugs. British J Anaesthesia 2000;84 (3): 367-71. PMID 10793599.

[30] Grøntved A, Hentzer E. Vertigo reducing effect of ginger root. A controlled clinical study. J Otorhinoryngol Relat Spec 1986;48:282-6.

[31] http://en.wikipedia.org/wiki/Ginger,. Ginger NCCAM Herbs at a Glance. Nccam. Nih.gov.

[32] Chen, Jaw-Chyun; Li-Jiau Huang, Shih- Lu Wu, Sheng-Chu Kuo, Tin-Yun Ho, Chien-Yun Hsiang. Ginger and Its Bioactive Component Inhibit Enter toxigenic Escherichia coli Heat- Labile Enterotoxin- Induced Diarrhoea in Mice. Journal of Agricultural and Food Chemistry 2007;55 (21): 8390-8397. doi: 10.1021/jf071460f. PMID 17880155.

[33] http://en.wikipedia.org/wiki/Ginger, University of Meryland Medical Centre (2006). Ginger.

[34] O'Hara, Mary; Kiefer, David; Farrell, Kim; Kemper, Kathi. A Review of 12 Commonly Used Medicinal Herbs. Archives of Family Medicina 1998;7(7): 523-536. doi: 10.1001/archfami.7.6.523. PMID 9821826.

[35] Rhode, J.; Fogoros, S.; Zick, S.; Wahl, H.; Griffith, K.A.; Huang, J.; Liu, J. R. Ginger inhibits cell growth and modulates angiogenic factres in ovarian cancer cells. BMC Complementary & Alternative Medicine 2007;7: 44. doi: 10.1186/1472-6882-7-44. PMC 2241638. PMID 18096028.

[36] Kim, J.S.; et al., Sa Im; Park, Hye Won; Yang, Jae Heon; Shin, Tae-Yong; Kim, Youn-Chul; Baek, Nam=In; Kim, Sung-Hoon et al. Cytotoxic components from the dried rhizomes of Zingiber officinale Roscoe. Archeves of pharmacal Research 2008;31 (4): 415-418. doi: 10.1007/s12272-001-1172-y. PMID 18449496.

[37] Choudhury, D.; Amlan; Bhattacharya, Abhijit; Chakrabarti, Gopal. Aqueous extract of ginger shows antiproliferative activity through disruption of microtubule network of cancer cells. Food Chem Toxicol. 2010;48(10): 2872-2880. doi10.1016/j.fct. 2010.07.020.

[38] Oyagbemi, A.A.; Saba, A. B.; Azeez, O.I. Molecular targets of [6]- gingerol: Its potential roles in cancer chemoprevention. Biofactors 2010;36(3): 169- 178. doi: /Pp. 425-426. ISBN 0-684-80001-2.

[39] Jakes, Susan. Beverage of Champions. Times on- line.

[40] MDidea Extracts Professional. Dosage and Administration of Ginger.2010.

[41] www.webcrawler.com/ Mayo Clinic (1 May 2006). "drugs & Supplements: Ginger (Zingiber officinale Foscoe)".

[42] http://Jumblebox.Webs.com.

[43] Ueda H., Ippoushi K, Takeuchi A. Repeated oral administration of a squeezed ginger (Zingiber officiale) extract augmented the serum corticosterone level & had anti- inflammatory properties. Biosci Biotechnol Biochem. 2010; 74(11): 2248-52.

[44] Ahui ML, champy, Ramadan A, pham van L, Araujo L, Brou Andre K., Diem S, Damotte D, Kati- conlibaly S, Offoumou MA, Dym, Thieblemant N, Herbelin A. Ginger prevents Th$_2$- mediated immune response in a mouse model of airway inflammation, Int. Immuno pharmacol.2008 ;8 (12): 1626-32.

[45] Dykeewicz M, Fineman S, Skoner D, et.al. Diagnosis and management of rhinitis. Complete guidelines of the joint task fore on practice parameters in allergy, asthma, and immunology. Ann Allergy, Asthma, Immunol 1998; 81:478.

[46] Durham SR, Jories AS. Mechanisms & treatment of allergic rhinitis & intrinsic rhinitis in Jans. Mackay and T.R> Bull "Scott- Brown's" otolaryngo- logngology 1997, 6th eition, part 4: ch: 6: 4/6/1- 4/6/16, ch.9:4/9/1- 4/9/7.

[47] Abba I. Terr, A topic disease in Danial P. stites, Abba I. Terr, Tristram G. Basic & clinical Immunology G. parslow 1994 8th edition, ch. 25:327-345.

[48] Isabella A., Eli O., Peter H. Management of allergic rhinitis & it's impact on asthma A pocked Guide for physician & nurse 2001, 3-15.

[49] King H C. An Otolaryngologist's Guide to allergy. New York: 1990: 54.

[50] Barker JR. (ed) primer on allergic & immunologic diseases JAMA 1997;278, 1804-2025.

[51] Durham S. ABC of allergies BMJ 1998.

[52] Warren CPW, Holford- Strevens V, Wang C, Manfreda J. The relationship between smoking & total IgE levels, Journal of allergy & clinical Immunology, Vol. 69, issue 4, April 1982, P. 370-375.

[53] Badreldin H. Ali, Gerald Blunded, Musbah O., Tanira Abderrahim Nemmar. Some phyto chemical, pharmacological & toxicological properties of ginger (Zingiber Officinale) A review of recent research, Food Chemical Toxicology, 2008; 46:409-420.

[54] Maeda- Yamamoto M, Emak, Shibuichi L, In vitro and in vivo anti allergic effects of benifuuki green tea containing O-Methylated catechin & ginger extract enhancement. Cytotechnology 2007; 55 (2-3): 135-42, doi: 10.1007/s 10616- 007-9112-1 Epub 2007 Nov. 25.

4

Probiotics and Allergic Diseases — Usefulness of Animal Models — From Strains Selection to Mechanistic Studies

Elodie Neau, Marie-José Butel and
Anne-Judith Waligora-Dupriet

1. Introduction

The prevalence of allergies has dramatically and rapidly increased over the past decades in areas with a "westernized" or "industrialized" lifestyle. This increase and the dichotomy in the rate of allergic disease between industrialized and developing countries are two lines of evidence suggesting that environmental changes are a major factor in the development of allergies. There is mounting evidence that the microbiota is a key environmental factor that influences oral tolerance. Alterations in the sequential establishment of gut microbiota observed in western countries could therefore be responsible for a T-helper balance deviation toward a Th2 profile, a major factor in the rise of allergic diseases. Likewise treatment with broad spectrum antibiotics in infancy leading to microbiota alterations and dysbiosis, is associated with increased susceptibility to allergy [1]. Indeed recent epidemiological studies have linked factors influencing microbiota establishment and risk of allergy [2,3]. Hence, increasing evidences suggest that the composition of the microbiota influences intestinal barrier functions [4,5] and both local [6] and systemic immune responses [7]. A specific signature of the microbiota has been associated with allergy sensitivity [8-10]. This hypothesis has been confirmed by studies using mice models which have shown that the gut microbiota is likely to play a role in the development of oral tolerance. We and other have shown that the lack of gut microbiota in germ free mice is associated with the development of Th2 and IgE responses to dietary antigens [11,12]. The specific gut microbiota observed in mice with food allergy by Noval-Rivas *et al* was able of transmitting disease susceptibility to naive germ-free recipients [9]. In humans, several studies highlighted differences in the composition of bacterial communities in the feces of subject with or without allergic diseases; however, available epidemiological studies remain controversial [13]. Numerous studies support that a low diversity of the gut microbiota in infancy is important, more than the prevalence of specific bacterial taxa but this low diversity can also be attributed to specific bacterial group, such as *Bacteroidetes* and *Proteobacteria* [14-17]. Interestingly, Ling *et al* described distinct alterations of the gut microbiota in IgE and non-IgE mediated food allergy [18]. Despite discrepancies between clinical studies, the likely relationship between the intestinal microbiota and allergy assess the usefulness of modulation of the gut microbiota that may help prevent and manage allergic diseases. This notion supports the use of probiotics, prebiotics and symbiotics.

If present results of clinical trials do not allow concluding unambiguously in favor of probiotics, studies have shown the benefits of this approach, justifying further research in this direction [13,19-21]. Recent reviews reported studies showing the beneficial effects in the prevention of atopic dermatitis [19-21]. Prevention of respiratory allergies also seems possible [21]. Differences between studies are most likely due to differences in the populations studied - in terms of type of allergy, evolutionary stage of the disease, environment, genetic background - but also to the various probiotic used in terms of strain, dose, duration and time of administration in relation to the development of allergy, and finally the follow-up period [13, 19]. The combined prenatal and postnatal administration of probiotics appears more effective [21]. However, the conflicting results reported today do not allow the recommendation of the use of probiotics in prevention of allergy by expert committees. Despite the promising results on prevention and treatment of allergic diseases by various strains, EFSA did not delivered favorable opinions on requests. Progress in our basic knowledge of probiotic strains, in strain selection, and in understanding their mechanisms of action is needed to give credibility to the health claims made for probiotics and especially for the design of efficacious therapeutic agents. For these reasons, animal models constitute unavoidable tools for biomedical research. They are used for their potential to mimic the human disease process, and allow better understanding of key events of allergic disease development.

2. Animal models of food allergy, asthma and atopic dermatitis

In this chapter, only animal models that have been used to characterize the impact of probiotics on allergy will be described.

The impact of probiotics on allergy – including food allergy, asthma and atopic dermatitis – was mainly studied on small laboratory animals (mice and rats), but domestic animals, as dogs and piglets, were also used. It is important to carefully choose animal model because it can deeply affect the study. Indeed, genetic predispositions condition IgE responsiveness [22].

2.1. Rodent models

2.1.1. Mice model

Mice are the first model organism because of its easy reproduction and its low cost of maintenance. This model does not completely mirror the human but it shares with him similar mechanisms of immune regulation, notably in T cell polarization [23]. These animals have the

Other major allergens are peanut extract in food allergy [30,35,43,57], birch pollen from *Betula verrucosa* (Bet v 1) [58-60] and house dust mite *Dermatophagoides pteronyssinus* (Der p) [32,61,62] in asthma. The capacity to induce the immune system to produce IgE antibodies, elicit allergic symptoms, and bind to allergen-specific IgE depend of allergen [63]. For example, by oral route, the allergenic potential of peanut extract is far higher than the one of cow's milk [63], and egg, Brazil nut and spinach [64]. The different allergens induce different types of antibody isotype patterns, whether it be IgG1, IgG2a, IgE and IgA. The allergenic potential of these molecules depends on the size and physicochemical properties of the protein, the glycosylation status, the biologic and enzymatic activities and the way in which the protein is processed and presented to the immune system [64]. Moreover, all mice strains are not susceptible to the same allergens. For example, BALB/c genetic background is completely resistant to peanut-induced anaphylaxis unlike C3H strain [37]. Experimental and clinical data indicate a difference in gender susceptibility to allergic inflammation [65,66]. These differences appear to vary with the route of administration used (see 3.2).

The dose of allergen and its frequency of administration are also important parameters in the magnitude of the immune response. Kroghsbo *et al* [27] have orally immunized BALB/c mice with a low (0.5 mg) or a high (5 mg) dose of OVA. Results revealed that the OVA dose had no impact on the production of IgG1 and IgA, but had an impact on production of IgG2a and IgE, with a higher level obtained with the higher dose of allergen. Nevertheless, the allergen dose administered should not be too high. Indeed, a high-dose of allergen can be associated with an induction of tolerance, while low-dose is known to induce sensitization [51,67]. In addition to the dose, the frequency of antigen exposure plays also a role. Nelde *et al* have showed that, after intraperitoneal (IP) sensitization of BALB/c mice, IgE synthesis was best induced by increasing the frequency of OVA application with low-dose than with few exposures with high doses [68]. The magnitude of the sensitization therefore depends on the type and the dose of the used allergen, but also on the route of administration (see below).

3.2. Route of exposure

The route by which antigen is administered has its advantages and disadvantages, and affects both the magnitude and the type of response obtained. It must be chosen depending on the purpose of the study. The route of delivery to animals should closely look like about the projected route of administration to humans. The most common routes for allergen administration are oral, IP and epicutaneous (EC) routes. Intra-nasal (IN) - for administration of pneumallergen in model of asthma [69], intra-tracheal (IT) [55], and subcutaneous routes (SC) [55,59,60,62,70,71] are more rarely employed.

3.2.1. Oral route

To model food allergy, antigen administration via the gastrointestinal tract – in other words, by gavage (IG) – provides clear ties to the human condition, and it is thus very relevant for exposure to food antigens. Additionally, it has the advantage of being economical, convenient, and relatively safe. Oral route also allows testing different allergens to evaluate their allergenic potential [64]. Oral immunization does not discriminate between males versus females, with no differences in their level of Th1 (i.e. IgG2a) or Th2 -associated (i.e. IgE and IgG1) antibodies [65]. This route can be used for sensitization studies [30,33-35,43-45,72-75] but also for tolerance studies [76-78]. Consequently, this route is principally used to study the impact of probiotics on food allergy.

3.2.2. Intraperitoneal route

The intraperitoneal administration is a common technique in laboratory rodents. It can be used to administer large volumes of fluid safely, unlike oral route which only tolerate low volumes [79]. The pharmacokinetic of substances administered by this route is closed to those seen after oral administration, with a passage by the liver. Special care must be taken regarding the injected substances which should be sterile, isotonic and nonirritating. There are differences in sensitization according to the gender when this route is applied. Bonnegarde-Bernard *et al* have therefore showed that female mice C57BL/6 sensitized by intraperitoneal route develop higher level of allergen-specific IgE, IgG2a and IgA than males [65]. This route is used in experimental murine models of food allergy and asthma, in sensitization or tolerance induction studies [80-83].

3.2.3. Epicutaneous route

Some substances can also be administered directly to the skin surface (epicutaneous administration) for a topical affect. The allergen is captured by skin dendritic cells that migrate to the afferent lymph nodes and activate immune responses and allergen-specific cytokine production [84]. Several studies have demonstrated that this route allows to sensitize to various antigens, in the absence of adjuvant [85], with a strong Th2 response [86,87]. For that, they utilized occlusive dressings and/or prolonged exposure to the antigen. The extent of absorption of substances through the skin and into the systemic circulation depends on many parameters, as for example the surface area of application, the integrity of the skin and the contact time [79]. Contrary to the oral route, the epicutaneous administration is inadequate to discriminate the allergenic potential of proteins [64]. This route is very employed in atopic dermatitis model [52,53,66,88-95].

3.2.4. Comparison of routes of exposure

Several publications have compared the impact of these different routes of administration on sensitization. Animals can be sensitized to many allergens, but in an adjuvant-dependent manner, whatever the route practiced (IP, SC, IG, EC, and IN), with a significant production of allergen-specific IgE, IgG1 and IgG2a [49,64,85]. The maximal level of these immunologic markers is attained via the cutaneous route [85]. A mucosal administration (i.e. IG, SC or IN administrations) was shown to develop a robust allergen-specific IgA response by contrast with a cutaneous exposure [85]. The intraperitoneal route allowed a stronger IgE and IgG response compared with that obtained by oral route [49], but this response was weaker than the one observed with intranasal and epicutaneous allergen application [68]. Contrary to the oral route, intraperitoneal and epicutaneous administrations did not allow the induction of oral tolerance [87].

3.3. The use of adjuvant

Most proteins are poorly immunogenic or non-immunogenic when administered on their own. To increase the immune response and thus sensitize animals, the majority of experimental studies utilize an adjuvant. The latter leads to a Th2 skewing, and abrogates the establishment of oral tolerance [96, 97]. There are exogenous Th2 adjuvants as glycans, endogenous adjuvants as thymic stromal lymphopoietin (TSLP) and experimental adjuvants as cholera toxin, aluminum hydroxide and enterotoxin B from *Staphylococcus aureus*.

3.3.1. Cholera toxin

Cholera toxin (CT) is secreted by the bacterium *Vibrio cholerae*, which is responsible for aqueous diarrhea. The major effect of CT is to promote the uptake of antigen by antigen-presenting cells and to facilitate the presentation of antigen to T cells by favoring the intestinal permeability. Indeed, it induces *in vivo* the maturation and the migration of gastrointestinal dendritic cells (DCs) from the *lamina propria* to the mesenteric lymph nodes where they present antigen to naive T cells. CT also enhances the migration from the subepithelial dome region of Peyer's patches to the interfollicular T-cell areas. This maturation of DCs also includes the up-regulation of the co-stimulatory molecules OX40L and TIM-4, known to facilitate differentiation of responder T cells into Th2 cells. The neutralization of these two molecules has been shown to abrogate Th2 skewing in the gastrointestinal tract [96, 98].

3.3.2. Aluminum hydroxide

Aluminum hydroxide (alum) rarely induces cellular immune responses. However, it slows down the rate of release of the antigen and in this way increases the duration of antigen interaction with the immune system. It also promotes macrophage uptake. Therefore, it enhances the immune response against the antigen [97,99].

3.3.3. Enterotoxin B from Staphylococcus aureus

The enterotoxin B (SEB) is produced by *Staphylococcus aureus* in a variety of environments, including food substrates [97]. It causes severe diarrhea, nausea and intestinal cramping often starting within a few hours of ingestion. In the same way as the cholera toxin, the SEB induces the up-regulation of co-stimulatory molecules TIM-4, but also CD80 and CD86, which promotes the Th2 skewing.

3.3.4. Impact of dose of adjuvant

Few studies have focused on the impact of dose adjuvant on sensitization. Kroghsbo *et al* have tested three different CT doses (0.1, 1 or 10 µg) on BALB/c mice, sensitized to ovomucoid or ovalbumin [27]. They have observed a clear dose-dependent response on antibody induction, with the strongest response at the highest CT dose for any of the tested antibody isotypes (IgG1, IgG2a, IgE, and IgA). They were able to determine a threshold value (between 0.1 and 1 µg) for the lowest CT dose needed for sensitization. A weak dose of CT (0.1 µg) leads to initiation of IgG1 production. To observe an IgE production, a higher dose of CT (10 µg) is necessary.

4. Probiotic administration

Animal models can be used to select probiotic strains which can prevent or manage allergy, and to study their mechanism of action. Indeed, these animal models can be discriminant. For instance, if number of studies showed a positive impact of probiotic supplementation in their models of allergy (Tables 4 to 6), Meijerink *et* al showed a strain specific effect in a peanut allergy model [57]. Lee *et al* studied the protective impact on OVA sensitization of four strains of *Lactobacillus* [100]. None of them induced a change in IgE levels. Moreover, one of them led to an increase in allergic response. Likewise, de Jonge *et al* have found similar levels of IgG1 and IgG2a in Brown Norway rats sensitized to peanut extract, receiving or not a strain of *L. casei* Shirota by gavage [43]. A lack of benefit of supplementation was also observed in three models of asthma [62,70,71,101]. Sometimes, an improvement of symptoms, with a decrease of clinical signs after oral challenge, but without correlation with a decrease in markers of sensitization can be also observed [54,58,59].

4.1. Evaluation of beneficial effect of probiotic

The beneficial effect of probiotic supplementation is evaluated according to the model used.

4.1.1. Models of anaphylaxis

In models of anaphylaxis, clinical markers are analyzed after challenge by allergen, according to a scale score based on observed clinical symptoms (number of itches, mobility during the experiment, swelling of eyes and/or noise, aspect of hair, and body temperature). Thang *et al* and Schouten *et al* have scored symptoms of systemic anaphylaxis as follows: 0=no symptoms; 1=pilar erecti, scratching and rubbing around the nose and head; 2=pilar erecti, reduced activity; 3=activity after prodding and lowered body temperature; 4=no activity after prodding, labored respiration, and lowered body temperature; 5=death [28,74]. There are other models of anaphylaxis, in particular murine models of intestinal anaphylaxis induced by OVA. Food allergy symptoms are then scored by the criteria of diarrhea and rectal temperature [102,103]. However, this model has not been used yet to evaluate the impact of probiotic.

4.1.2. Models of asthma

In models of asthma, there is no scale of scores. The impact of probiotic is estimated by the determination of the cellular composition of bronchoalveolar fluid (total cell count and proportion of each cell type – lymphocytes, neutrophils, eosinophils and monocytes), the evaluation of number of infiltrated inflammatory cells in lung, and by the measurement of bronchial hyperresponsiveness [70,81,104].

4.1.3. Models of atopic dermatitis

As in models of food allergy, a scale of scores can be used in models of atopic dermatitis. Matsuda *et al* have estimated clinical skin condition after sensitizations as follows: 0=none, 1=mild, 2=moderate, 3=severe, for each of these symptoms: itch, erythema/hemorrhage, edema, excoriation/erosion and scaling/dryness [105]. The frequency and the duration of scratching, the numbers of infiltrated cells and the epidermal/auricular thickening can be also measured [88,90,105].

The limit of all these evaluations lies in its subjectivity despite a blind evaluation system. This subjectivity results in a problem of reproducibility of the method. An analysis of biological markers of allergic reaction, i.e. the dosage in plasma of mast cell protease-1 (MCP-1) and/or histamine release during mast cell degranulation, provides less subjective data than clinical score [30,34,35]. These models also allow evaluating sensitization through dosage of allergen-specific and total IgE, IgG1 and IgG2a [60,92,100].

4.2. Route and dose of probiotic supplementation

The dose of probiotic is often comprised between 10^6 and 10^9 CFU. When the dose of probiotic is tested, the highest dose shows, most of the time, better results [35,62,89,94,106]. Jan et al have tested three increasing doses of Lactobacillus gasseri (1, 2 and 4.10^6 CFU) in BALB/c mice, in a model of asthma. Only the highest dose (4.10^6 CFU) caused a significant decrease in the number of monocytes, lymphocytes and neutrophils in bronchoalveolar lavage fluid [62].

In oral administration, we distinguish the intra-gastric (IG) administration, in other words the gavage (with a needle), from oral administration (PO) (probiotic mixed in water or food). These two routes of exposure are principally used for the probiotic supplementation and whatever the types of allergy study. Gavage allows giving a precise dose of bacteria, but it is constraining because each animal must be handled individually leading to an additional stress in animals. Administration of the probiotic strains in drinking water or food avoids these problems of stress, but it raises the problem of their stability. Moreover, it does not allow knowing precisely the amount of bacteria received per day per animal. Probiotic can also be given by intranasal administration in models of asthma, or by epicutaneous exposure in models of atopic dermatitis. Intranasal administration allows a contact more extended with the probiotic, and therefore a longer action. However, according to the protocols, an anesthesia is necessary [107,108]. It could affect the lung antigen deposition by changing the breathing pattern and airway reflexes in animal [109]. Pellaton et al have demonstrated that intranasal exposure is more effective than gavage, with a lesser infiltration of eosinophils, in a model of asthma [106].

4.3. Window and frequency of probiotic administration

In the window of administration, we will consider the number of weeks of supplementation as well as the number of administration per week. According to studies, the probiotic is administered between 1 to 15 weeks, during 3 to 7 days per week.

The term "prevention" refers to an administration of the probiotic that starts prior to sensitizations and continues throughout the experiment. On the contrary, the term "management/treatment" refers to an administration of the probiotic that starts after sensitizations until the end of protocol.

In studies, probiotic is mainly tested for prevention and therefore administrated until two weeks before the start of sensitizations. Meijerink et al began administration of probiotic by gavage 14 days prior to sensitizations [57]. Each of the three strains of *Lactobacillus* had a different impact on allergy. The strain of *L. plantarum* WCFS1 have promoted allergic response (increase of IgE, IgG1 and MCP-1), the strain of *L. casei* Shirota had no impact on allergy, while the strain of *L. salivarius* HMI001 allowed the decrease of peanut-specific IgE and MCP-1. Yu *et al*, in a model of asthma, have given a strain of *L. rhamnosus* Lcr35 in BALB/c mice, 7 days before sensitizations. They observed a decrease in both bronchial hyperresponsiveness and number of cells in bronchoalveolar fluid [110]. Some studies have administered the probiotic in treatment, i.e. after the last sensitization, in models of food allergy and asthma, with a positive impact of supplementation. Schiavi *et al* have demonstrated, in a model of shrimp tropomyosin allergy, that the administration of VSL#3 during 20 days after the fourth sensitization allowed a decrease of clinical scoring and specific IgE, together with an induction of IgA on C3H/HeJ mice [34]. Similar results have been found in studies of Zhang *et al* [35], and Forsythe *et al* [111], with the administration of ImmuBalance™ in a model of food allergy, and with the gavage of strain *L. reuteri* ATCC 23272 in a model of asthma, respectively.

This high heterogeneity in the different protocols of probiotic administration make difficult, even impossible, comparisons between studies, and prevents establishment of an optimal administration scheme of probiotic. Comparison between prevention and management protocols shows that the window of administration plays a key role in the efficiency of probiotic, with a better effect in prevention. Indeed, in a model of food allergy, Kim *et al* [33] have showed, on C3H/HeJ mice sensitized to OVA, an improvement of allergic symptoms on the tail associated with a decrease of specific IgE in prevention, more important than those observed in treatment. Tanaka *et al* [42] in a model of atopic dermatitis and Yu *et al* [110] in a model of asthma have obtained comparable results. On the contrary, Bickert *et al* revealed a positive impact of probiotic, with an IP administration of *Escherichia coli* Nissle 1917 mixed with OVA, at the same time of sensitizations [31]. In study of Huang *et al*, similar effects of probiotics in prevention and treatment have been observed, suggesting that a long-term supplementation was not necessary [45]. Zuercher *et al* have obtained more contrasted results. They have observed that an oral administration of *Lactococcus lactis* NCC 2287 was effective in the management of food allergy symptoms in sensitized BALB/c mice, with a decrease in symptoms upon OVA challenge. However, this administration had no effect on the prevention of sensitization, with similar levels of OVA-specific IgE and IgG1, and MCP-1 [75].

4.4. Age and sanitary status of animals

The age and the sanitary status of animals have also an influence. In study of Lyons *et al*, the strain of *Bifidobacterium* AH1205 led to an increase of the percentage of CD4/CD25⁺cells in spleen and Peyer's patches in pups but not in adult mice. The strain of *Bifidobacterium* AH1206 had the same impact, but in both pups and adult mice. These two strains were then tested in models of asthma and food allergy. Only the strain AH1206, which had an impact on pups and adult mice, showed a positive impact on allergy, with a decrease in bronchoalveolar cell number and OVA-specific IgE [112]. Similarly, depending on whether mice are germ-free or conventional, the induction of CD4/CD25/Foxp3⁺cells in spleen was not the same, with a lower induction in germ free, whatever the strain studied [112].

5. Concluding remarks

At a time when probiotics seem promising products for the prevention and treatment of allergy, fundamental and clinical studies failed the issuance of health claims and the implementation of recommendations by expert committees. The use of animal models is an essential step in the selection of strains of interest. However, such a use must be part of a rationalization process taking into account the 3Rs (Reduce, Reuse and Recycle) and ethical rules. *In vitro* models can bring the prior information on the behavior of the strains with respect to immunostimulary capacities. For instance, Foligne *et al* have discriminated pro- and anti-inflammatory strains in a model of human peripheral blood mononuclear cells according to their cytokine profile [113]. Dendritic cells model can also allow selecting probiotic strains able to prime monocyte-derived DCs to drive the development of Treg cells [114]. Based on this first strain selection, animal models allow analyzing their mechanism of action. Indeed, probiotics can act on various actors of immunity. They can improve the barrier integrity [115], induce IgA secretion [28], and/or modulate T-helper balance, switching from Th2 to Th1 response [116] or enhancing Treg activity [34]. However, one should consider carefully the choice of the model and the design of probiotic administration to provide results which could be considered predictive for benefits in human and support the design of clinical studies.

Strain	Age	Allergen	Route	Adjuvant	Window	References
BALB/c	6 wks	BLG	IP	alum	1/wk, x1 wk	[80]
BALB/c male	3 wks	BLG	IP	alum	1/wk, x3 wks	[28]
BALB/c female	6 wks	OVA	IP	alum	1/2wks, x2	[100]
OVA-TCR female	8 wks	OVA	IG	/	4/wk, x2 wks	[73]
C3H/HeOuJ female	6 wks	peanut extract	IG	CT	3/wk then 1/wk, x3 wks	[57]
BALB/c	6 wks	OVA	IG	CT	4/wk then 1/wk	[75]
Swiss Albino	6-8 wks	OVA	IP	alum	1/wk, x2 wks	[116]
C3H/HeJ female	8 wks	shrimp tropomyosin	IG	CT	1/wk, x4 wks	[34]
BALB/c female	18-22g	OVA	IP	SEB	3/wk, x1 wk	[115]
C3H/HeJ female	5 wks	peanut extract	IG	CT	1/wk, x8 wks	[35]
BALB/c male	7 wks	OVA	IP	alum	1/wk, x2 wks	[83]
C3H/HeJ	5 wks	OVA	IG	CT	3/wk then 1/2wks, x2	[72]

Strain	Age	Allergen	Route	Adjuvant	Window	References
female						
C3H/HeOuJ female	3 wks	whey protein	IG	CT	1/wk, x6 wks	[74]
BALB/c	8 wks	OVA	IP	CT	1/wk, x3 wks	[112]
C57BL/6 female	8 wks	peanut extract	IG	CT	1/wk, x4 wks	[30]
C3H/HeJ female	3 wks	OVA	IG	CT	3/wk then 1/2wks, x2	[33]
Sprague-Dawley male	150-180g	OVA	IG and IP	Freund	4/wk then 1/wk	[44]
Brown-Norway female	3 wks	OVA	IG	/	7/wk, x6 wks	[45]
Brown-Norway female	3-4 wks	peanut extract	IG	/	7/wk, x6 wks	[43]
Yorkshire	birth	ovomucoid	IP	CT	1/wk, x3 wks	[54]

Table 1. Protocols of sensitizations in food allergy

Strain	Age	Allergen	Route	Adjuvant	Window	References
GF BALB/c female	8 wks	Bet v 1	SC	alum	1/2wks, x3	[60]
BALB/c female	5 wks	cedar pollen	SC	/	5/2wks	[70]
GF BALB/c	birth	Bet v 1	SC	alum	1/2wks, x3	[59]
BALB/c female	6 wks	OVA	IP	alum	1/wk, x2 wks	[91]
BALB/c male	20-25g	OVA	IP	alum	1/wk, x2 wks	[104]
BALB/c female	6-8 wks	Der p	SC	Freund	1/wk, x2 wks	[62]
BALB/c female	6-10 wks	Bet v 1 + *Phleum pretense* 1 and 5	IP	alum	1/2wks, x3	[58]
BALB/c male	5 wks	OVA	IP and IN	alum	1/2wks (IP) then 3/wk, x4 wks (IN)	[69]
BALB/c female	3 wks	cedar pollen	SC	/	4/wk then 1/wk	[71]
BALB/c female	6-8 wks	OVA	IP	alum	1/2wks, x4	[82]
BALB/c male	5-8 wks	OVA	IP	alum	1/wk, x2 wks	[81]
C57BL/6 female	6-8 wks	OVA	IP	alum	1/2wks, x2	[31]
BALB/c	20-25g	OVA	IP	alum	2/wk, x1 wk	[111,117]

Strain	Age	Allergen	Route	Adjuvant	Window	References
male						
C57BL/6 female	3-4 wks	Der p2	EC	/	1/2wks, x3	[32]
BALB/c	20-25g	OVA	IP	CT	2/wk, x1 wk	[112]
BALB/c	-	Der p1	IP	alum	1/wk, x3 wks	[61]
BALB/c female	6 wks	OVA	IP	alum	1/wk, x2 wks	[110]
BALB/c female	4 wks	OVA	IP	alum	1/2wks, x2	[106]
BALB/c female	8 wks	OVA	IP	/	3/wk, x2 wks	[118]
BALB/c female	6-8 wks	OVA	IP	alum	1/2wks, x2	[119]
BALB/c female	8 wks	Par j 1	IP	alum	1/3wks, x2	[101]
Duroc x Landrace	3 wks	*Ascaris suum*	SC et IT	alum	1/2wks, x3 (SC) then 1/2wks, x2 (IT)	[55]

Table 2. Protocols of sensitizations in asthma

Strain	Age	Allergen	Route	Adjuvant	Window	References
NC/Nga	-	FITC	EC	dibutyl phtalate	1/wk, x3 wks	[92]
NC/Nga male	6 wks	DNCB	EC	/	2/wk, x2 wks	[120]
NC/NgaTnd	8 wks	/	/	/	/	[105]
SKH-1/fr female	4 wks	OVA	EC	/	1/3wks, x3	[90]
NC/Nga	6 wks	Df	EC	SDS	1/wk, x5 wks	[95]
NC/NgaTndCrlj female	10 wks	Df	EC	SDS	2/wk, x4 wks	[88]
BALB/c female	8-10 wks	OVA	IP and EC	alum	1/2wks, x2 then 7/2wk, x3	[94]
NC/NgaTnd	5 wks	/	/	/	/	[42]
NC/Nga male	4 wks	DF	IP	/	1/wk, x14 wks	[121]
NC/Nga female	6 wks	DNCB	EC	/	2/wk, x3 wks	[89]
NC/Nga female	birth	/	/	/	/	[122]
NC/Nga	6 wks	Df	EC	/	3/wk, x5 wks	[66]
NC/Nga male	6 wks	PCl	EC	/	1x	[93]
Beagle	birth	Df	EC	/	3/wk, x1 wk	[53]
Beagle	birth	Df	EC	/	2/wk, x12 wks	[52]

Table 3. Protocols of sensitizations in atopic dermatitis

Probiotic	Route	Window	Dose	Impact		References
L. plantarum NRIC0380	IG	3/wk, x4 wks	200µg or 2mg	sensitization	↘	[80]
VSL#3	IG	7/wk, x5 wks	15.10^9 CFU	clinic sensitization	↘ ↘	[28]
L. casei YIT9029 (L1) *L. casei* HY7201 (L2) *L. brevis* HY7401 (L3) *L. plantarum* HY20301 (L4)	IG	7/wk, x3 wks	2mg	sensitization	L1, L3, L4, ↗ L2	[100]
L. brevis HY7401 (LB) *L. casei* Shirota YIT9029 (LC) *L. longum* HY8001 (BL)	IG	4/wk, x2 wks	2mg	clinic sensitization	↘ LB, LC, BL ↘ LB, LC, BL	[73]
L. plantarum WCFS1 (LP) *L. salivarius* HMI001 (LS) *L. casei* Shirota (LC)	IG	3/wk, x6 wks	10^9 CFU	sensitization	↗ LP, ↘ LS, LC	[57]
L. lactis NCC2287	PO	7/wk, x1 (M) or 8 (P) wks	5.10^8 CFU/mL	clinic sensitization	P, ↘ M P, M	[75]
Dahi	PO	7/wk, x1,2 or 3 wk(s)	-	sensitization	↘	[116]
VSL#3	IG	7/wk, x3 wks	7,5.10^8 CFU	clinic sensitization	↘ ↘	[34]
Bifidobacterium	IG	7/wk, x1 wk	10^8 CFU/mL	sensitization	↘	[115]
ImmuBalance™	PO	7/wk, x4 wks	0,5 or 1%	clinic sensitization	↘ ↘	[35]
L. pentosus S-PT84	PO	7/wk, x5 wks	0,075%	sensitization	↘	[83]
B. bifidum BGN4	PO	7/wk, x7 wks (P) or 7/wk, x2 wks (M)	0,2%	clinic sensitization	↘ P, M ↘ P, M P > M	[72]
Immunofortis (IF) *B. breve* M-16V (BB) symbiotic (SY)	PO	7/wk, x10 wks	2%	clinic sensitization	↘ IF, BB, SY ↘ SY, IF, BB	[74]
B. breve AH1205 (BB). *B. longum* AH1206 (BL) *L. salivarius* AH102 (LS)	IG	7/wk, x5 wks	2.10^9 CFU	sensitization	↘ BL, BB, LS	[112]
VSL#3	IG	7/wk, x3 wks	7,5.10^8 CFU	clinic	↘	[30]
B. bifidum BGN4 (BB) *L. casei* 911 (LC) *E. coli* MC4100 (EC)	PO	7/wk, x7 wks	0,2%	sensitization	↘ BB, LC, EC BB, LC > EC	[33]
LGG *B. animalis* MB5	IG	7/wk, x4 wks	10^9 CFU	-		[44]

Probiotic	Route	Window	Dose	Impact		References
LGG + *B. longum* BB536	IG	7/wk, x2, 3 or 10 wks	0,5.10^9 CFU	sensitization	↘	[45]
L. casei Shirota	IG	7/wk, x8 wks	10^9 CFU	sensitization		[43]
L. lactis MG1363	IG	7/wk, then 3/wk then 1/wk, x3 wks	10^9 CFU	clinic sensitization	↘	[54]

Table 4. Protocols of probiotic administration in models of food allergy

Probiotic	Route	Window	Dose	Impact		References
B. longum ssp. *longum* CCM7952	IG	1x (parents before coupling)	2.10^8 CFU	sensitization	↘	[60]
E. faecalis FK-23	IG	7/wk, x3 wks	60mg	infiltration sensitization		[70]
L. paracasei NCC2461	PO	7/wk, x4 wks	2.10^9 CFU/mL	clinic sensitization	↘	[59]
L. rhamnosus Lcr35	IG	7/wk, x3 wks	10^9 CFU/ 600μL	infiltration	↘	[91]
E. faecalis FK-23	IG	7/wk, x4 wks	60mg	infiltration	↘	[104]
L. gasseri A5	IG	7/wk, x4 wks	1,2 or 4.10^6 CFU	sensitization		[62]
L. paracasei NCC2461 *B. longum* NCC3001	IN	day of sensitization (M) or 3/wk, x2 wks (P)	5.10^8 CFU	sensitization	↘ M, P NCC3010 > NCC2461	[58]
L. crispatus KT-11 (LC) LGG (LG)	PO	7/wk, x8 wks	5.10^7 CFU/g	clinic sensitization	↘ LC, LG ↘ LC, LG	[69]
E. faecalis FK-23	IG	7/wk, x3 wks	30mg	sensitization		[71]
L. salivarius PM-A0006	IG	7/wk, x8 wks	2,6 or 5,5.10^6 CFU, or 3,6.10^7 CFU	infiltration sensitization	↘ ↘	[82]
B. breve M16V	IG	7/wk, x2 wks	10^9 CFU	infiltration sensitization	↘ ↘	[81]
E. coli Nissle 1917	IG	day of sensitization (M) or 7/wk, x4 wks (P)	10^8 CFU	infiltration sensitization	↘ M, P ↘ M, P	[31]
L. reuteri ATCC23272	IG	7/wk, x1 wk	10^9 CFU	infiltration sensitization	↘ ↘	[111,117]
L. casei Shirota	IG	3/wk, x4 wks	10^9 CFU	sensitization	↘	[32]
B. breve AH1205 (BB) *B. longum* AH1206 (BL)	IG	7/wk, x2 wks	2.10^9 CFU	infiltration	↘ BL, BB, LS	[112]

Probiotic	Route	Window	Dose	Impact		References
L. salivarius AH102 (LS)						
E. coli Nissle 1917	IN	3/wk, x2 wks	10^9 CFU	sensitization	↘	[61]
L. rhamnosus Lcr35	IG	7/wk, x3 wks (P) or 1 wk (M)	10^9 CFU	infiltration sensitization	↘ P, M ↘ P, M	[110]
L. paracasei NCC2461 (A) *L. plantarum* NCC1107 (B)	IN or IG	7/wk, x1 wk	10^9 CFU	infiltration	↘ A, B IN > IG	[106]
LGG (LG) *B. lactis* Bb-12 (BB)	IG	4/wk, x8 wks	10^9 CFU	infiltration sensitization	↘ LG, BB ↘ LG, BB	[118]
L. rhamnosus HN001	PO	7/wk, x7 wks	10.10^{10} CFU	clinic	↘	[55]

Table 5. Protocols of probiotic administration in models of asthma

Probiotic	Route	Window	Dose	Impact		References
Vitreoscilla filiformis	CUT	1/wk, x4 wks	20% v/v	clinic sensitization	↘	[92]
L. sakei probio 65	IG	7/wk, x2 wks	5.10^9 CFU/mL	clinic sensitization	↘ ↘	[120]
ImmuBalance™	PO	7/wk, x2 wks	$1,8.10^8$/g	clinic infiltration sensitization	↘ ↘ ↘	[105]
L. rhamnosus Lcr35	IG	7/wk, x8 wks	10^9 CFU/ 600µL	clinic infiltration sensitization	↘ ↘ ↘	[90]
L. plantarum CJLP55 (A) *L. plantarum* CJLP133 (B) *L. plantarum* CJLP136 (C)	PO	7/wk, x8 wks	10^{10} CFU	clinic infiltration sensitization	↘ A, B, C ↘ A, B, C ↘ A, B, C	[95]
B. subtilis JCM20036	IG	6/wk, x4 wks	$1,2.10^{17}$ CFU	clinic infiltration	↘ ↘	[88]
E. coli Nissle 1917	PO	7/wk, x4 wks	10^7 or 10^8 CFU	clinic infiltration sensitization	↘ ↘	[94]
L. rhamnosus CGMCC1.3724	PO	7/wk, x12 wks (P) or 7/wk, x7 wks (M)	5.10^8 CFU/mL	clinic sensitization	↘ P, M ↘ P, M	[42]
L. crispatus KT-11 (A) *L. crispatus* KT-23 (B) *L. crispatus* KT-25 (C)	PO	7/wk, x15 wks	1mg	clinic sensitization	↘ A, B, C ↘ A, B, C	[121]
B. subtilis KCTC1666 + *L. acidophilus* KCTC3155	PO	7/wk, x3 wks	1 or 2%	clinic sensitization	↘ 2% > 1%	[89]

Probiotic	Route	Window	Dose	Impact		References
LGG	PO	7/wk, x10 wks	4.10^4 CFU/g	clinic infiltration sensitization	↘ ↘	[122]
L. johnsonii NCC533	IG	2 days	$1,5.10^{11}$ CFU/mL	clinic sensitization	↘	[66]
L. paracasei KW3110 + LGG	PO	7/wk, x11 wks	0,03% or 0,3%	clinic sensitization	↘ 0,3% > 0,03%	[93]
LGG Culturelle®	IG	7/wk, x6 months	20.10^9 CFU	-		[53]
LGG	IG	7/wk, x6 months		clinic	↘	[52]

Impact of probiotic by comparison with control mice, in term of clinical score (clinic); markers of sensitization, i.e. allergen-specific and total IgE and IgG1 (sensitization); and infiltration of inflammatory cells, i.e. lymphocytes, neutrophils, eosinophils and monocytes, in lung and/or bronchoalveolar fluid (infiltration).

↗ increase in symptoms or negative effect; ↘ decrease in symptoms or positive effect; → no change in symptoms or no effect

Table 6. Protocols of probiotic administration in models of atopic dermatitis

Author details

Elodie Neau, Marie-José Butel and Anne-Judith Waligora-Dupriet[*]

*Address all correspondence to: anne-judith.waligora@parisdescartes.fr

EA 4065, DHU Risques et Grossesse, Faculté des Sciences Pharmaceutiques et Biologiques, Université Paris Descartes, Sorbonne Paris-Cité, France

References

[1] Foliaki S, Pearce N, Bjorksten B, Mallol J, Montefort S, von ME. Antibiotic use in infancy and symptoms of asthma, rhinoconjunctivitis, and eczema in children 6 and 7 years old: International Study of Asthma and Allergies in Childhood Phase III. J Allergy Clin Immunol 2009 Nov;124(5):982-9.

[2] Jaakkola JJ, Ahmed P, Ieromnimon A, Goepfert P, Laiou E, Quansah R, et al. Preterm delivery and asthma: a systematic review and meta-analysis. J Allergy Clin Immunol 2006 Oct;118(4):823-30.

[3] Liem JJ, Kozyrskyj AL, Huq SI, Becker AB. The risk of developing food allergy in premature or low-birth-weight children. J Allergy Clin Immunol 2007 May;119(5): 1203-9.

[4]   Macpherson AJ, Slack E, Geuking MB, McCoy KD. The mucosal firewalls against commensal intestinal microbes. Semin Immunopathol 2009 Jul;31(2):145-9.

[5]   Slack E, Hapfelmeier S, Stecher B, Velykoredko Y, Stoel M, Lawson MA, et al. Innate and adaptive immunity cooperate flexibly to maintain host-microbiota mutualism. Science 2009 Jul 31;325(5940):617-20.

[6]   Gaboriau-Routhiau V, Rakotobe S, Lecuyer E, Mulder I, Lan A, Bridonneau C, et al. The key role of segmented filamentous bacteria in the coordinated maturation of gut helper T cell responses. Immunity 2009 Oct 16;31(4):677-89.

[7]   Round JL, Mazmanian SK. The gut microbiota shapes intestinal immune responses during health and disease. Nat Rev Immunol 2009 May;9(5):313-23.

[8]   Mortha A, Chudnovskiy A, Hashimoto D, Bogunovic M, Spencer SP, Belkaid Y, et al. Microbiota-dependent crosstalk between macrophages and ILC3 promotes intestinal homeostasis. Science 2014 Mar 28;343(6178):1249288.

[9]   Noval RM, Burton OT, Wise P, Zhang YQ, Hobson SA, Garcia LM, et al. A microbiota signature associated with experimental food allergy promotes allergic sensitization and anaphylaxis. J Allergy Clin Immunol 2013 Jan;131(1):201-12.

[10] Rodriguez B, Prioult G, Hacini-Rachinel F, Moine D, Bruttin A, Ngom-Bru C, et al. Infant gut microbiota is protective against cow's milk allergy in mice despite immature ileal T-cell response. FEMS Microbiol Ecol 2012 Jan;79(1):192-202.

[11] Rodriguez B, Prioult G, Bibiloni R, Nicolis I, Mercenier A, Butel MJ, et al. Germ-free status and altered caecal subdominant microbiota are associated with a high susceptibility to cow's milk allergy in mice. FEMS Microbiol Ecol 2011 Apr;76(1):133-44.

[12] Sudo N, Sawamura S, Tanaka K, Aiba Y, Kubo C, Koga Y. The requirement of intestinal bacterial flora for the development of an IgE production system fully susceptible to oral tolerance induction. J Immunol 1997 Aug 15;159(4):1739-45.

[13] Waligora-Dupriet AJ, Butel MJ. Microbiota and Allergy: From Dysbiosis to Probiotics. In: Celso Pereira, editor. Allergic Diseases-Highlights in the Clinic, Mechanisms and Treatment. InTech; 2012. p. 413-34.

[14] Abrahamsson TR, Jakobsson HE, Andersson AF, Bjorksten B, Engstrand L, Jenmalm MC. Low gut microbiota diversity in early infancy precedes asthma at school age. Clin Exp Allergy 2014 Jun;44(6):842-50.

[15] Bisgaard H, Li N, Bonnelykke K, Chawes BL, Skov T, Paludan-Muller G, et al. Reduced diversity of the intestinal microbiota during infancy is associated with increased risk of allergic disease at school age. J Allergy Clin Immunol 2011 Sep;128(3): 646-52.

[16] Forno E, Onderdonk AB, McCracken J, Litonjua AA, Laskey D, Delaney ML, et al. Diversity of the gut microbiota and eczema in early life. Clin Mol Allergy 2008;6:11.

[17] Wang M, Karlsson C, Olsson C, Adlerberth I, Wold AE, Strachan DP, et al. Reduced diversity in the early fecal microbiota of infants with atopic eczema. J Allergy Clin Immunol 2008 Jan;121(1):129-34.

[18] Ling Z, Li Z, Liu X, Cheng Y, Luo Y, Tong X, et al. Altered fecal microbiota composition associated with food allergy in infants. Appl Environ Microbiol 2014 Apr;80(8): 2546-54.

[19] Castellazzi AM, Valsecchi C, Caimmi S, Licari A, Marseglia A, Leoni MC, et al. Probiotics and food allergy. Ital J Pediatr 2013;39:47.

[20] Kim HJ, Kim HY, Lee SY, Seo JH, Lee E, Hong SJ. Clinical efficacy and mechanism of probiotics in allergic diseases. Korean J Pediatr 2013 Sep;56(9):369-76.

[21] Kuitunen M. Probiotics and prebiotics in preventing food allergy and eczema. Curr Opin Allergy Clin Immunol 2013 Jun;13(3):280-6.

[22] Herz U, Renz H, Wiedermann U. Animal models of type I allergy using recombinant allergens. Methods 2004 Mar;32(3):271-80.

[23] Shay T, Jojic V, Zuk O, Rothamel K, Puyraimond-Zemmour D, Feng T, et al. Conservation and divergence in the transcriptional programs of the human and mouse immune systems. Proc Natl Acad Sci U S A 2013 Feb 19;110(8):2946-51.

[24] Bix M, Wang ZE, Thiel B, Schork NJ, Locksley RM. Genetic regulation of commitment to interleukin 4 production by a CD4(+) T cell-intrinsic mechanism. J Exp Med 1998 Dec 21;188(12):2289-99.

[25] McIntire JJ, Umetsu SE, Akbari O, Potter M, Kuchroo VK, Barsh GS, et al. Identification of Tapr (an airway hyperreactivity regulatory locus) and the linked Tim gene family. Nat Immunol 2001 Dec;2(12):1109-16.

[26] Akiyama H, Teshima R, Sakushima JI, Okunuki H, Goda Y, Sawada JI, et al. Examination of oral sensitization with ovalbumin in Brown Norway rats and three strains of mice. Immunol Lett 2001 Aug 1;78(1):1-5.

[27] Kroghsbo S, Christensen HR, Frokiaer H. Experimental parameters differentially affect the humoral response of the cholera-toxin-based murine model of food allergy. Int Arch Allergy Immunol 2003 Aug;131(4):256-63.

[28] Thang CL, Boye JI, Zhao X. Low doses of allergen and probiotic supplementation separately or in combination alleviate allergic reactions to cow beta-lactoglobulin in mice. J Nutr 2013 Feb;143(2):136-41.

[29] Morafo V, Srivastava K, Huang CK, Kleiner G, Lee SY, Sampson HA, et al. Genetic susceptibility to food allergy is linked to differential TH2 -TH1 responses in C3H/HeJ and BALB/c mice. J Allergy Clin Immunol 2003 May;111(5):1122-8.

[30] Barletta B, Rossi G, Schiavi E, Butteroni C, Corinti S, Boirivant M, et al. Probiotic VSL#3-induced TGF-beta ameliorates food allergy inflammation in a mouse model of

peanut sensitization through the induction of regulatory T cells in the gut mucosa. Mol Nutr Food Res 2013 Dec;57(12):2233-44.

[31] Bickert T, Trujillo-Vargas CM, Duechs M, Wohlleben G, Polte T, Hansen G, et al. Probiotic Escherichia coli Nissle 1917 suppresses allergen-induced Th2 responses in the airways. Int Arch Allergy Immunol 2009;149(3):219-30.

[32] Lim LH, Li HY, Huang CH, Lee BW, Lee YK, Chua KY. The effects of heat-killed wild-type Lactobacillus casei Shirota on allergic immune responses in an allergy mouse model. Int Arch Allergy Immunol 2009;148(4):297-304.

[33] Kim H, Kwack K, Kim DY, Ji GE. Oral probiotic bacterial administration suppressed allergic responses in an ovalbumin-induced allergy mouse model. FEMS Immunol Med Microbiol 2005 Aug 1;45(2):259-67.

[34] Schiavi E, Barletta B, Butteroni C, Corinti S, Boirivant M, Di FG. Oral therapeutic administration of a probiotic mixture suppresses established Th2 responses and systemic anaphylaxis in a murine model of food allergy. Allergy 2011 Apr;66(4):499-508.

[35] Zhang T, Pan W, Takebe M, Schofield B, Sampson H, Li XM. Therapeutic effects of a fermented soy product on peanut hypersensitivity is associated with modulation of T-helper type 1 and T-helper type 2 responses. Clin Exp Allergy 2008 Nov;38(11): 1808-18.

[36] Bashir ME, Louie S, Shi HN, Nagler-Anderson C. Toll-like receptor 4 signaling by intestinal microbes influences susceptibility to food allergy. J Immunol 2004 Jun 1;172(11):6978-87.

[37] Berin MC, Zheng Y, Domaradzki M, Li XM, Sampson HA. Role of TLR4 in allergic sensitization to food proteins in mice. Allergy 2006 Jan;61(1):64-71.

[38] Shinagawa K, Kojima M. Mouse model of airway remodeling: strain differences. Am J Respir Crit Care Med 2003 Oct 15;168(8):959-67.

[39] Van Hove CL, Maes T, Cataldo DD, Gueders MM, Palmans E, Joos GF, et al. Comparison of acute inflammatory and chronic structural asthma-like responses between C57BL/6 and BALB/c mice. Int Arch Allergy Immunol 2009;149(3):195-207.

[40] Matsuda H, Watanabe N, Geba GP, Sperl J, Tsudzuki M, Hiroi J, et al. Development of atopic dermatitis-like skin lesion with IgE hyperproduction in NC/Nga mice. Int Immunol 1997 Mar;9(3):461-6.

[41] Suto H, Matsuda H, Mitsuishi K, Hira K, Uchida T, Unno T, et al. NC/Nga mice: a mouse model for atopic dermatitis. Int Arch Allergy Immunol 1999;120 Suppl 1:70-5.

[42] Tanaka A, Jung K, Benyacoub J, Prioult G, Okamoto N, Ohmori K, et al. Oral supplementation with Lactobacillus rhamnosus CGMCC 1.3724 prevents development of atopic dermatitis in NC/NgaTnd mice possibly by modulating local production of IFN-gamma. Exp Dermatol 2009 Dec;18(12):1022-7.

[43] de Jonge JD, Ezendam J, Knippels LM, Penninks AH, Pieters R, van LH. Lactobacillus casei Shirota does not decrease the food allergic response to peanut extract in Brown Norway rats. Toxicology 2008 Jul 30;249(2-3):140-5.

[44] Finamore A, Roselli M, Britti MS, Merendino N, Mengheri E. Lactobacillus rhamnosus GG and Bifidobacterium animalis MB5 induce intestinal but not systemic antigen-specific hyporesponsiveness in ovalbumin-immunized rats. J Nutr 2012 Feb; 142(2):375-81.

[45] Huang J, Zhong Y, Cai W, Zhang H, Tang W, Chen B. The effects of probiotics supplementation timing on an ovalbumin-sensitized rat model. FEMS Immunol Med Microbiol 2010 Nov;60(2):132-41.

[46] de Jonge JD, Knippels LM, Ezendam J, Odink J, Penninks AH, van LH. The importance of dietary control in the development of a peanut allergy model in Brown Norway rats. Methods 2007 Jan;41(1):99-111.

[47] Atkinson HA, Miller K. Assessment of the brown Norway rat as a suitable model for the investigation of food allergy. Toxicology 1994 Aug 12;91(3):281-8.

[48] Knippels LM, Penninks AH, Spanhaak S, Houben GF. Oral sensitization to food proteins: a Brown Norway rat model. Clin Exp Allergy 1998 Mar;28(3):368-75.

[49] Dearman RJ, Caddick H, Stone S, Basketter DA, Kimber I. Characterization of antibody responses induced in rodents by exposure to food proteins: influence of route of exposure. Toxicology 2001 Oct 30;167(3):217-31.

[50] Dearman RJ, Kimber I. Animal models of protein allergenicity: potential benefits, pitfalls and challenges. Clin Exp Allergy 2009 Apr;39(4):458-68.

[51] Helm RM, Ermel RW, Frick OL. Nonmurine animal models of food allergy. Environ Health Perspect 2003 Feb;111(2):239-44.

[52] Marsella R, Santoro D, Ahrens K. Early exposure to probiotics in a canine model of atopic dermatitis has long-term clinical and immunological effects. Vet Immunol Immunopathol 2012 Apr 15;146(2):185-9.

[53] Marsella R, Santoro D, Ahrens K, Thomas AL. Investigation of the effect of probiotic exposure on filaggrin expression in an experimental model of canine atopic dermatitis. Vet Dermatol 2013 Apr;24(2):260-e57.

[54] Rupa P, Schmied J, Wilkie BN. Prophylaxis of experimentally induced ovomucoid allergy in neonatal pigs using Lactococcus lactis. Vet Immunol Immunopathol 2011 Mar 15;140(1-2):23-9.

[55] Thomas DJ, Husmann RJ, Villamar M, Winship TR, Buck RH, Zuckermann FA. Lactobacillus rhamnosus HN001 attenuates allergy development in a pig model. PLoS One 2011;6(2):e16577.

[56]   Lunney JK. Advances in swine biomedical model genomics. Int J Biol Sci 2007;3(3): 179-84.

[57]   Meijerink M, Wells JM, Taverne N, de Zeeuw Brouwer ML, Hilhorst B, Venema K, et al. Immunomodulatory effects of potential probiotics in a mouse peanut sensitization model. FEMS Immunol Med Microbiol 2012 Aug;65(3):488-96.

[58]   Schabussova I, Hufnagl K, Wild C, Nutten S, Zuercher AW, Mercenier A, et al. Distinctive anti-allergy properties of two probiotic bacterial strains in a mouse model of allergic poly-sensitization. Vaccine 2011 Feb 24;29(10):1981-90.

[59]   Schabussova I, Hufnagl K, Tang ML, Hoflehner E, Wagner A, Loupal G, et al. Perinatal maternal administration of Lactobacillus paracasei NCC 2461 prevents allergic inflammation in a mouse model of birch pollen allergy. PLoS One 2012;7(7):e40271.

[60]   Schwarzer M, Srutkova D, Schabussova I, Hudcovic T, Akgun J, Wiedermann U, et al. Neonatal colonization of germ-free mice with Bifidobacterium longum prevents allergic sensitization to major birch pollen allergen Bet v 1. Vaccine 2013 Nov 4;31(46):5405-12.

[61]   Adam E, Delbrassine L, Bouillot C, Reynders V, Mailleux AC, Muraille E, et al. Probiotic Escherichia coli Nissle 1917 activates DC and prevents house dust mite allergy through a TLR4-dependent pathway. Eur J Immunol 2010 Jul;40(7):1995-2005.

[62]   Jan RL, Yeh KC, Hsieh MH, Lin YL, Kao HF, Li PH, et al. Lactobacillus gasseri suppresses Th17 pro-inflammatory response and attenuates allergen-induced airway inflammation in a mouse model of allergic asthma. Br J Nutr 2012 Jul 14;108(1):130-9.

[63]   Adel-Patient K, Bernard H, Ah-Leung S, Creminon C, Wal JM. Peanut-and cow's milk-specific IgE, Th2 cells and local anaphylactic reaction are induced in Balb/c mice orally sensitized with cholera toxin. Allergy 2005 May;60(5):658-64.

[64]   Bowman CC, Selgrade MK. Differences in allergenic potential of food extracts following oral exposure in mice reflect differences in digestibility: potential approaches to safety assessment. Toxicol Sci 2008 Mar;102(1):100-9.

[65]   Bonnegarde-Bernard A, Jee J, Fial MJ, Steiner H, DiBartola S, Davis IC, et al. Routes of allergic sensitization and myeloid cell IKKbeta differentially regulate antibody responses and allergic airway inflammation in male and female mice. PLoS One 2014;9(3):e92307.

[66]   Inoue R, Nishio A, Fukushima Y, Ushida K. Oral treatment with probiotic Lactobacillus johnsonii NCC533 (La1) for a specific part of the weaning period prevents the development of atopic dermatitis induced after maturation in model mice, NC/Nga. Br J Dermatol 2007 Mar;156(3):499-509.

[67]   Yamanaka K, Nakanishi T, Watanabe J, Kondo M, Yamagiwa A, Gabazza EC, et al. Continuous high-dose antigen exposure preferentially induces IL-10, but intermittent antigen exposure induces IL-4. Exp Dermatol 2014 Jan;23(1):63-5.

[68] Nelde A, Teufel M, Hahn C, Duschl A, Sebald W, Brocker EB, et al. The impact of the route and frequency of antigen exposure on the IgE response in allergy. Int Arch Allergy Immunol 2001 Apr;124(4):461-9.

[69] Tobita K, Yanaka H, Otani H. Anti-allergic effects of Lactobacillus crispatus KT-11 strain on ovalbumin-sensitized BALB/c mice. Anim Sci J 2010 Dec;81(6):699-705.

[70] Shimada T, Cheng L, Yamasaki A, Ide M, Motonaga C, Yasueda H, et al. Effects of lysed Enterococcus faecalis FK-23 on allergen-induced serum antibody responses and active cutaneous anaphylaxis in mice. Clin Exp Allergy 2004 Nov;34(11):1784-8.

[71] Shimada T, Kondoh M, Motonaga C, Kitamura Y, Cheng L, Shi H, et al. Enhancement of anti-allergic effects mediated by the Kampo medicine Shoseiryuto (Xiao-Qing-Long-Tang in Chinese) with lysed Enterococcus faecalis FK-23 in mice. Asian Pac J Allergy Immunol 2010 Mar;28(1):59-66.

[72] Kim H, Lee SY, Ji GE. Timing of bifidobacterium administration influences the development of allergy to ovalbumin in mice. Biotechnol Lett 2005 Sep;27(18):1361-7.

[73] Lee J, Bang J, Woo HJ. Effect of orally administered Lactobacillus brevis HY7401 in a food allergy mouse model. J Microbiol Biotechnol 2013 Nov 28;23(11):1636-40.

[74] Schouten B, van Esch BC, Hofman GA, van Doorn SA, Knol J, Nauta AJ, et al. Cow milk allergy symptoms are reduced in mice fed dietary synbiotics during oral sensitization with whey. J Nutr 2009 Jul;139(7):1398-403.

[75] Zuercher AW, Weiss M, Holvoet S, Moser M, Moussu H, van OL, et al. Lactococcus lactis NCC 2287 alleviates food allergic manifestations in sensitized mice by reducing IL-13 expression specifically in the ileum. Clin Dev Immunol 2012;2012:485750.

[76] Maciel M, Fusaro AE, Duarte AJ, Sato MN. Modulation of IgE response and cytokine production in Peyer's patches and draining lymph nodes in sensitized mice made tolerant by oral dust mite administration. J Interferon Cytokine Res 2000 Dec;20(12):1057-63.

[77] Meulenbroek LA, van Esch BC, Hofman GA, den Hartog Jager CF, Nauta AJ, Willemsen LE, et al. Oral treatment with beta-lactoglobulin peptides prevents clinical symptoms in a mouse model for cow's milk allergy. Pediatr Allergy Immunol 2013 Nov;24(7):656-64.

[78] Qu C, Srivastava K, Ko J, Zhang TF, Sampson HA, Li XM. Induction of tolerance after establishment of peanut allergy by the food allergy herbal formula-2 is associated with up-regulation of interferon-gamma. Clin Exp Allergy 2007 Jun;37(6):846-55.

[79] Turner PV, Brabb T, Pekow C, Vasbinder MA. Administration of substances to laboratory animals: routes of administration and factors to consider. J Am Assoc Lab Anim Sci 2011 Sep;50(5):600-13.

[80] Enomoto M, Noguchi S, Hattori M, Sugiyama H, Suzuki Y, Hanaoka A, et al. Oral administration of Lactobacillus plantarum NRIC0380 suppresses IgE production and

induces CD4(+)CD25(+)Foxp3(+) cells in vivo. Biosci Biotechnol Biochem 2009 Feb; 73(2):457-60.

[81] Hougee S, Vriesema AJ, Wijering SC, Knippels LM, Folkerts G, Nijkamp FP, et al. Oral treatment with probiotics reduces allergic symptoms in ovalbumin-sensitized mice: a bacterial strain comparative study. Int Arch Allergy Immunol 2010;151(2): 107-17.

[82] Li CY, Lin HC, Hsueh KC, Wu SF, Fang SH. Oral administration of Lactobacillus salivarius inhibits the allergic airway response in mice. Can J Microbiol 2010 May;56(5): 373-9.

[83] Nonaka Y, Izumo T, Izumi F, Maekawa T, Shibata H, Nakano A, et al. Antiallergic effects of Lactobacillus pentosus strain S-PT84 mediated by modulation of Th1/Th2 immunobalance and induction of IL-10 production. Int Arch Allergy Immunol 2008;145(3):249-57.

[84] Dioszeghy V, Mondoulet L, Dhelft V, Ligouis M, Puteaux E, Benhamou PH, et al. Epicutaneous immunotherapy results in rapid allergen uptake by dendritic cells through intact skin and downregulates the allergen-specific response in sensitized mice. J Immunol 2011 May 15;186(10):5629-37.

[85] Dunkin D, Berin MC, Mayer L. Allergic sensitization can be induced via multiple physiologic routes in an adjuvant-dependent manner. J Allergy Clin Immunol 2011 Dec;128(6):1251-8.

[86] Hsieh KY, Tsai CC, Wu CH, Lin RH. Epicutaneous exposure to protein antigen and food allergy. Clin Exp Allergy 2003 Aug;33(8):1067-75.

[87] Strid J, Hourihane J, Kimber I, Callard R, Strobel S. Epicutaneous exposure to peanut protein prevents oral tolerance and enhances allergic sensitization. Clin Exp Allergy 2005 Jun;35(6):757-66.

[88] Goto K, Iwasawa D, Kamimura Y, Yasuda M, Matsumura M, Shimada T. Clinical and histopathological evaluation of Dermatophagoides farinae-induced dermatitis in NC/Nga mice orally administered Bacillus subtilis. J Vet Med Sci 2011 May;73(5): 649-54.

[89] Jung BG, Cho SJ, Koh HB, Han DU, Lee BJ. Fermented Maesil (Prunus mume) with probiotics inhibits development of atopic dermatitis-like skin lesions in NC/Nga mice. Vet Dermatol 2010 Apr;21(2):184-91.

[90] Kim HJ, Kim YJ, Kang MJ, Seo JH, Kim HY, Jeong SK, et al. A novel mouse model of atopic dermatitis with epicutaneous allergen sensitization and the effect of Lactobacillus rhamnosus. Exp Dermatol 2012 Sep;21(9):672-5.

[91] Kim HJ, Kim YJ, Lee SH, Kang MJ, Yu HS, Jung YH, et al. Effects of Lactobacillus rhamnosus on asthma with an adoptive transfer of dendritic cells in mice. J Appl Microbiol 2013 Sep;115(3):872-9.

[92] Volz T, Skabytska Y, Guenova E, Chen KM, Frick JS, Kirschning CJ, et al. Nonpathogenic bacteria alleviating atopic dermatitis inflammation induce IL-10-producing dendritic cells and regulatory Tr1 cells. J Invest Dermatol 2014 Jan;134(1):96-104.

[93] Wakabayashi H, Nariai C, Takemura F, Nakao W, Fujiwara D. Dietary supplementation with lactic acid bacteria attenuates the development of atopic-dermatitis-like skin lesions in NC/Nga mice in a strain-dependent manner. Int Arch Allergy Immunol 2008;145(2):141-51.

[94] Weise C, Zhu Y, Ernst D, Kuhl AA, Worm M. Oral administration of Escherichia coli Nissle 1917 prevents allergen-induced dermatitis in mice. Exp Dermatol 2011 Oct; 20(10):805-9.

[95] Won TJ, Kim B, Lim YT, Song DS, Park SY, Park ES, et al. Oral administration of Lactobacillus strains from Kimchi inhibits atopic dermatitis in NC / Nga mice. J Appl Microbiol 2011 May;110(5):1195-202.

[96] Berin MC, Shreffler WG. T(H)2 adjuvants: implications for food allergy. J Allergy Clin Immunol 2008 Jun;121(6):1311-20.

[97] Mohan T, Verma P, Rao DN. Novel adjuvants & delivery vehicles for vaccines development: a road ahead. Indian J Med Res 2013 Nov;138(5):779-95.

[98] Blazquez AB, Berin MC. Gastrointestinal dendritic cells promote Th2 skewing via OX40L. J Immunol 2008 Apr 1;180(7):4441-50.

[99] Janeway C, Travers P, Walport M, Shlomchik MJ. Immunobiology-The Immune System in Health and Disease. 6th ed. Garland Science Publishing; 2004.

[100] Lee J, Bang J, Woo HJ. Immunomodulatory and anti-allergic effects of orally administered Lactobacillus species in ovalbumin-sensitized mice. J Microbiol Biotechnol 2013 May;23(5):724-30.

[101] Mastrangeli G, Corinti S, Butteroni C, Afferni C, Bonura A, Boirivant M, et al. Effects of live and inactivated VSL#3 probiotic preparations in the modulation of in vitro and in vivo allergen-induced Th2 responses. Int Arch Allergy Immunol 2009;150(2): 133-43.

[102] Shin HS, Bae MJ, Jung SY, Shon DH. Preventive effects of skullcap (Scutellaria baicalensis) extract in a mouse model of food allergy. J Ethnopharmacol 2014 May 14;153(3):667-73.

[103] Wang JH, Fan SW, Zhu WY. Development of Gut Microbiota in a Mouse Model of Ovalbumin-induced Allergic Diarrhea under Sub-barrier System. Asian-Australas J Anim Sci 2013 Apr;26(4):545-51.

[104] Zhang B, An J, Shimada T, Liu S, Maeyama K. Oral administration of Enterococcus faecalis FK-23 suppresses Th17 cell development and attenuates allergic airway responses in mice. Int J Mol Med 2012 Aug;30(2):248-54.

[105]   Matsuda A, Tanaka A, Pan W, Okamoto N, Oida K, Kingyo N, et al. Supplementation of the fermented soy product ImmuBalance effectively reduces itching behavior
of atopic NC/Tnd mice. J Dermatol Sci 2012 Aug;67(2):130-9.

[106]   Pellaton C, Nutten S, Thierry AC, Boudousquie C, Barbier N, Blanchard C, et al. In-
tragastric and Intranasal Administration of Lactobacillus paracasei NCC2461 Modulates Allergic Airway Inflammation in Mice. Int J Inflam 2012;2012:686739.

[107]   Farraj AK, Harkema JR, Jan TR, Kaminski NE. Immune responses in the lung and local lymph node of A/J mice to intranasal sensitization and challenge with adjuvant-
free ovalbumin. Toxicol Pathol 2003 Jul;31(4):432-47.

[108]   McCusker C, Chicoine M, Hamid Q, Mazer B. Site-specific sensitization in a murine
model of allergic rhinitis: role of the upper airway in lower airways disease. J Allergy
Clin Immunol 2002 Dec;110(6):891-8.

[109]   Southam DS, Dolovich M, O'Byrne PM, Inman MD. Distribution of intranasal instil-
lations in mice: effects of volume, time, body position, and anesthesia. Am J Physiol
Lung Cell Mol Physiol 2002 Apr;282(4):L833-L839.

[110]   Yu J, Jang SO, Kim BJ, Song YH, Kwon JW, Kang MJ, et al. The Effects of Lactobacillus rhamnosus on the Prevention of Asthma in a Murine Model. Allergy Asthma Immunol Res 2010 Jul;2(3):199-205.

[111]   Forsythe P, Inman MD, Bienenstock J. Oral treatment with live Lactobacillus reuteri
inhibits the allergic airway response in mice. Am J Respir Crit Care Med 2007 Mar
15;175(6):561-9.

[112]   Lyons A, O'Mahony D, O'Brien F, MacSharry J, Sheil B, Ceddia M, et al. Bacterial
strain-specific induction of Foxp3+T regulatory cells is protective in murine allergy
models. Clin Exp Allergy 2010 May;40(5):811-9.

[113]   Foligne B, Nutten S, Grangette C, Dennin V, Goudercourt D, Poiret S, et al. Correlation between in vitro and in vivo immunomodulatory properties of lactic acid bacteria. World J Gastroenterol 2007 Jan 14;13(2):236-43.

[114]   Smits HH, Engering A, van der Kleij D, de Jong EC, Schipper K, van Capel TM, et al.
Selective probiotic bacteria induce IL-10-producing regulatory T cells in vitro by
modulating dendritic cell function through dendritic cell-specific intercellular adhesion molecule 3-grabbing nonintegrin. J Allergy Clin Immunol 2005 Jun;115(6):
1260-7.

[115]   Zhang LL, Chen X, Zheng PY, Luo Y, Lu GF, Liu ZQ, et al. Oral Bifidobacterium
modulates intestinal immune inflammation in mice with food allergy. J Gastroenterol
Hepatol 2010 May;25(5):928-34.

[116]   Jain S, Yadav H, Sinha PR, Kapila S, Naito Y, Marotta F. Anti-allergic effects of probiotic Dahi through modulation of the gut immune system. Turk J Gastroenterol 2010
Sep;21(3):244-50.

[117] Karimi K, Inman MD, Bienenstock J, Forsythe P. Lactobacillus reuteri-induced regulatory T cells protect against an allergic airway response in mice. Am J Respir Crit Care Med 2009 Feb 1;179(3):186-93.

[118] Feleszko W, Jaworska J, Rha RD, Steinhausen S, Avagyan A, Jaudszus A, et al. Probiotic-induced suppression of allergic sensitization and airway inflammation is associated with an increase of T regulatory-dependent mechanisms in a murine model of asthma. Clin Exp Allergy 2007 Apr;37(4):498-505.

[119] Blumer N, Sel S, Virna S, Patrascan CC, Zimmermann S, Herz U, et al. Perinatal maternal application of Lactobacillus rhamnosus GG suppresses allergic airway inflammation in mouse offspring. Clin Exp Allergy 2007 Mar;37(3):348-57.

[120] Kim JY, Park BK, Park HJ, Park YH, Kim BO, Pyo S. Atopic dermatitis-mitigating effects of new Lactobacillus strain, Lactobacillus sakei probio 65 isolated from Kimchi. J Appl Microbiol 2013 Aug;115(2):517-26.

[121] Tobita K, Yanaka H, Otani H. Heat-treated Lactobacillus crispatus KT strains reduce allergic symptoms in mice. J Agric Food Chem 2009 Jun 24;57(12):5586-90.

[122] Sawada J, Morita H, Tanaka A, Salminen S, He F, Matsuda H. Ingestion of heat-treated Lactobacillus rhamnosus GG prevents development of atopic dermatitis in NC/Nga mice. Clin Exp Allergy 2007 Feb;37(2):296-303.

5

Airborne Allergens

Olga Ukhanova and Evgenia Bogomolova

1. Introduction

A huge number of substances of various origin forming atmospheric aerosols constantly circulates in the atmospheric air (Table 1). One of the most important components of such aerosols are airborne allergens. Airborne allergens are substances of biological origin, which getting into the human body promote the induction of the immune response with the subsequent development of an allergic disease. Allergic reaction is directly caused by proteins and glycoproteins forming the airborne allergen.

Type of particles	Diameter (mkm)
Smoke, smog	0, 001-0, 1
Dust	0, 1
Bacteria	0, 3-10
Fungi spores / conidia	1, 0-100, 0
Algae / seaweed	0, 5
Fragments of lichen	1, 0
Protozoa	2, 0
Spores of mosses	6, 0-30, 0
Pollen	10, 0-100, 0
Fragments of plants and animals, seeds, insects	>100

Table 1. The components of the atmospheric aerosols and their size [4].

More than 15 million people in Europe suffer from allergic rhinitis, conjunctivitis, bronchial asthma, atopic dermatitis and food allergy. Climatic and geographic features of the Russian Federation (its Northern and Southern parts, as well as European and Asian territories) contribute to a different sickness rate among the population [1, 2].

So far there are many questions concerning monitoring and a variety of the airborne allergens, and especially their influence on the human body. The study of the airborne allergens is of theoretical and practical interest for many specialists (allergists, laboratorians, ecologists, biologists). The biological study of the airborne allergens is connected with the problem of the origin, transport, protein structure and protein interaction with the macroorganism. Under the influence of the environment the airborne allergens may be a subject to significant changes and they may change their properties.

This chapter presents the main types of the airborne allergens: their origin, transport, properties, monitoring, etc.

2. Classification of the airborne allergens

The most common airborne allergens are pollen, fungal spores, house dust, house dust mites, animal allergens, insect allergens, industrial allergens, food and drug allergens.

Origin	Types of the allergens		
Noninfectious allergens			
Animals	Epidermal	Food-borne	Insect
	Hair/wool epithelium feather saliva excrements	Fish and cancroid protein Honey	Chitinous cover and products of insects vital activity
Plants	Pollen	foodstuffs	
Drugs	antibiotics, sulfanilamides, immunological drugs		
Industrial substances	polymers, pesticides, metalls		
Dust	house, library, archive dust		
Infectious allergens			
Phycomycetes	spores, products of fungi vital activity		

Table 2. Classification of the airborne allergens.

The scientific line-molecular allergology-intensively develops in modern allergology for the last 10-15 years. The modern allergen nomenclature adopted and approved in 2013 by WAO is now becoming routine in practice of the allergist [3].

We will present the most well-known and popular airborne allergens in applied medicine which are used for the diagnosis and treatment of allergic diseases of reaginic type (IgE-dependent allergic reactions or type I of immune response). Such diseases include allergic rhinitis, allergic conjunctivitis, atopic dermatitis, bronchial asthma, urticaria, etc.

The knowledge of the airborne allergens types is very useful in routine practice of a medical specialist for the purpose of individual selection of methods of diagnosis and treatment of patients with respiratory allergosis, as well as for the prevention of allergic diseases in genetically predisposed to atopy or already sensitized patients.

3. Pollen allergens

3.1. Aeropalynology

Aeropalynology is a part of aerobiology studying pollen grains and spores of plants passively circulating in the atmosphere. Also, it is a branch of modern biology that studies the structure and laws of formation of the pollen rain. Aeropalynology is closely connected with allergology as pollen of plants and fungal spores belong to the most widespread airborne allergens causing diseases of the upper airways [4]. Aeropalynologists are the experts engaged in identification of qualitative and quantitative structure of a pollen rain. They study features of its daily rhythms and seasonal dynamics, compile a calendar of allergenic plants dusting and sporulation of mycelial fungi. These data are necessary for various experts (allergists, otorhinolaryngologists, general practitioners) and patients to predict exacerbations of allergic diseases and to take preventive measures.

Long-term observations over the years are the most informative for identifying patterns of plants dusting over large areas with different climate and landscapes.

Currently there is a single international aeropalynology service that possesses information about the dynamics of the pollen concentrations of the most common allergenic taxa in the air and the bank of these data. Since 1993, the database provides information on the dusting of different plants in Europe and forecasts the dusting based on the current and long-term aeropalynological observations [5, 6].

The program of aeropalynological research was launched in Russia in 2007. Several cities with installed pollen monitoring stations (volumetric Burkard SporeWatch sampler) had been included in this program (Fig. 1-3). These cities are Moscow, St. Petersburg, Saratov, Stavropol, Astrakhan, Rostov-on-Don, Krasnodar, Yaroslavl, Novosibirsk, Yekaterinburg, Ryazan, Smolensk, and others. The aeropalynological stations start working from 15 of April to 15 of September every year (the period of active flowering of wind-pollinated plants in Russia). The aeropalynological monitoring is carried out the year-round in Moscow and St. Petersburg. The studies of pollen are carried out by the Russian allergists and laboratory technicians, who were trained under the guidance of Severova E.A. at the Department of Palynology, Faculty of Biology of Moscow State University. The station in Moscow is the curator of a national Russian network of aeropalynological monitoring and represents Russia in the European and International association of aeropalinologists.

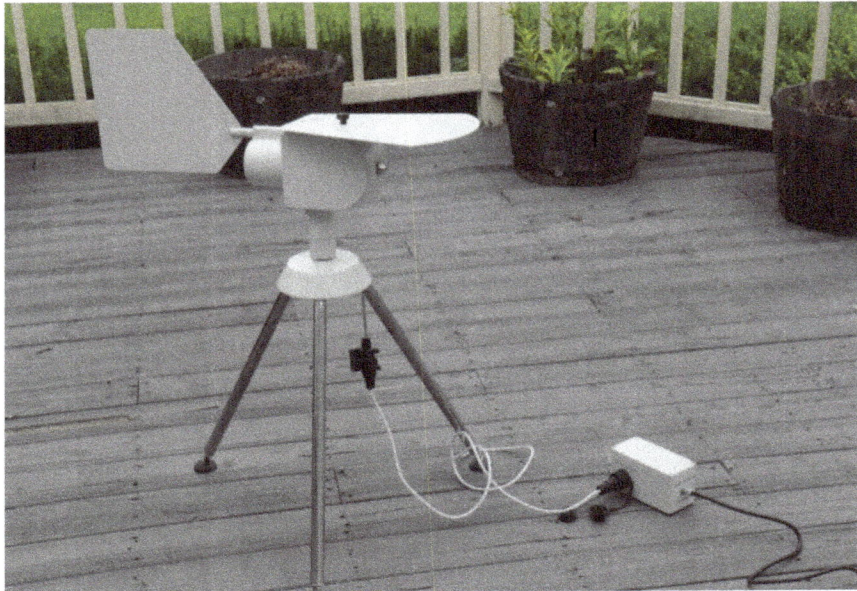

Figure 1. Burkard SporeWatch sampler

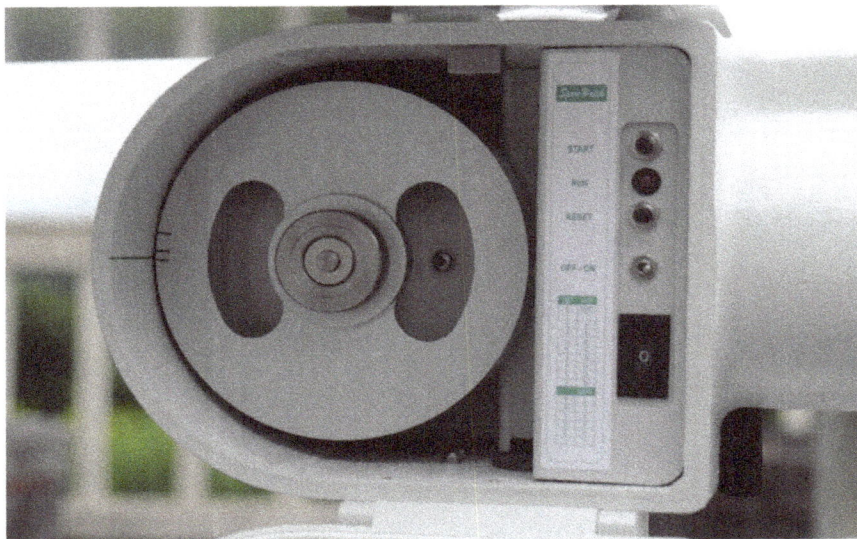

Figure 2. Burkard SporeWatch sampler Cylinder with 7-days or 24-hours periods of selection in Krasnodar

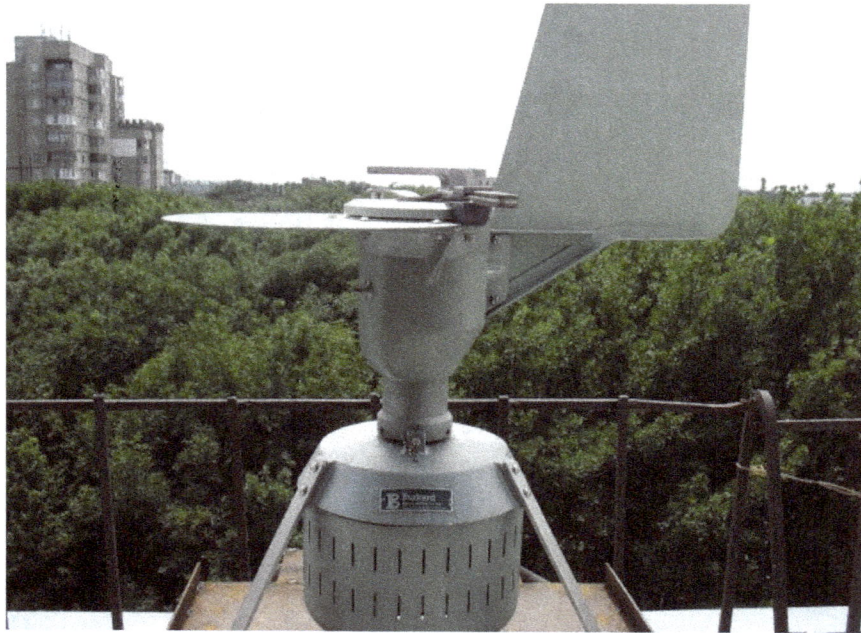

Figure 3. Burkard-Hirst SporeWatch in Moscow, Saratov, Pyatigorsk, Rostov-on-Don, St. Petersburg, Stavropol

The measurement of the concentration of mycelial fungi spores in the atmospheric air is carried out by means of the automatic Burkard sampler on the Petri dish with Czapek agarized medium (Fig. 4).

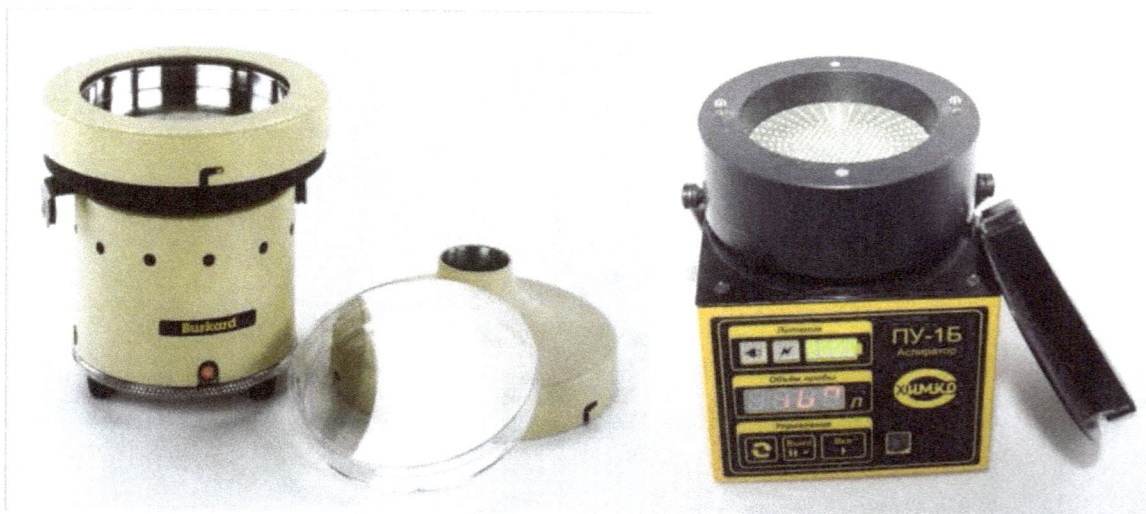

Figure 4. Burkard SporeWatch sampler and sampler (St. Petersburg) PU-1B The determination of the spores concentration (colony forming units-CFU) in the atmospheric air of the premises, parks and industrial areas is also very informative for collecting the patient's medical history and selection of diagnostic tests in vivo and in vitro.

3.2. Pollen-grain morphology

For allergology the greatest interest is represented by pollen grains of wind-pollinated plants (angiosperms and gymnosperms) because pollen is spread by wind over hundreds of kilometers from the habitats of plants. Most of the entomogenous plants are not allergenic for human.

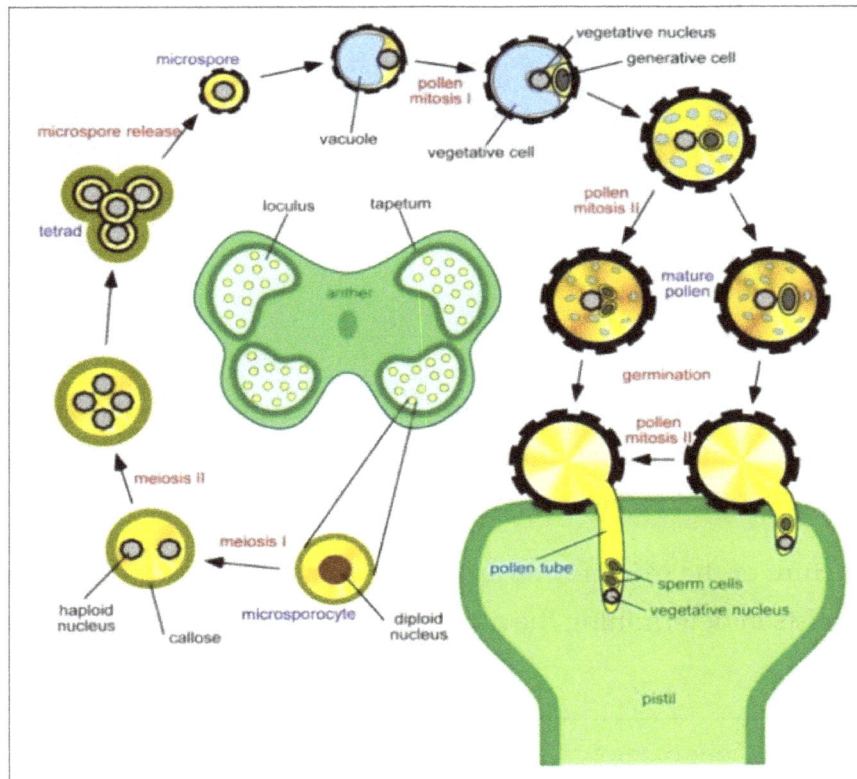

Figure 5. The pollen grain development and its participation in fertilization

Pollen grains are reduced male gametogophytes developing inside the microspore shell. Pollen grains of the angiosperms are formed from microspores (mother cells) in microsporangia which represent anther nests.

Each pollen grain consists of the vegetative cell, and the generative cell is immersed in the cytoplasm of the vegetative cell (Fig. 5). During the germination the vegetative cell forms a pollen tube, and the nucleus of the generative cell forms 2 sperm cells involved in fertilization [4].

3.3. Sporoderma

Sporoderma is a shell of pollen grains (Fig. 6).

Sporoderma is a set of morphologically different layers: perispory (Perina=trifina), exine (exosporium), and intine (endosporium) which protect the cytoplasm of the pollen grain from the external influence. The sporoderma layer structure is specific to orders, families, genera and species of higher plants.

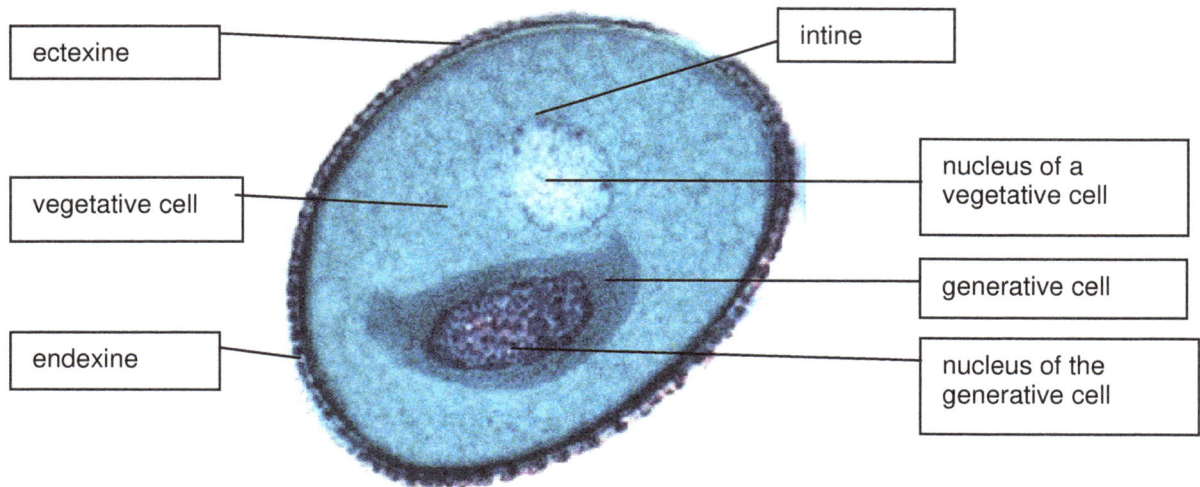

Figure 6. Pollen grain structure

The exine is the outer part of the pollen grain shell of most seed plants. The structure of the exine includes sporopollenin. It is a biopolymer that can withstand the high temperature, and is insoluble in alkalis and acids (Fig. 7).

The internal structure of the exine forms texture and sculpture. And that is a main point for the aeropalynologists in determining the morphological type of pollen grains.

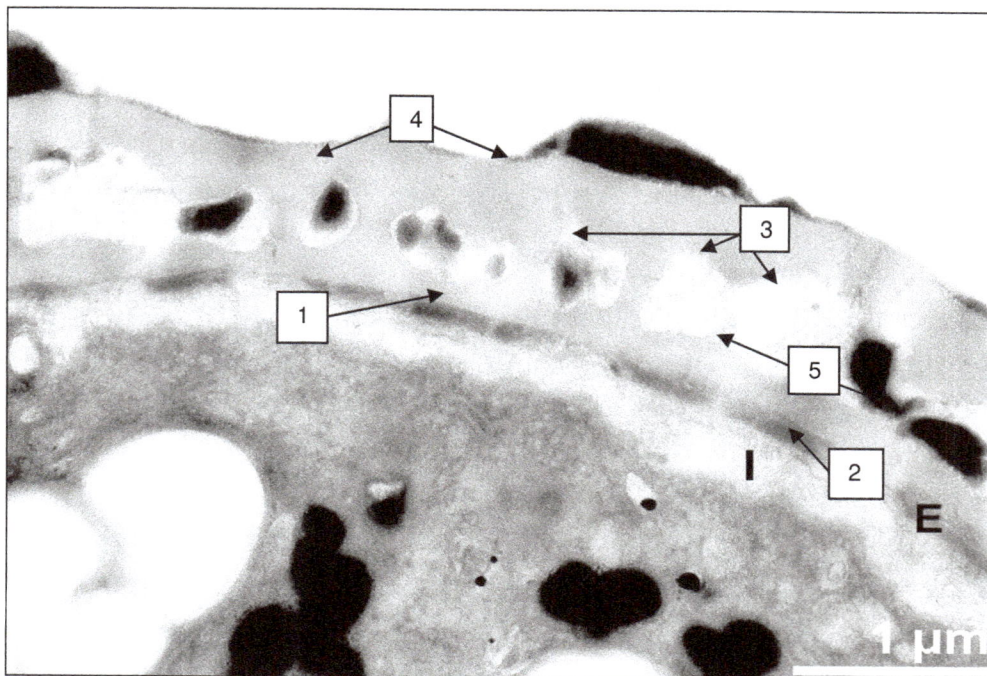

Figure 7. The structure of angiosperm sporoderma: 1-endexine, 2 – intine, 3-styles, 4-integument, 5-underlaying layer.

Intine is the inner layer of sporoderma bordering with cytoplasm and collapsing in acytolysis processing.

Trifina is a thin squamous layer of wind-pollinated plants. It is poorly visible in contrast to the pollen of the entomophilous plants.

The complex morphology and molecular composition of pollen helps to activate the immune system of a human for the purpose of elimination of airborne allergens from mucosa of the respiratory tract [4].

3.4. The main plants the pollen of which causes an allergy

In the central Europe, the most common cause of pollinosis is the pollen of wind-pollinated plants: trees, cereals and weeds. Their pollen is volatile, and during flowering of these plants the pollen accumulates in the air in quantity sufficient enough to create a relatively high concentration.

As a result of the aeropalynological researches the calendars of dusting are compiled annually. The calendars containing 15 taxa of plants are compiled for Europe.. However, in the North and the South of Russia (the European part of it) a range of airborne allergens is larger and depends on the trajectory of the distribution of pollen (Fig. 8) [4].

During the examination and management of patients with pollinosis, the seasonal and daily changes of the pollen content should also be taken into account.

The allergy to pollen of grasses and trees grows only in the period of their flowering. So each region has its own seasonal peaks of incidence. The maximum concentration of pollen in the air is in the early morning hours, from dawn until 12 p.m.

Among deciduous trees the allergic diseases are caused most often by pollen of birch, alder, hazel, maple, oak, and others. We present the main taxa of trees which are determined in the atmospheric air:

1. Alnus incana (Grey alder) (Fig.9)

2. Betula verrucosa (Common silver birch) (Fig.10)

3. Corylus avellana (Hazel) (Fig.11)

4. Quercus alba (Oak) (Fig.12)

5. Ulmus americana (Elm) (Fig.13)

6. Salix caprea (Willow) (Fig.14)

7. Populus deltoides (Cottonwood) (Fig.15)

8. Acer negundo (Fig.16)

9. Fraxinus americana (White ash) (Fig.17)

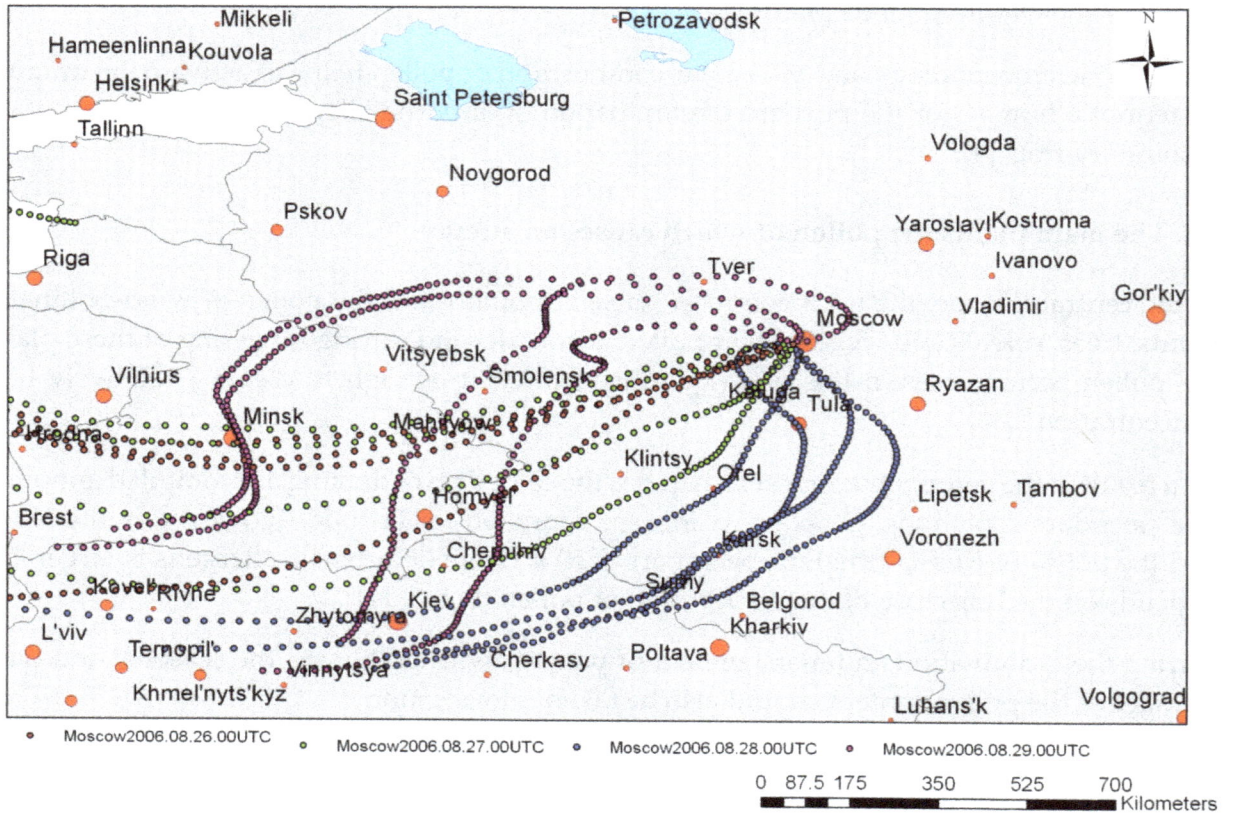

Figure 8. The trajectory of the distribution of pollen from Moscow.

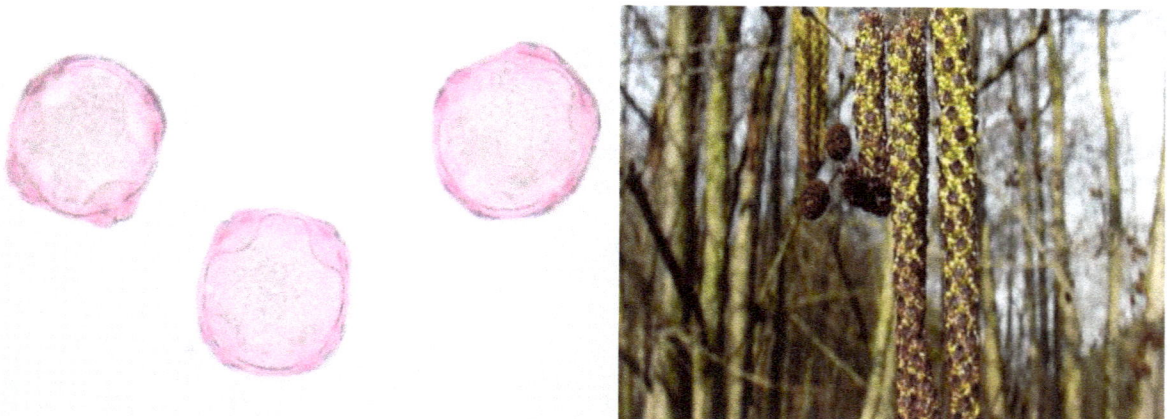

Figure 9. Alnus incana

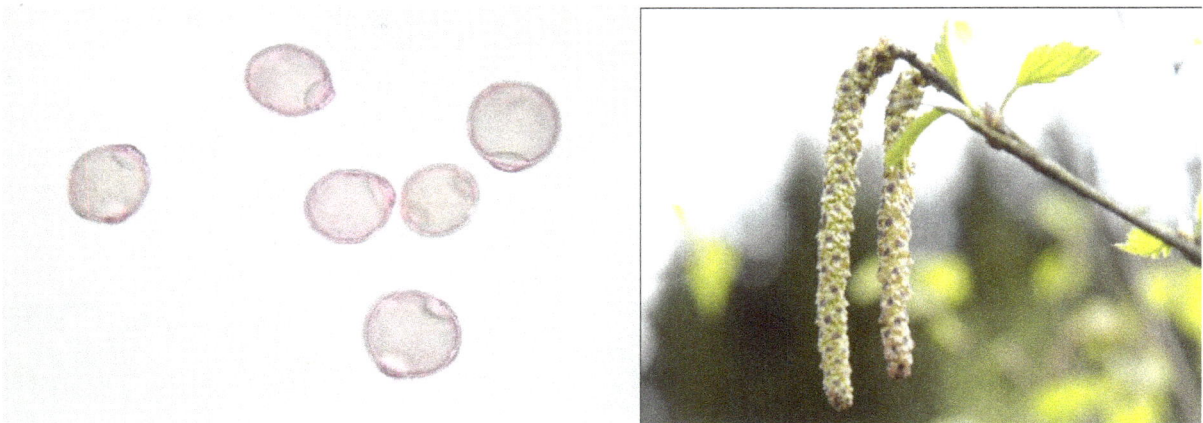

Figure 10. Betula verrucosa

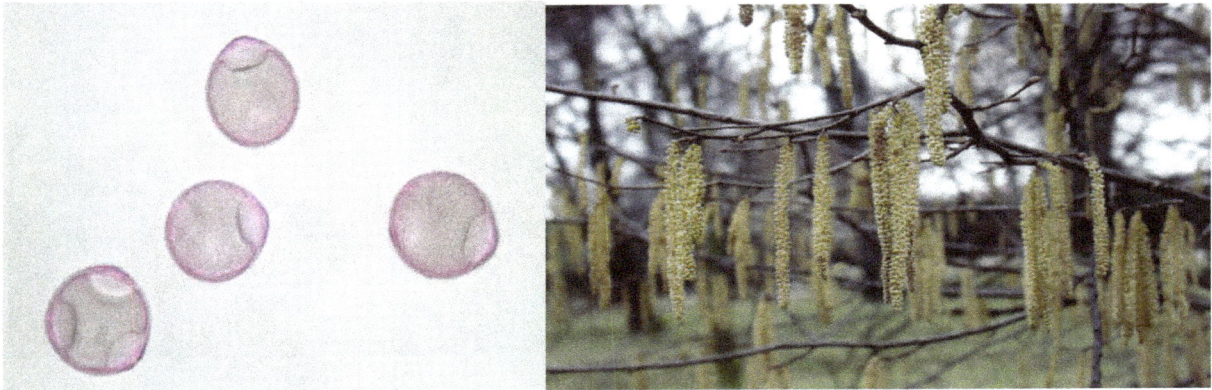

Figure 11. Corylus avellana

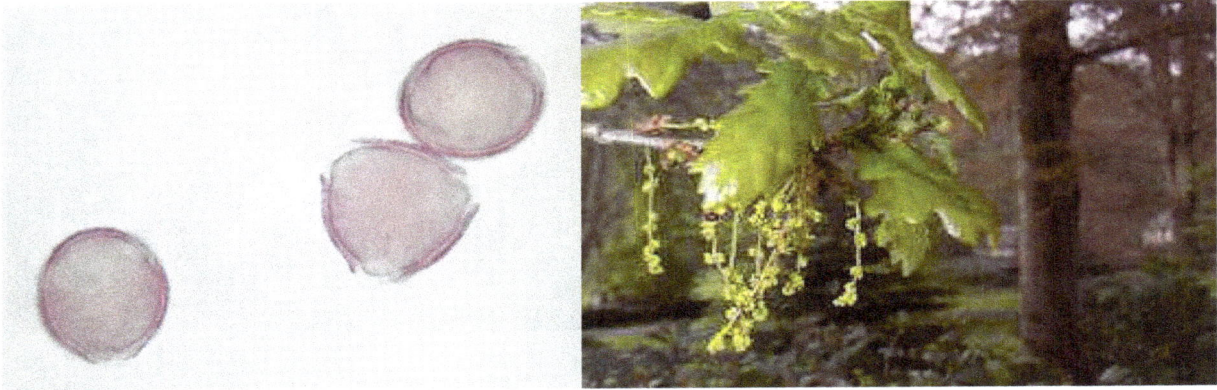

Figure 12. Quercus alba

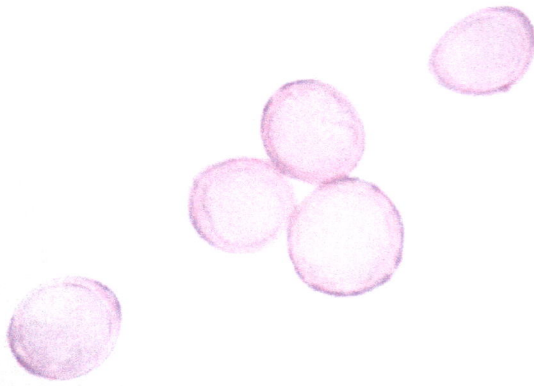

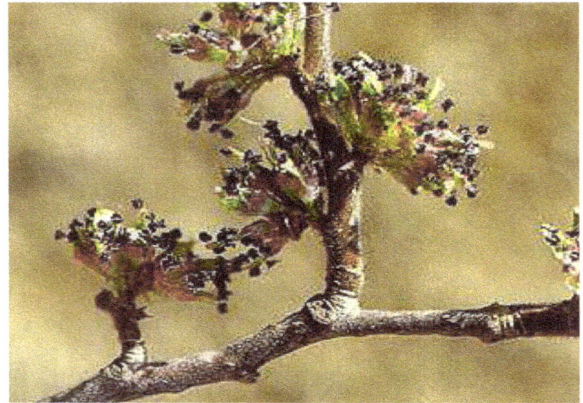

Figure 13. Ulmus Americana

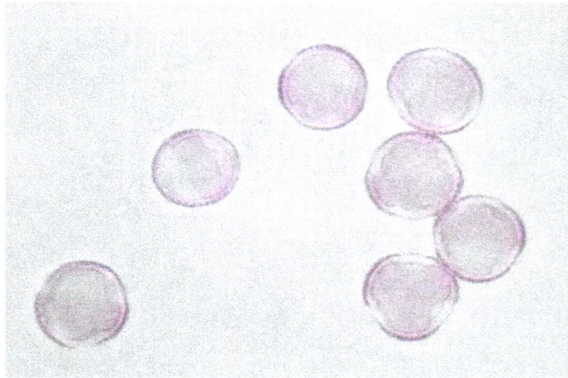

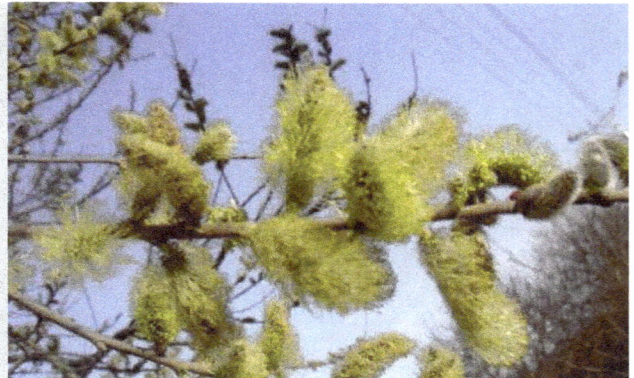

Figure 14. Salix caprea

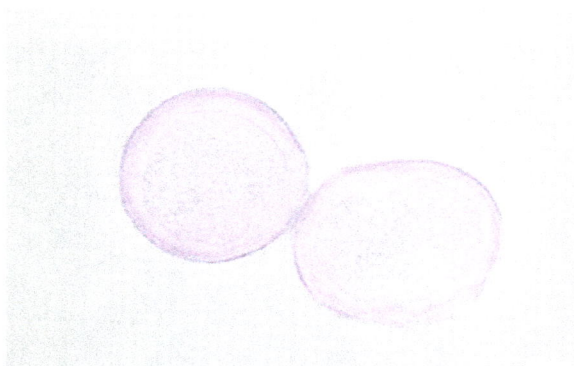

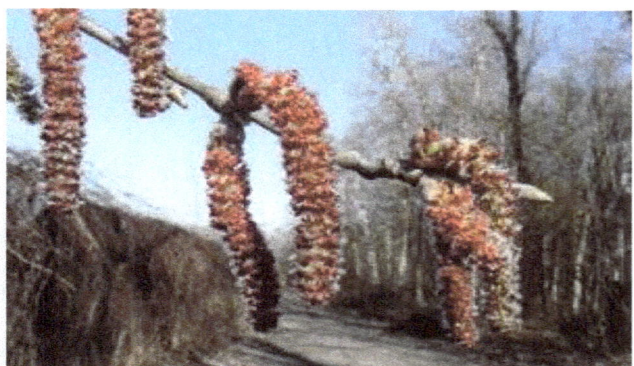

Figure 15. Populus deltoids

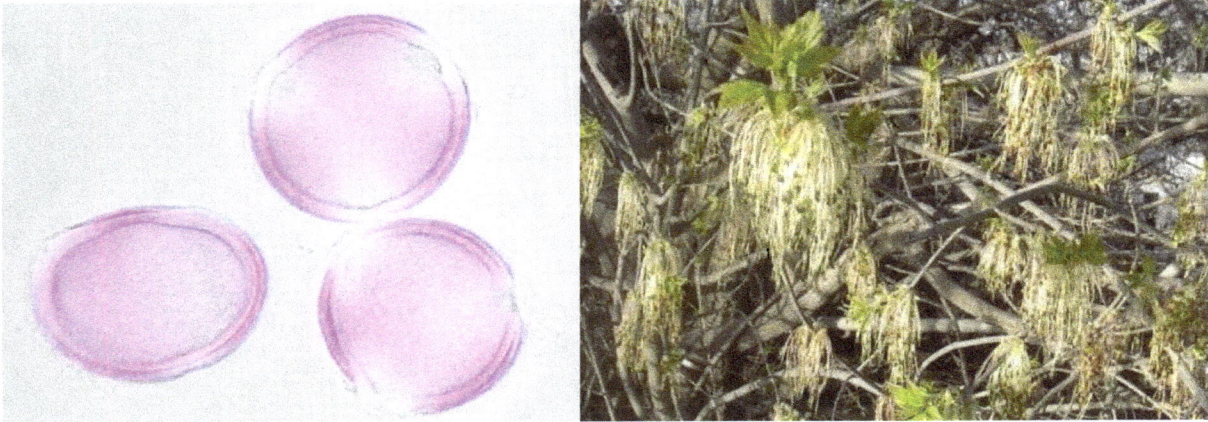

Figure 16. Acer negundo

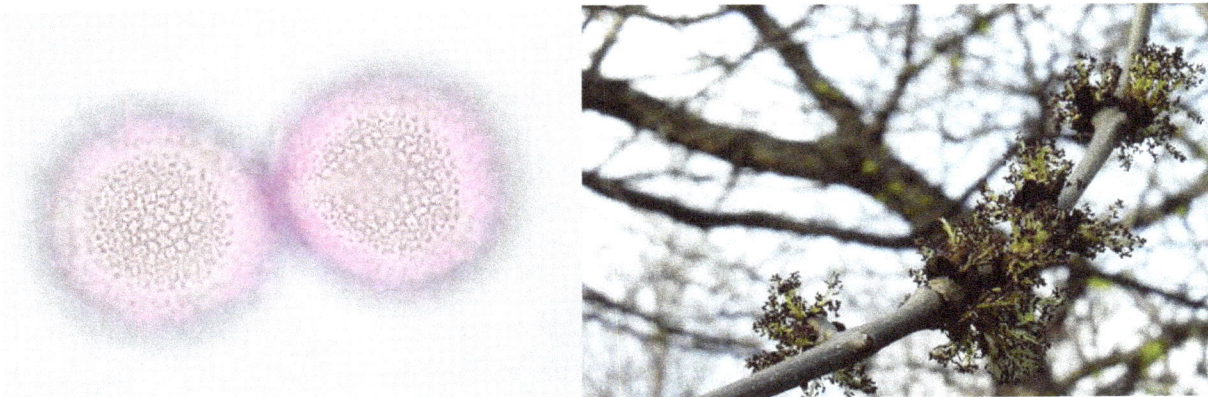

Figure 17. Fraxinus Americana

There is a structural homology between allergens of trees pollen, and it is expressed much more weakly, than the existing affinity of allergens of grass pollen. Therefore, the patients who have an increased sensitivity to the birch pollen react at the same time to the pollen of hazel and alder.

The coniferous plants produce the pollen in large quantities, but its allergenicity is lower because the diameter of pollen grains is 30 to 100 microns.

The birch pollen has the most evident allergenic activity among the analogs – the pollen of deciduous wind-pollinated plants-because it contains about 40 proteins, the 6 of which have the properties of allergens [11].

The development of technology of various recombinant allergens production has revealed that the common allergens of protein nature (e.g. "panallergens", Bet v 1 protein and Bet v 2 birch profilin) are responsible for cross-reacting of allergens of spring trees pollen [11].

The main taxa of cereals (Poaceae) (Fig.18):

1. Dactylis glomerata (Cocksfoot)

2. Festuca elatior (Meadow fescue)

3. Phleum pratense (Timothy)

4. Poa pratensis (Meadow grass)

5. Agrostis stolonifera (Redtop, Bentgrass)

6. Bromus inermis (Brome grass)

7. Secale cereale (Cultivated rye)

8. Holcus lanatus (Velvet grass)

9. Alopecurus pratensis (Meadow foxtail)

10. Maize (Corn)

11. Arrhenatherum elatius

The main characteristic of the cereals pollen is its spherical, oval or elliptical shape. There are no many detailed species and genera definitions. But pollen grain has always one pore (Fig. 18) and a smooth surface. The size of the cultivated cereals pollen is usually larger than of wild one and ranges from 25 to 75 microns [4].

Eleven groups of major and minor allergens could be defined among the cereals [12, 13].

The allergens of the 1st group (Dac g 1, Poa p1, Phi p 1, Hol I 1) are glycoproteins with a molecular weight of 31-35 kD, and they represent major allergens with a high immunogenicity. They are homologous between different types of the cereal herbs in 90%. They bind with high affinity with asIgE (allergen-specific immunoglobulin E) and cause severe sensitization of the patient.

The allergens of the 5th group (Dac g 5, Poa p 5, Phi p 5, Hol I 5) have molecular weight of 27-33 kD. They are identical to the 1st group on a spatial configuration of amino acids (isoforms) and are major, because of their cross-stimulation of asIgE synthesis from 65% to 85%.

The allergens of the 2, 3, 4, 6, 7, 10, 11, 12 and 13 groups are the minor allergens of the cereals pollen. They are also homologous to each other. The sizes of the allergens of the 2 and 3 groups (Dac g 2, Dac g 3, Poa p 2, Phi p 2, Phi p 3, Hol I 2) to 1-12 kD are non-glycosylated proteins, which are homologous in 85-90% between species and have 15% of immunogenicity, causing the expression of asIgE in 40-60% of patients.

The 4th group of allergens (Poa p 4, Phi p 4) is represented by glycoproteins with α-helical and β-foliated structure having a molecular weight of up to 50-67 kD. Sensitization to them is detected in 80% of patients, but quantitatively the asIgE synthesis is less than to allergens of the 1st and 5th groups. The group Poa p 6 and Phi p 6 have cross-activity with Poa p 5 and Phi p 5 in 60-70% of patients, but they are not allergen-specific for the grass family.

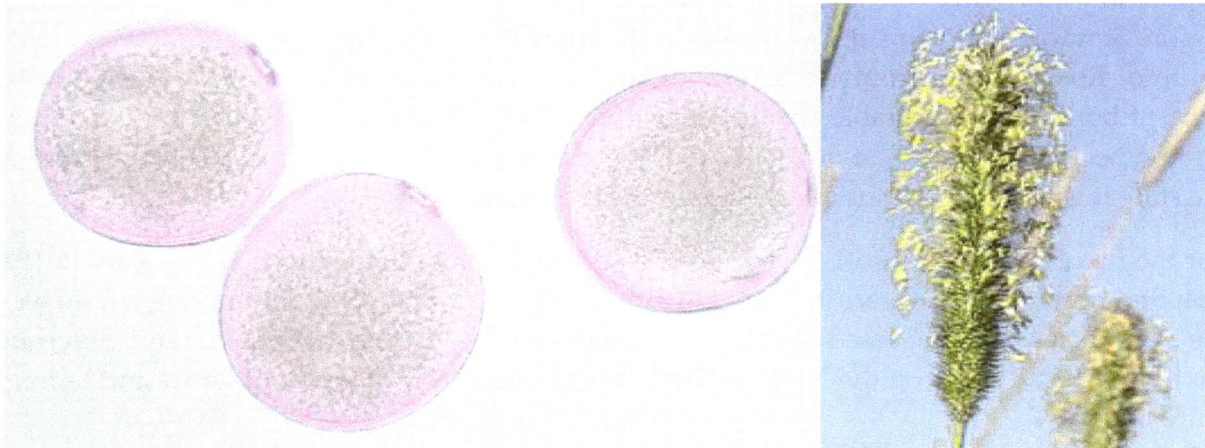

Figure 18. Poaceae. Phleum pratense.

The 7th group of allergens (Dac g CBP, Poa p CBP, Phi p 7) has a molecular weight of 8-12 kD, causes a sensitization in 10% of patients, and has a high immunogenicity. However, they are not very often recognized as minor allergens in the periodical literature. The minority of the allergens of the 10th group is associated with a low molecular weight of 12 kD. Less than 5% of patients are sensitive to them (Lol p 10, Poa p 10). The 11-13 groups of proteins (Dac g 11, Phi p 11, Poa p 12, Phi p 12, Phi p 13, Lol p 12, Fes p 13 et al.) The 12th group is represented by profillins. They have low allergenicity due to the molecular weight of 18 to 50 kD. From 15 to 55% of patients are sensitized to them [14, 15, 16].

The main taxa of weeds (Chemopodiaceae+Amaranthaceae):

1.   Ambrosia elatior (Common ragweed)

2.   Ambrósia artemisiifólia (Radweed) (Fig.18)

3.   Ambrosia psilostachya (Western ragweed)

4.   Ambrosia trifida (Gigant ragweed)

5.   Artemisia absinthium (Wormwood) (Fig.20)

6.   Artemisia vulgaris (Mugwort)

7.   Atriplex canescens(Orach) (Fig.21)

8.   Taraxacum vulgare (Dandelion)

9.   Helianthus annuus (Sunflower)

10. Matricaria chamomilla (Camomille)

11. Urtica dioica (Nettle) (Fig.22)

The most aggressive allergen in the southern part of Europe and Russia is ragweed (Fig.19). It is also common in the North, South, Central America, Japan, Africa and the CIS countries. The population morbidity of the ragweed pollinosis in the Southern regions of Russia (Rostov region, Stavropol and Krasnodar territories)is from24% to38%. The spread of ragweed in the South of Russia began from the Stavropol territory. The Stavropol territory is located in the zone of boundaries favorable for the development of the quarantine weed of ragweed. 2.5 million hectares of land had been affected in the Stavropol territory since 1999 (according to the state inspection for plant quarantine of the Stavropol territory).

For the first time in the USSR the ragweed was found by the botanist S.G. Kolmakov in 1918 near Stavropol. Its seeds were brought in 1916-1917 by the railway builders among whom were the Americans. The ragweed spreads extremely quickly in the Krasnodar and Stavropol territories. Its advance on the North is limited by the duration of daylight hours and temperature factors.

In its homeland, this plant has more than 30 species. There are several varieties of ragweed: dwarf Ambrosia elatior, giant Ambrosia tritida and Ambrosia psilostachya. There are 2 common types on the Stavropol territory: Ambrósia artemisiifólia and three-separate and Ambrosia trifida. This annotinous spring weed, reproducing by seeds, is a light-, heat-loving, and wind-pollinated plant. This plant produces up to 1, 000 seedlings per 1 square meter. One bush can give 88.000 seeds which remain in the soil till 4-5 years. The windy weather, typical for Stavropol territory, contributes to the spread of pollen over distances of 20-30 km.

The ragweed pollen grains are round, of prickly sculpture, with the size of 23-24 microns and a molecular weight of 37 kD (Dalton), and they contain 5 major allergens (epitopes). For comparison, the orach pollen is 35 kD, the wormwood pollen is 19 kD, and the sunflower pollen is 14 kDa. The ragweed pollen contains two main antigens – the antigen E and the antigen K. The antigen E is 200 times more active than the antigen K [4].

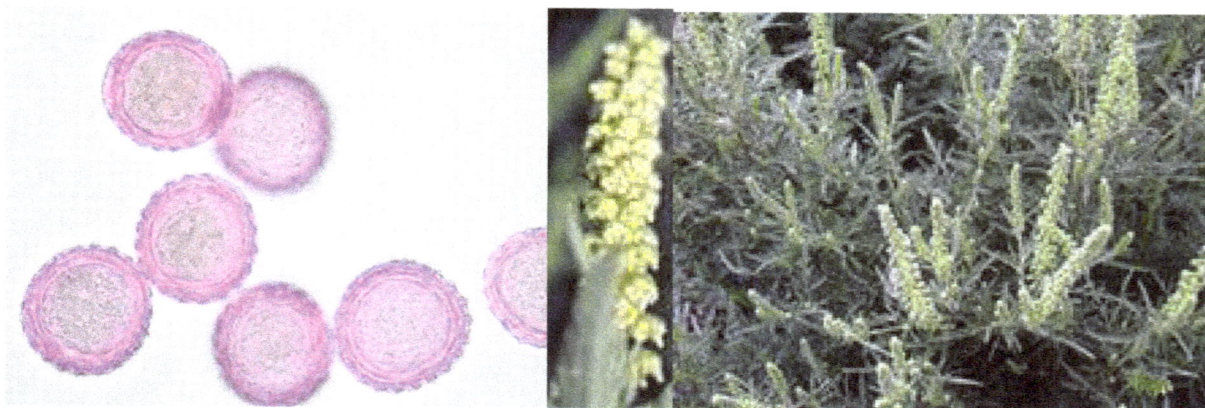

Figure 19. Ambrósia artemisiifólia

The weed pollen has also high homology and cross-allergenic properties. The co-sensitization between ragweed and wormwood among the patients is characteristic in 93% of cases. The major allergen of ragweed is Amb a 1 (E) and Amb a 2 (K) with a molecular weight of 38 kD. The minor allergen of ragweed is profilin with low Mm=11 kD. The major allergens of wormwood include Art v 1, Art v 2, Art v 4, Art v 5 and Art v 6 (Mm=35-67 kD). 62% of the

patients with ragweed pollinosis are sensitized to them [17].

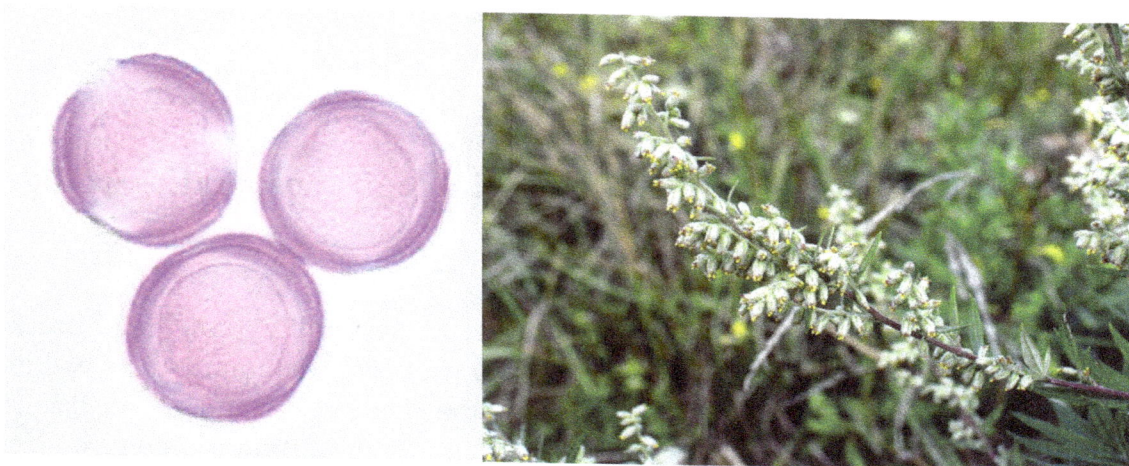

Figure 20. Artemisia absinthium

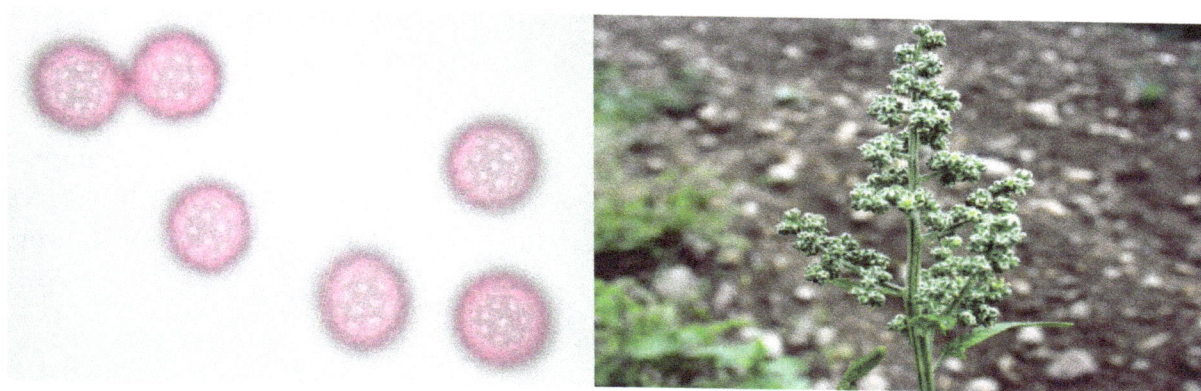

Figure 21. Atriplex canescens

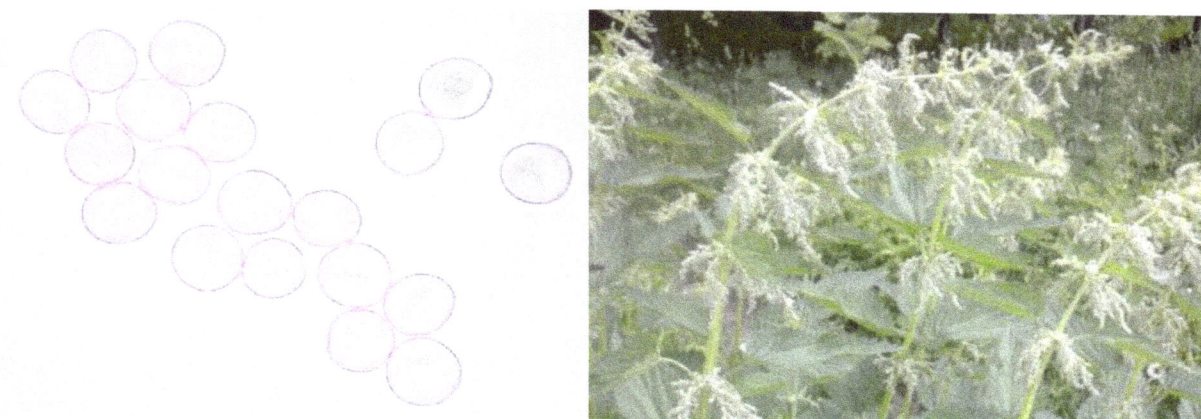

Figure 22. Urtica dioica

Depending on the climatic and geographic features of the region, it is appropriate to include in the calendar more information about plants flowering, the pollen of which is logged in the air in significant quantities. The calendars of plants flowering help the allergist to compare the clinical symptoms that develop in a patient depending on the season of the year and the place where he resides, rests or works.

4. The influence of ecology on morphopalinological properties of the airborne allergens

Due to the deteriorating environmental situation, there is a variability of allergenic properties of pollen. In recent years, there is evidence that the chemical compounds that pollute the environment, can change the allergenic properties of the plants pollen and, as a consequence, lead to the formation of new properties and combinations of the airborne allergens.

The major pollutants contained in the air are nitrogen oxides (32.3%) and hydrocarbons (24%). Harmful emissions from motor transport made 359 thousand tons or 85% of the total emissions in 2007-2008, and increased by 20% in comparison with 2006 [19]. In the structure of emissions from motor transport 75.4% accounts for carbon monoxide, 13.7% for hydrocarbons, 7.9% for nitrogen oxides, 1.2% for carbon black [19].

In 2011 we estimated the presence in the tests of spring atmospheric rain the changes in morphological features of pollen and technogenic particles. The changes were mainly observed in the pollen of Acer n. and Salix l, the trees growing along the motorway of the city of Stavropol (Fig. 23) [18].

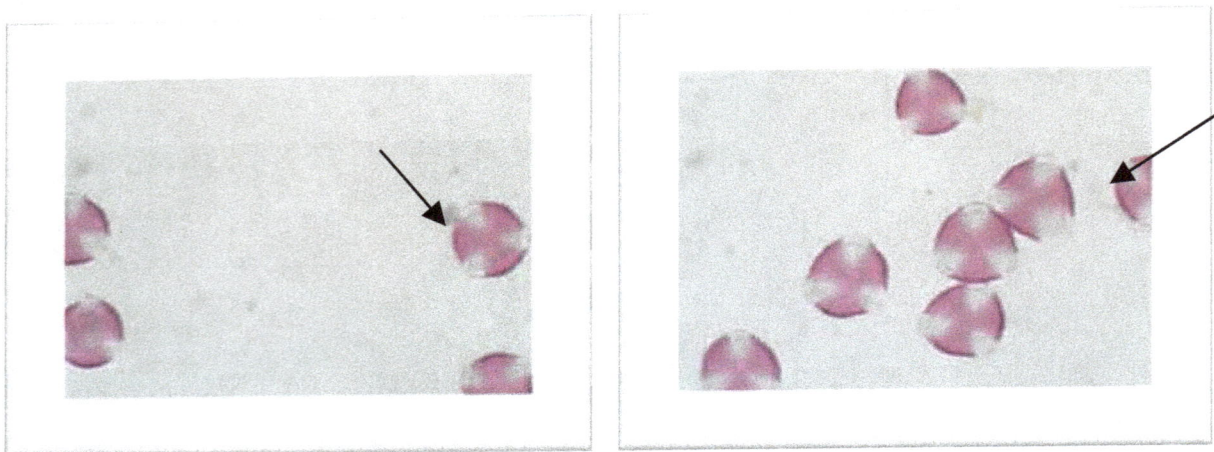

Figure 23. Salix sp. along the motorway. The arrow indicates the pollutants.

The same morphological changes of pollen are shown by Dr. Dzyba O. F. on the pollen of gymnosperms (Pinus sylvestris) growing in the city of St. Petersburg (Fig.24) [20].

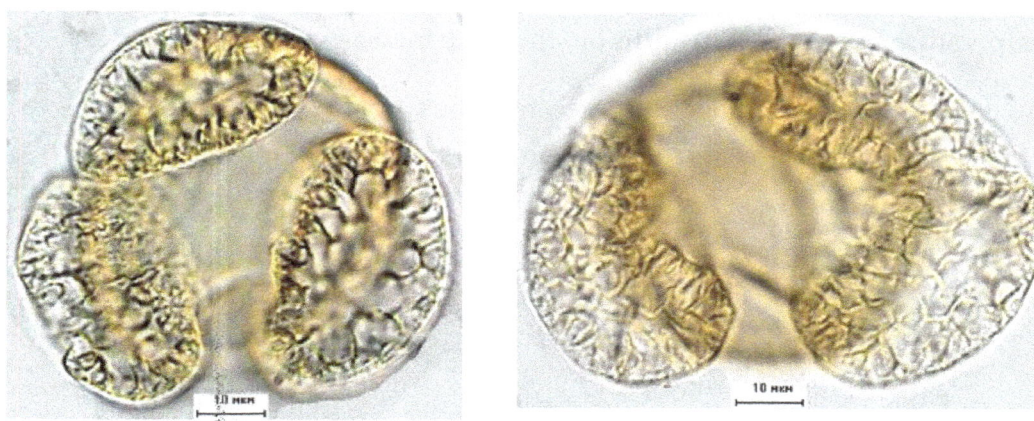

Figure 24. The polymorphism of Pinus sylvestris.

In the conditions of the environmental pollution the plants pollen dominating during a pallination season, is capable to transfer microcells of a technogenic origin, forming the increased antigenic activity. The severity of clinical symptoms of respiratory allergies in patients, in addition to the weather conditions, is caused by the simultaneous effect of non-specific trigger and specific cause-significant factors on the upper airways mucosa. Thus, the safety of the living environment is an essential component of human ecology, as a key factor in reducing the risk of development of allergic diseases.

5. The insect allergens

5.1. House dust mites (Acarida)

Dust is the main multicomponent inhalation allergen. The allergen from house dust is distinguished by the complexity in antigenic composition. It consists of fungi, pollen particles, metabolic products of insects, epidermis particles of animals and humans. A powerful component of house dust allergen is also micromites Dermathophagoides pteronyssimus and Dermathophagoides farinae – the tiny arthropods like Arthropoda, invisible to the naked eye, the body diameter of which is about 0.3 mm. The number of micromites increases in autumn. These mites feed on flakes of desquamated corneal layer of human skin which is the largest part of the house dust components, and live in symbiosis with the microscopic mold fungi living in mattresses and other bedding. Mite excrements are also ideal allergens. Anti-genes of pincers rather large therefore allergic reactions to them arise not so quickly as on epidermis of cats. Mites antigens are large enough so allergic reactions to them do not occur as fast as to the cats epidermis. The allergy to house dust most often manifests itself in the form of bronchial asthma, rhinitis, and rarely-conjunctivitis. House dust and barns mites are microscopic arthropods invisible to the naked eye (). Their excrements, body parts are airborne allergens of the living premises, warehouses, barns, archives and libraries. The body diameter of an insect is about 0.3 mm. They have full-blown allergenic activity. The size of mites varies from 0.1 to 0.5 mm. They are widely spread around the globe. The normal cycle of their life is about

65-80 days. The female mite oviposits about 60 eggs at once. The ideal habitat is an apartment with a temperature of 18-25 °C. In addition, they like increased humidity [21, 22].

House dust mite: Dermatophagoides pteronyssinus (Fig.25), Dermatophagoides farinae, Dermatophagoides microceras, Euroglyphus maynei, Blomia Tropicalis.

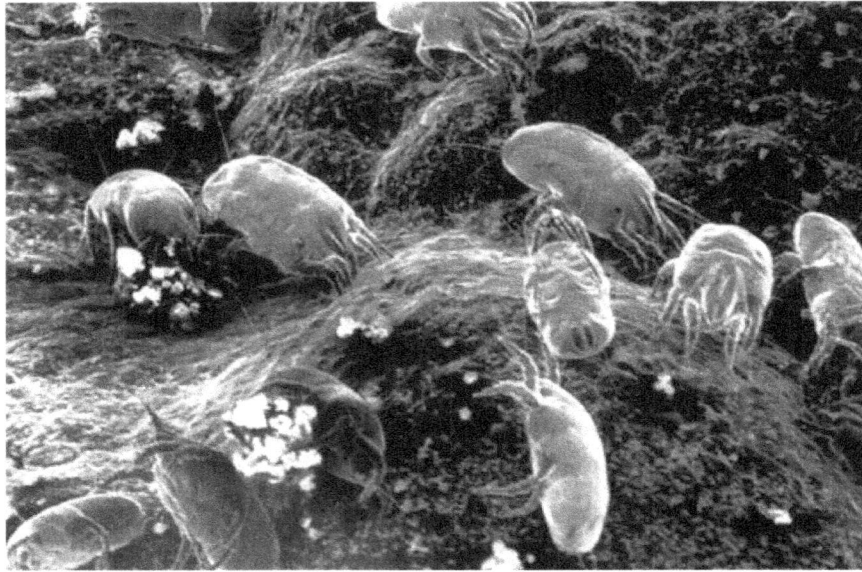

Figure 25. House dust mite. Dermatophagoides pteronyssinus

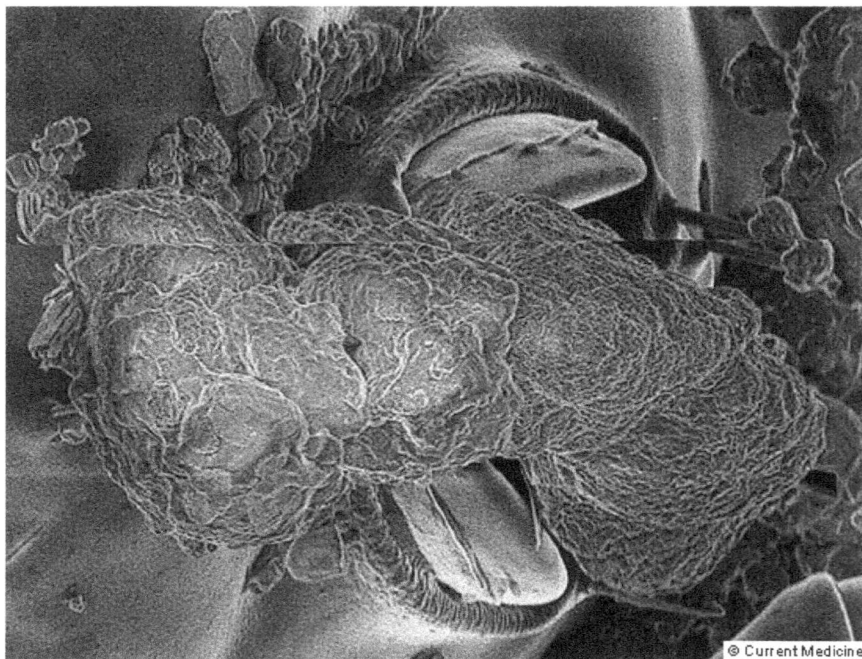

Figure 26. Mites excrements

Dermatophagoides pteronyssinus feed on flakes of desquamated epidermis of human skin which is the largest part of the house dust. Small fragments of mites (from 10 to 40 microns) and their metabolic products (especially fecal particles) have a remarkable ability to cause allergies: respiratory allergosis, bronchial asthma, allergic conjunctivitis and angioneurotice-dema. The fecal balls of house dust mites contain about 13 different groups of major and minor allergens that come from the intestinal tract of insects. The most studied are the major allergens Dermatophagoides pteronyssinus-Der p 1 and Dermatophagoides farinae-Der f 1. The polypeptide chain of the main allergen consists of 216 amino-acid remains with a N-terminal threonine. The threshold concentration for the development of sensitization in genetically predisposed to atopy patients, is the content of 92 µg/g of dust of the major allergens of mites. Approximately 500 mites per 1 gram of dust provoke attacks of bronchial asthma in sensitized patients.

Storage mite: Acarus siro (Fig.27), Lepidoglyphus destructor, Tyrophagus putrescentiae, Glycyphagus domesticus.

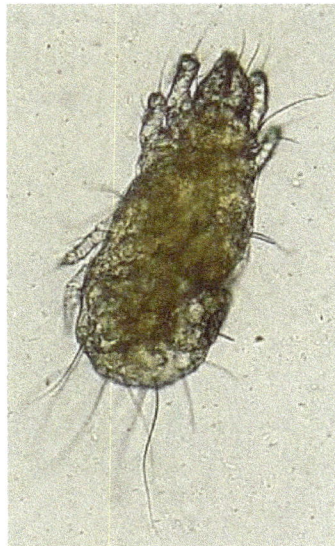

Figure 27. Acarus siro

The flour mite damages grains of cereals, oil-bearing plants, legumes, preferring flour to cereals, fodder and dried vegetables, fruits, medical and tobacco raw materials, spices, leather, cheese, sausage, egg powder, fish and meat bone flour. Its body is oval and whitish, the body surface is shiny, legs and mouthparts are brownish-red. The body length of male mite is up to 0.5 mm, female mite is up to 0.7 mm [23]. The mite often penetrates into the embryo, forming a latent form of infection, and, first of all, dangerous for seed grain. In most cases, the patients sensitized to flour mites work in the agricultural industry and/or directly with the grain. A detailed medical history is very important to clarify the diagnosis, since a particular profession (a librarian, an archivist, an agronomist or a housewife) promotes sensitization to different kinds of mites and, therefore, the individual selection of immunotherapy.

Other representatives of Arthropoda are stinging and not stinging insects. As the airborne allergens, the insect allergens can be fragments and products of insects' vital activity. The patients, whose professional activity is connected with insects, are usually sensitized to them: the beekeepers, the persons living near apiaries, the workers of fish-farms, insectaries and granaries, entomologists and other. The known insects causing an allergy are cockroaches, gnats, caddis flies, moth, flies, mosquitoes, Daphnia. Very often the patients sensitized to mites can cross-react to the above-mentioned allergens.

The cross sensitization can be caused by Der p 10 (tropomyosine), the minor allergen for patients with the allergy to the house dust mites [22]. However it may point to risk of development of allergic reactions to Crustacea or snails. The cockroaches also have a major allergen Bla g 2 and cross-allergen tropomyosine Bla g 7 which indicates the risk of allergic reactions to Crustacea (most often to the shrimps) [24]. In their turn, shrimps and other Crustacea also contain other clinically relevant allergens: sarcoplasmatic calcium-binding protein and argininekinase [25]. The most important airborne allergens for such patients are parvalbumins (Gad c 1, Cyp c 1). These are major allergens of fish, stable to the action of temperatures and digestive enzymes. Parvalbumins have a high degree of cross-reactivity in which patients sensitized to one of parvalbumin may react to other fish parvalbumin. It may be a river, sea, ocean, white or red fish. There are cases of severe allergic reactions of patients on inhalation of vapours with fish parvalbumin through casual contact in everyday life (eating places, hotels, etc.) [26].

The special populations of patients with frequent and prolonged contact with hymenopterous insects are beekeepers, their families and their neighbors. The systemic allergic reactions may be developed not only after insects stinging, but also on inhalation of the body parts and the products of their activity [27]. As a rule, these reactions are caused in patients sensitized to the major allergens Api m 1 of a honey bee, Ves v 5 and/or Ves v 1 of a wasp. The allergic cross reaction between the bees and wasps allergen may be due to the carbohydrate part of glycoproteins (CCD)[28]. The poison and bodies allergens of the most Hymenoptera contain the CCD, which are responsible for the cross-IgE-reactivity between bees and wasps allergens [29].

6. The main fungal allergens

The role of fungal allergens in the structure of allergic diseases is very important. The mycogenic sensitization arising due to the long contact of a human body with allergens of microscopic fungi, plays an increasingly important role in people's lives, particularly the residents of megapolises [30]. Aeroallergens, which include fungal spores and fungal cell wall components, surround us everywhere in everyday life, at work places, in nature. By means of scratch test method, the frequency of sensitization to allergens of house dust mites, mycelial and yeast fungi was investigated among the patients of the allergic center. It was revealed that 12, 69% of patients showed hypersensitivity only to one of the allergens. 87, 31 % of patients had combined forms of sensitization to two or more allergens. It is noted that the sensitization to fungi allergens (82, 84%) in comparison with the occurrence of the sensitization to house dust mite allergens (67, 16%) is found more often [32, 33, 34, 35, 36].

All stages of micromycetes allergens intake into the organism have been studied up to the present day, and the mechanisms of their influence on the immune system have been proposed. There also have been conducted large-scale epidemiological researches; the role of fungal allergens in the pathogenesis of a number of allergic diseases was established.

Microscopic fungi are widespread in nature, they are capable to colonize all substrates and absorb almost any organic substance. The main reservoir for microscopic fungi is soil and plant remains, where the number of fungal propagules can be up to several hundreds of thousands of CFU per gram of substrate. Due to their small size, they easily enter the bioaerosols and can be transferred in the atmosphere over long distances. The concentration of fungal spores in the air may be 2-3 orders greater than the one of pollen [38]. In certain periods of the year (from spring to autumn) the total number of fungal propagules in the air bioaerosol can be 1-2 orders greater. However, not only quantitative but also qualitative composition of fungal allergens is of great importance for the development of mycogenic sensitization. There are new ecological niches for fungi habitat due to human activities in large cities. This is mainly organic waste in landfills and production as well as bioaffected objects of urban infrastructure (emergency buildings and facilities for various purposes).

The allergy to fungi is known for a long time. For example, hay fever had been described in detail in 1819, the role of micromycetes in its etiology was shown in 1873 [31]. Currently, numerous studies have proven the value of mycogenic sensitization in the pathogenesis of allergic rhinitis, bronchial asthma, allergic bronchopulmonary mycosis, exogenous allergic alveolitis, atopic dermatitis [32, 33, 34, 35, 36]. Epidemiological researches have shown that the level of mycogenic sensitization is very significant and varies depending on the genetic characteristics of the surveyed groups of population, climatic and geographical features of their habitats-from 5% (southern Europe) to 40% (Portland, USA) for patients with bronchial asthma [32]. And in the desert environment (Kuwait) there was the indicator of 46% among the surveyed patients with asthma [37].

In July 2014 the number of registered non-food fungi allergens, the list of which is available on the website www.allergen.org, reached 108, according to the Subcommittee on Nomenclature of allergens of International Union of Immunological Societies (IUIS).

Some strains of micromycetes can synthesize up to 40 macromolecules connecting IgE [39]. The vast number of the registered allergens belongs to 5 genera-Aspergillus, Alternaria, Cladosporium, Penicillium, Malassezia (Fig. 28-31), while the symptoms of respiratory allergies are connected with about 80 genera of fungi [40].

The sensitization of a macroorganism occurs, in particular, due to the action of proteases which can degrade proteins providing the impenetrability of the epithelial cell barrier. Partial proteolysis of these proteins causes a disturbance of the monolayer structure and the flow of allergenic material through it. The desquamation of epithelial cells was observed in the processing of cell cultures by means of proteases A. fumigatus. Using various inhibitors, the researchers defined a role of serine proteases in the process of destruction of the cell layer [41]. Also, the influence of fungi allergens on the immunological mechanisms operating on the principle of negative feedback is mentioned in a number of works.

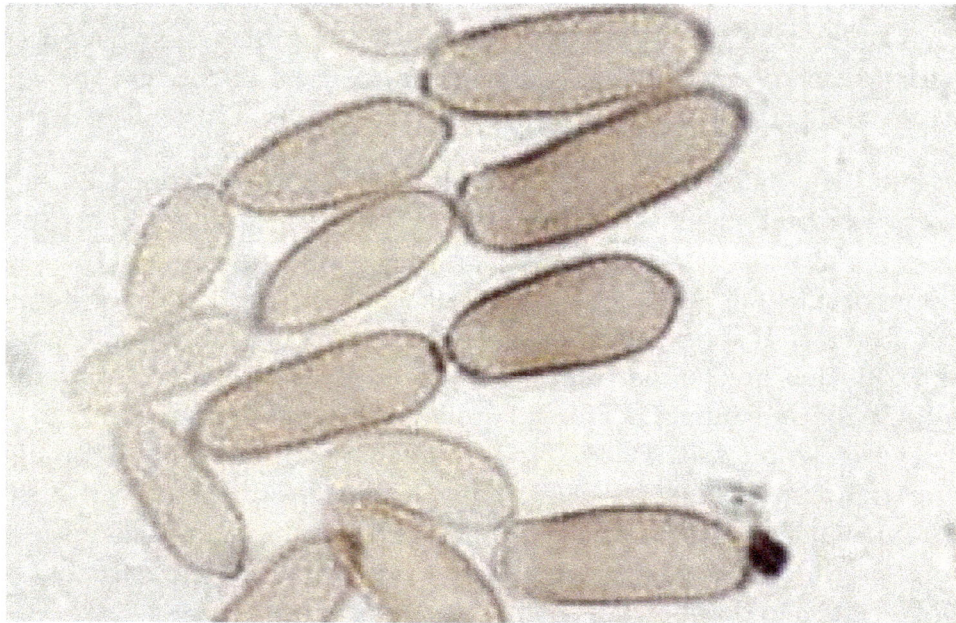

Figure 28. Cladosporium

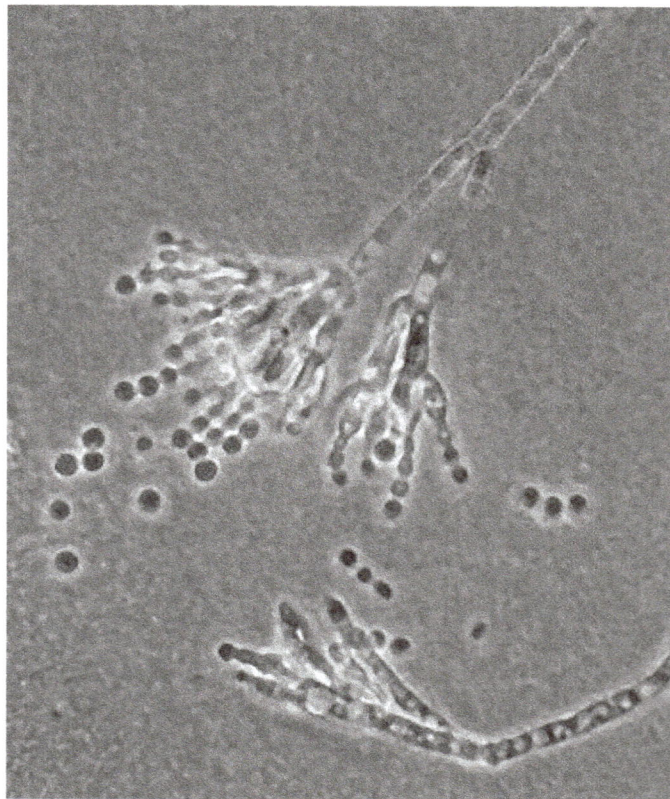

Figure 29. Penicillium

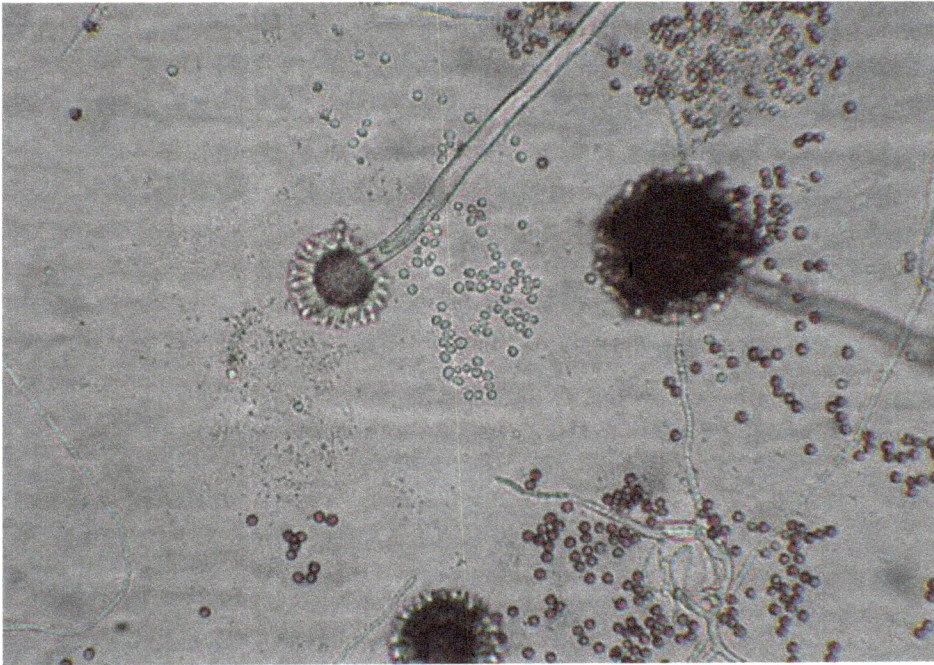

Figure 30. Aspergillus

Fungi allergens possessing the proteolytic activity, as well as proteases of dermatophagoidic mite allergens are capable to break protective barriers of an organism independently. They are able to overcome the immunological tolerance, and are recognized by immunocompetent cells, followed by the elaboration of specific reaginic antibodies and the induction of release of the allergic reaction mediators. In this regard, we should note the difference of fungal and plant allergens. It is known that there is an absence of proteases among known plant allergens. At the same time it is also known about high proteolytic activity of pollen plant extracts [42]. Obviously, there are unidentified proteases in the composition of these extracts and, presumably, they provide transportation and adjuvant functions, but they are not allergens.

To understand the features of a mycogenic sensitization we should into consideration the form in which allergens get into the respiratory tract. The inhaled allergens of plants and fungi, as opposed to domestic or epidermal ones, are present in the aerosol products primarily in encapsulated form. They are the pollen of grasses and trees, spores / conidia of fungi. Exceptions arise after the rain when there might be emission of contents of the swollen pollen grains in the form of submicroscopic particles [43] and in cases of technogenic emissions. Conidia, on the average, have much smaller size than pollen grains. The diameter of micromycete conidia of such widespread genera as Penicillium and Aspergillus doesn't exceed 2-5 microns. The exception is Alternaria with its large macroconidia, which, however, may be found in aerosols in segmented form (Fig. 30).

The antigen-presenting function is poorly expressed in pulmonary macrophage. To initiate an immune response, spores enclosed in hard envelope must have time to release a sufficient amount of sensitizing material into the environment before macrophages phagocytize them. This material containing the protease must penetrate the epithelial barrier and reach the

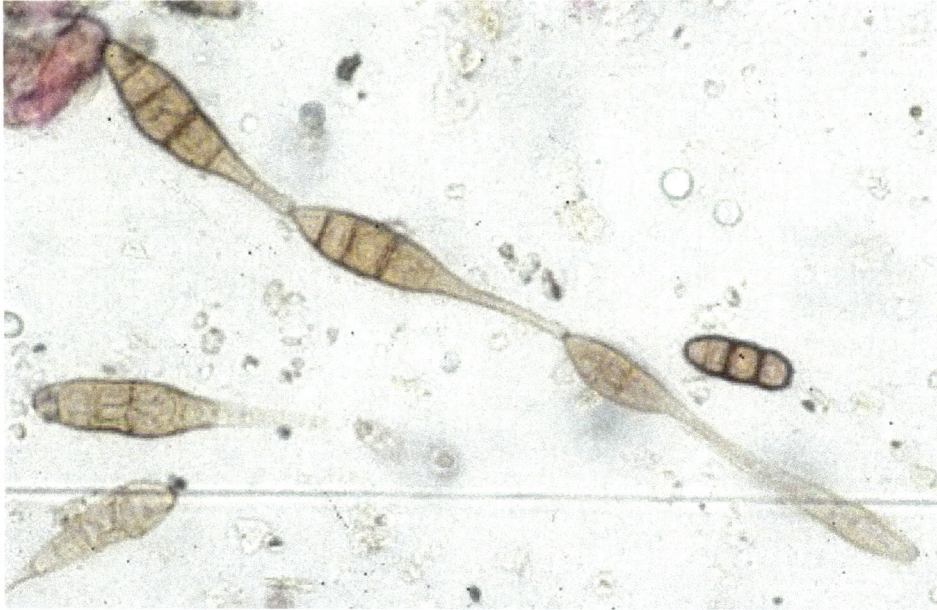

Figure 31. Alternaria

dendritic cells and Langerhans cells in the airways or dendritic cells in the alveolar epithelium. It is necessary to take into account that the respiratory part of the lungs is the most tolerant due to the small number of antigen-presenting cells. At the massive inflow of antigenic material, the condition of tolerance can be overcome with the emergence of IgG-mediated exogenous allergic alveolitis. As for the speed of extraction of allergenic material from the spores, it was shown during the study of bazidiospores that it depends primarily on the thickness of the envelope [44].When studying the effect of conidia germination of several mitospore fungi on their excretion of detected immunochemical allergens into the environment, the Australian authors found that small and durable conidia of such fungi as A. fumigatus and P. chrysogenum, only slightly produce allergens without prolonged pre-incubation in a humid environment [45, 46].

In conclusion, it should be noted that, despite the pronounced "aggressiveness" of fungal allergens, there are constraints allowing a healthy organism to stand a natural background of mycoallergens with no harm. In case of the allergen load rise or in the development of atopic states the risk of a mycogenic sensitization significantly increases.

7. The airborne allergens of animals

The airborne allergens of animals are wool (hair), epidermis (Fig. 32), dried urine, saliva, and feces. The prevalence of an allergy to epidermis of pets is a worldwide growing problem of public health as a death rate in consequence of allergic diseases has disproportionate impact on socially and economically unprotected populations, in particular, on children [48].

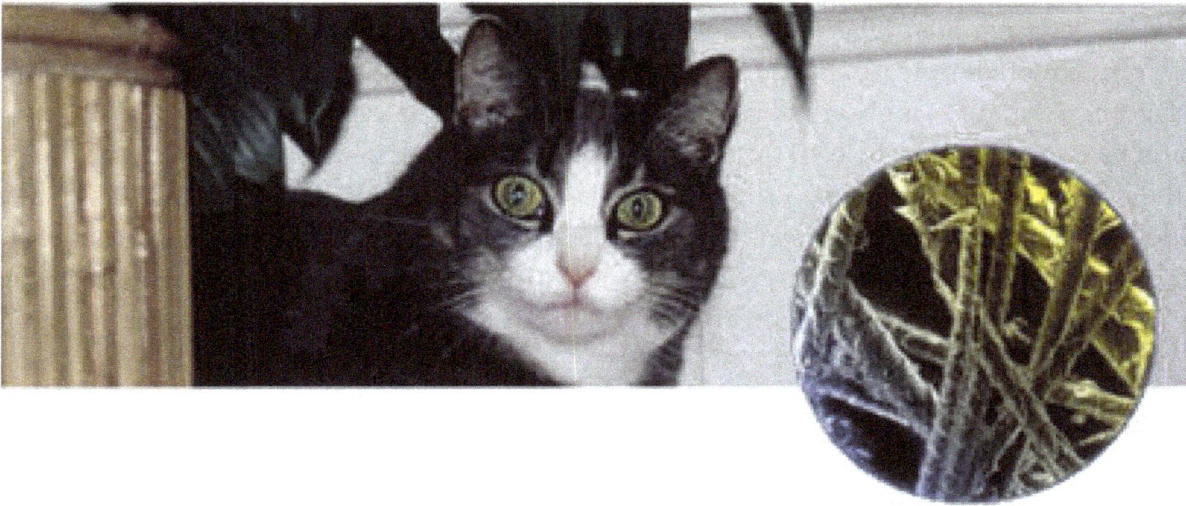

Figure 32. Cat's hair

The allergy to cats epidermis is one of the most widespread forms of allergic diseases in the USA and Europe in 10-15% of patients suffering from allergic rhinitis and (or) bronchial asthma (WAO 2011). Cats are the major source of the allergen Fel d 1. Though there are few molecules of the allergens in the extract of cat dandruff. The most significant of them is the Fel d 1. At the same time, approximately 90% of people with allergies to cats have an increased level of IgE specific for the protein. The level of allergen (secretoglobin) Fel d 1 is significantly higher in houses where the cats live [47]. In houses where the cats have never lived, there is a direct relationship between the level of allergen in the house and the number of domestic cats in the immediate environment, in general. The allergen Fel d 1 is also present in many public places in a concentration that may cause the development or worsening of symptoms among the people with allergies. This is particularly relevant and problematic for school children (Morris 2010). The other allergen associated with asthma patients is lipocalin Fel d 4 [47, 48].

Typically, many patients are co-sensitized to several species of animals. The cross activity of pets is caused by the following main allergens: Mus m 1, Equ with 1, Can f 1, Can f 2 and Can f 5 [50]. However, the cross-reactivity between animals is poorly understood on the molecular level. The biological variability of a source of animal allergens does not always allow to identify the cause-significant allergen of the patient by means of a simple skin test. 38% of patients were revealed sensitivity to Can f 5-allergen from male dogs prostate (33) and approximately 60% of patients are sensitized to Can f 1, Can f 2-epidermal allergens of animals. As Can f 5 in low concentration may be found in the dog's hair, it is difficult to reveal the sensitivity of the patient to this allergen by means of skin tests [49]. That explains the doctor's recommendations to remove completely an animal and the products of its life activity from premises and the surrounding territory whenever possible, and the absence or existence of hair on an animal doesn't matter. The airborne allergens of animals are conservative (stable) and even after the elimination they are present in the premises for a long period of time, both independently and as a part of house dust.

The special place is given to the study of a professional allergy of persons employed with animals: veterinarians, laboratory and vivarium staff, factory workers, farmers, etc. The development of allergic reactions (allergic rhinitis, conjunctivitis, urticaria, bronchial asthma and atopic dermatitis) is observed in 10-30% of workers. All of them have contacts with animal allergens on production. In 2010 the Spanish scientists showed a high sensitization of workers to the hair of various animals (a rat, a mouse, a guinea pig, a rabbit, a hamster, a dog, a cat, cattle, a goat and a horse) by means of the skin test. 62% of them had at least one positive skin test to the hair of various animals. Thus, the statistically significant association with the age, the length of service, the allergic history, the clinical manifestations and the level of serumal IgE wasn't proved [51].

8. Toxicoallergic aerosols

One of the reasons for the growth of new cases of respiratory allergies among people of working age is the occupational exposure to toxic and allergenic aerosols. Toxic airborne allergens are able to penetrate into the respiratory system in the form of vapor and smoke in the pre-heating, grinding to dust or in combination with gas components and polymeric binders. These methods are applied on production and service for packaging food products, construction, welding, production of household chemicals and many other things.

For example, a special place is occupied by phthalates formed from polyvinyl chloride (PVC), the products of which are widely distributed in living and working environment. During the processing, packaging and stacking of various materials the high concentrations of mono-and diphthalates in combination with formaldehyde, formic acid, acetaldehyde, acetic acid and benzoic acid penetrate in the breathing zone of workers. These substances are known for their toxic and allergenic properties. Getting into the respiratory tract, they can cause irritation of the mucous membrane as well as the damage of the epithelium of the upper airways, the bronchial tree, the mucous membrane of the eye, development of edema, inflammation, and violation of the mucociliary clearance. This leads to the diseases of the upper airways, the formation of the syndrome of bronchial obstruction and bronchial asthma (BA).

The mechanism of development and the peculiarities of the clinical course of respiratory diseases caused by toxicoallergic aerosols are still not clear. This is due to the low molecular weight and the interaction with proteins of the skin and mucous membranes. The experimental data in animals demonstrate the ability of toxicoallergic aerosols to cause the development of airway inflammation of immune and non-immune nature (Larsen ST, 2004; Frederiksen H, 2007). The in-depth study in this area has not been conducted [51].

The most well-known toxico-allergic substances (low-molecular weight substances, haptens) which may contribute to the development of allergic respiratory diseases of humans are given below (Table 3).

Name of the group	Airborne allergens	Items containing this substance
Aldehydes	Formaldehyde, acetaldehyde, Formaldehyde resin, para-tert-butylbenzaldehyde	Means for processing of fabrics, preservatives, solutions for metal processing, adhesive substances/glue, plastic, detergents, construction materials, corrosion inhibitors; fillers used in industry; chemicals used in flooring; paints, varnishes, impregnating products; printing ink, polishing materials, binders, surfactants, deodorants
Dichromate	Potassium dichromate	Cement, chrome leather, petroleum products, textile paint, antiseptics, preservatives, cosmetics, mortar, printing industry, detergents, concrete, photoreactants
Aromatic substancec	Cinnamaldehyde (1%)Cinnamic alcohol (1%)Eugenol (1%)Geraniol (1%)Hydroxycitronellal (1%)Isoeugenol (1%)Evernia Prunastri (1%)	Perfumes, eau de toilettes, colognes, powder, soap, shampoos, shower gels. Essential oil. Detergents. Aromatic candles. Spices, seasonings
Rosin, turpentine		Perfumes and cosmetics, glue, spices, wood resin. Rosin containing dental materials. Glue, paints, varnishes
Metals:, cobalt, chromium, palladium and their connections, nickel	Nickel sulfate, Cobaltchloride, Palladium chloride	Nickel plated items used in shipbuilding, aerospace and automobile industries
Derivative thyuram	Tetramethylthiuram disulfide (0, 25%)Tetraethylthiuram disulfide (0, 25%)Tetramethylthiuram monosulfide (0, 25%)	Catalysts used in the vulcanization process in the production of rubber items. Pesticides, prints, tubes, glue. Emulsion for the treatment of scabies. Fungicides, adhesive substances, paints; pharmaceutical substance used in veterinary medicine
A mixture of mercaptans	N-cyclohexen-sotatila sulfenamid (0, 5%)Mercaptobenzothiazoles (0, 5%)Morpholinyl mercaptobenzothiazoles (0, 5%)	The catalysts used in the vulcanization process in the production of rubber items
Phenylendiamine	Paraphenylenediamine	Hair dye, textile paint, ink for printers, photoreactants, lubricants, oil, gasoline (petrol); antioxidants and catalysts used in the manufacture of resins and plastics
Quaternium-15	Quaternium-15	Cleaning and polishing substances. Cosmetics, skin care and hair care products, latex paint, the solutions used in the processing of metals
Ethylendiamine	Ethylenediamine dihydrochloride, hexa-methylenediamine	Corrosion-resistant materials

Name of the group	Airborne allergens	Items containing this substance
Epoxy resin	Epoxy resin	Materials of plastic, adhesive materials. Covering of household items, adhesive tape, paint, corrosion-resistant, water-resistant, insulating materials, sports goods. The materials used in shipbuilding, aerospace and automobile industries. It Can be used in the preparation of specimen for electron microscopy
Esters of phthalic acid	phthalics	Plastic, polyethylene
Antibiotic drugs	Penicillin, neomycin,	antibiotic production

Table 3. The list of toxico-allergic substances in aerosols

Author details

Olga Ukhanova[2*] and Evgenia Bogomolova[1]

*Address all correspondence to: uhanova_1976@mail.ru

1 Komarov Botanical Institute of the Russian Academy of Sciences, St. Petersburg, Russia

2 Department of Allergology-Immunology, Ministry of Medical Care of the Stavropol Territory, Stavropol, Russia

References

[1] Ilyina N.I. Allergopathology in different regions of Russia according to the results of clinical and epidemiological studies: author. of thesis. - M., 1996. – p. 240

[2] Bousquet J., Khaltaev N., Cruz A.A. et al. Allergic Rhinitis and its Impact on Asthma (ARIA) 2008 update (in collaboration with the World Health Organization, GA(2)LEN and AllerGen). Allergy.v. 63 (Suppl. 86) 8-160.

[3] Severova E.A. Principles and methods of research aeropalynology. Moscow, 1999. 40 p.

[4] Polleninfo.org

[5] http://pollen.fmi.fi

[6]   Sastre J., Landivar M.E., Ruiz-García M. et al. How molecular diagnosis can change allergen-specific immunotherapy prescription in a complex pollen area. Allergy. 2012 v. 67, p.709-711.

[7]   Valenta R, Kraft D.Recombinantallergens: from production and characterization to diagnosis, treatment, and prevention of allergy. Methods. 2004 v. 32, p.207-208.

[8]   Ayuso R., Sánchez-Garcia S., Lin J. et al. Greater epitope recognition of shrimp allergens by children than by adults suggests that shrimp sensitization decreases with age. J Allergy Clin. Immunol. 2010 v. 125 p.1286-1293

[9]   http://www.allergen.org

[10] Ebo D.C., Bridts C.H. Verweij M.M. Sensitization profiles in birch pollen-allergic patient with and without oral allergy syndrome to apple^ lessons from multiplexed component-resolved allergy diagnosis. Clin. Exp. Allergy.2010 v.40, p.339-347.

[11] Constantin C., Quirce S., Poorafshar M. et al. Micro-arrayed wheat seed and grass pollen allergens for component-resolved diagnosis. Allergy. 2009, v.64. p.1030-1037.

[12] Weber RW. Cross-reactivity of pollen allergens. Curr Allergy Asthma Rep 2004 v. 4, p. 401-408.

[13] Andersson K, Lidholm J. Characteristics and immunobiology of grass pollen allergens. Int Arch Allergy Immunol 2003, v.130, p.87-107.

[14] Larsen J.N., Lowenstein H. Allergen nomenclature. J Allergy Clin Immunol 1996, v. 97, p.577-578.

[15] Cases B, Ibañez MD, Tudela J.I. et al. Immunological cross-reactivity between olive and grasspollen: implication of major and minor allergens.World Allergy Organ J. 2014 v. 8, p. 1-11.

[16] Boehme MW, Kompauer I, Weidner U. Respiratory symptoms and sensitization to airborne pollen of ragweed and mugwort of adults in Southwest Germany. Dtsch Med Wochenschr.2013, v.138, p.1651-1658.

[17] Ukhanova OP, Shishalova T.N., Ivanova O.S. The study of surface structure of pollen for quality assessment the environment in Stavropol. Herald MANEB. v.16. №2, p. 69-72.

[18] Severova EA, : OV, Polenova SV analysis of the characteristics dusting some taxa aeropalynology spectrum / proceedings of the I International seminar "Pollen as an indicator of environmental condition and paleoecological reconstruction", St.-Petersburg, 2001. S. 177-186.

[19] Dzyuba O.F. Palynology. [Electronic resource]: an Encyclopedic Fund. URL: http://russika.ru/ (date of access: 25.12.2008).

[20] Bronnert M, Mancini J, Birnbaum Jet al. Component-resolved diagnosis with commercially available D. pteronyssinus Der p 1, Der p 2 and Der p 10: relevant markers for house dust mite allergy. Clin Exp Allergy. 2012 v. 42, p.1406-1415.

[21] Resch Y, Weghofer M, Seiberler S. Molecular characterization of Der p 10: a diagnostic marker for broad sensitization in house dust mite allergy. Clin Exp Allergy. 2011, v.41, 1468-1477.

[22] Iraola V, Prados M, Pinto H. Allergological characterisation of the storage miteAcarus gracilis (Acari: Acaridae).Allergol Immunopathol (Madr). 2014 v. 31. [Epub ahead of print].

[23] Lee M.F. Song P.P. Sensitisation to Per a 2 of the American cockroach correlates with more clinical severity among airway allergic patients in Taiwan. Ann Allergy Asthma Immunol.2012, v.108, p.243-248.

[24] Lopata A.L., Lehrer S.B.Newinsights into seafood allergy. Curr Opin Allergy Clin Immunol. 2009 v. 9, p-270-277.

[25] Perez-Gordo M, Cuesta-Herranz J, Maroto A.S. et al. Identification of sole parvalbumin as a major allergen: study of cross-reactivity between parvalbumins in a Spanish fish-allergic population.Clin Exp Allergy. 2011, v. 41, p.750-758.

[26] Müller UR. Bee venom allergy in beekeepers and their family members.Curr Opin Allergy Clin Immunol. 2005. v. 5(4), p.343-347, Por S., Karakaya G., Yurtsever N. Bee and bee products allergy in Turkish beekeepers: determination of risk factors for systemic reactions. AllergolImmunopathol. 2006. v.34, p.180-184.

[27] Jin C, Hantusch B, Hemmer W. et al. Affinity of IgE and IgGagainstcross-reactive carbohydrate determinants on plant and insect glycoproteins. J Allergy Clin Immunol. 2008, v.121, p.185-190

[28] Müller U, Schmid-Grendelmeier P, Hausmann O, Helbling A. IgE to recombinant allergens Api m 1, Ves v 1, and Ves v 5 distinguish double sensitization from crossreaction in venom allergy. Allergy. 2012 v. 67, p.1069-1073.

[29] Kryakunov KN. History of Allergy// Total Allergology. Vol. 1. Ed. Gbedema. - SPb: "Normed-Izdat", 2001.-P.19-41.

[30] Frew A.J. Mold allergy: Some progress made, more needed //J.Allergy Clin.Immunol.-2004.-Vol.113, №2.-P.216-218.

[31] Zureik M., Neukirch C., Leynaert B., et al. Sensitisation to airborne moulds and severity of asthma: cross sectional study from European Community respiratory health survey // Brit.Med.J.-2002.-Vol.325.-P.411-414.

[32] Kurup V.P., Shen H.-D., Vijay H. Immunobiology of fungal allergens // Int.Arch.Allergy Immunol.- 2002.- Vol.129.- P.181-188.

[33] Greenberger P.A. Allergic bronchopulmonary aspergillosis //J.Allergy Clin.Immunol.- 2002.-Vol.110, №5.-P.685-692.

[34] Lee S.K., Kim S.S., Nahm D.H., et al. Hypersensitivity pneumonitis caused by Fusarium napiforme in a home environment //Allergy.-2000.-Vol.55.-P.1190-1193.

[35] Faergemann J. Atopic dermatitis and fungi //Clin.Microbiol.Rev.-2002.-Vol.15, №4.-P. 545-563.

[36] Ezeamuzie C.I., Al-Ali S., Khan M., et al.IgE-mediated sensitization to mould allergens among patients with allergic respiratory diseases in a desert environment // Int.Arch.Allergy Immunol.- 2000.-Vol.121.-P.300-307.

[37] Horner W.E., Levetin E., Lehrer S.B. Basidiospore allergen release: elution from intact spores.// J. Allergy Clin. Immunol.-1993.-Vol.92, №2.-P.306-312.

[38] Frew A.J. Mold allergy: Some progress made, more needed //J.Allergy Clin.Immunol.-2004.-Vol.113, №2.-P.216-218.

[39] Horner W.E., Helbling A., Salvaggio J.E., Lehrer S.B. Fungal allergens //Microbiol.Rev.-1995.-Vol.8, №2.- P.161-179.

[40] Tomee J.F., Wierenga A.T., Hiemstra P.S., Kauffman H.K. Proteases from Aspergillus fumigatus induce release of proinflammatory cytokines and cell detachment in airway epithelial cell lines.// J. Infect. Dis. – 1997.-Vol.176, №1.-P. 300-303.

[41] Kheradmand F., Kiss A., Xu J., et al. A protease-activated pathway underlying Th cell type 2 activation and allergic lung disease.// J. Immunol.-2002.-Vol. 169.-P.5904–5911.

[42] Grote M., Vrtala S., Niederberger V., et al. Release of allergen-bearing cytoplasm from hydrated pollen: A mechanism common to a variety of grass (Poaceae) // J. Allergy Clin.Immunol.-2001.-Vol.108, №1.-P.109-115.

[43] Horner W.E., Levetin E., Lehrer S.B. Basidiospore allergen release: elution from intact spores.// J. Allergy Clin. Immunol.-1993.-Vol.92, №2.-P.306-312.

[44] Mitakakis T.Z., Barnes C., Roger E. Spore germination increases allergen release from Alternaria // J. Allergy Clin.Immunol.-2001.-Vol.107, №2.-P.388 -390.

[45] Green B.J., Mitakakis T.Z., Tovey E.R. Allergen detection from 11 fungal species before and after germination // J. Allergy Clin.Immunol.-2003.-Vol.111, №2.-P.285 -289.

[46] Terada T, Zhang K, Belperio J, Londhe V, Saxon A. A chimeric human-cat Fcgamma-Feld1 fusion protein inhibits systemic, pulmonary, and cutaneous allergic reactivity to intratracheal challenge in mice sensitized to Feld1, the major cat allergen.Clin Immunol. 2006 v.120, p. 45-56.

[47] Nilsson O.B, Binnmyr J, Zoltowska A Characterization of the dog lipocalin allergen Can f 6: the role in cross-reactivity with cat and horse. Allergy. 2012 v. 67, p.751-757.

[48] Nordlund B, Konradsen JR, Kull I IgE antibodies to animal-derived lipocalin, kallik-rein and secretoglobin are markers of bronchial inflammation in severe childhood asthma. Allergy. 2012 v. 67, p.661-669.

[49] Grönlund H, Adédoyin J, Reininger R. Higher immunoglobulin E antibody levels to recombinant Fel d 1 in cat-allergic children with asthma compared with rhinocon-junctivitis. Clin Exp Allergy. 2008 v. 38, p.1275-1281.

[50] Macías Weinmann A, Escamilla Weinmann C, Pazos Salazar NG Sensitivity to ani-mals' allergens in people working with animals. Rev Alerg Mex. 2010, v.57, p. 185-189.

[51] Vasilyeva O., KuleminaE., Kolyaskina M.. Genetic risk factors for meat wrapper's asthma // Eur. Resp. J. vol.38. suppl.55 (2011) p. 4189.

6

Risk Factors for Allergy in Secondary School Girls

Ramla Hamed Ahmed Alobaidi,
Amina Hamed Ahmed Alobaidi and
Abdulghani M. Alsamarai

1. Introduction

Ambient air is identified by the World Health Organization as a high public health priority, since air pollution associated with increase in mortality and morbidity of disease [1,2]. Respiratory disorders are the most important health problems in Iraq [3] The reported studies indicated a high prevalence rate of allergic diseases in Iraqi population.[4] In addition, respiratory infection in children represent one of the major infectious problems in Iraq [5]. The community health research that were performed by Tikrit University College of Medicine [TUCOM] have estimated that more than a fourth of Iraqi children with asthma report weekly wheeze and cough. Two-thirds of report school absences and one-third report frequent sleep disturbances due to asthma. [5]

Respiratory and asthma symptoms are public health challenges in the area of secondary school student's health and are the leading cause of school absenteeism in children, and result in missed workdays and lost productivity in adults as well [6]. The evidence strongly suggests that poor indoor air quality in schools can impact on the respiratory health of students. Children are at greater risk of the development of respiratory diseases in poor environmental conditions because their immune system is still developing [7-9].

Even though poor indoor air quality (IAQ) may have a role in exacerbation of allergic disorders [10] the socio-economic status may also have a key role in the development and progress of respiratory symptoms and asthma, especially in school students [11-13]. The influence of socio-economic status could be explained by current and past individual exposures to lifestyle and environmental factors [13].

Globally allergic diseases form a major health problem with increased incidence with time and thus are with socioeconomic impact on individuals and community [14]. Health care delivery for individuals with allergic diseases is insufficient and/or inadequate. Although, in the last decades there is progress in allergic diseases research, still there is a gap in information related to explore the underlying causes, therapies and eventual prevention [15-17]. Therefore, 'Global Allergy Forum'. participants concluded that *there are numerous unmet clinical needs and millions of patients are undertreated or not treated with the most appropriate methods.*[14]. In many countries, including Iraq, health care delivery accessibility to and affordability of effective therapeutic approaches are not provided. The development of novel effective therapies for allergic diseases is slow as compared to other medicine fields [14].

A new integrative approach is needed to understand how a complex network of immunological, genetic, and environmental factors leads to a complex allergic phenotype [15]. *There is a tremendous lack of knowledge regarding many unsolved issues, Apart from true lack of information, there is a tremendous gap between actual existing knowledge and its effective application for the millions of people in need [14].* Kirkuk, an area that characterised with high air pollution levels [18]. Since action should be taken at various levels and through existing doctors, scientists, and lay organizations to solve these problems, thus this study was performed to clarify the problem levels in the above context. Informed consent taken from all girls included in the study and the study protocol was approved by the ethical committee.

Objective: To:

Clarify the role of environmental and personal factors as risk factors for development of asthma and allergy in secondary school students.

2. Materials & methods

2.1. Site of the study

Kirkuk, an Iraqi governorate that is located North-Western to Baghdad, with 1.200 000 inhabitants. An area that is characterised by production of oil and its products. The governorate is with air pollution, which may be of health hazard in some areas of the governorate [18].

2.2. Study population

The study was carried out in two sites of Kirkuk Governorate. The first one was a secondary school in Kirkuk city center, while the others (3 schools) located in Kirkuk rural areas. A total of 594 girls included in the study, their age range from 12-22 years, with a mean age of 16.4 years. Of them, 387 (65.2%) were from urban and 207 (34.8%) were from rural areas.

2.3. Assessment of symptoms

The occurrence of symptoms and demographic characteristics was recorded by a self administered questionnaire given directly to each student. The questionnaire requested information on personal factors, health status, physical activities, environmental exposures at present and during childhood, and information on type of residence, type of ownership, house age, size of the dwelling, number of subjects living in the house, type of ventilation, type of cooling, type of heating, presence of animals in the house, presence of tree, grass, spider and wool in houses, presence of cockroach and wall painting.

2.4. Statistical methods

Chi square test was determined using SPSS (version 16) to clarify the significance of differences. Significance of differences in means were calculated by Students t test. In all statistical analyses, two tailed tests and 5% level of significance were used. The influence of different factors on the prevalence of asthma or allergy was analysed by both linear and logistic regression using SPSS statistical package. Odd ratios with 95% confidence interval were calculated from the logistic regression models.

3. Results

3.1. Asthma for whole study population

For all survey data (combined urban and rural), there was agreement between the two analysis methods in demonstrating significant association between asthma development and risk factors such as oil drinking; oil heating; fan cooling; child respiratory tract infection; child exposure to agricultural dust and work; family history of asthma; child playing; menses irregularity; depression; food allergy; heartburn; IBS; stress; house presence of wool, grass and tree; family history of atopy; and presence of water cycle within house. However, there was agreement between the two methods in relation to negative significant association between crowding index; house ownership; air condition heating; electricity heating and asthma development. Table 1

Variable	Regression		Logistic regression	
	B	P value	B	P value
Oil drinking	0.272	0.000	1.544	0.000
BMI	**0.012**	**0.015**	-0.057	0.068
Crowding index	-0.050	0.000	-0.274	0.002
House ownership	-0.297	0.000	-1.626	0.000
Oil heating	0.119	0.007	0.900	0.000
Gas heating	0.017	0.803	-0.014	0.973
Air condition heating	-0.146	0.000	-0.731	0.003
Electricity heating	-0.139	0.000	-0.483	0.037

Variable	Regression		Logistic regression	
	B	P value	B	P value
Fan cooling	0.164	0.002	1.003	0.007
Air condition cooling	**-0.085**	**0.035**	-0.418	0.067
Water cooling	-0.022	0.615	-0.141	0.555
Animal exposure	0.077	0.123	0.423	0.079
Child exposure to smoking	0.066	0.177	0.348	0.145
Child respiratory tract infection	0.186	0.000	0.988	0.000
Child exposure to cockroach	-0.022	0.566	0.061	0.766
Child residence	**0.111**	**0.023**	0.452	0.069
Child hitting	-0.062	0.157	-0.343	0.181
Child exposure agriculture dust	0.171	0.001	1.012	0.001
Child agriculture work	0.149	0.002	0.891	0.003
Child physical activity	0.055	0.139	0.283	0.145
Family history of asthma	0.169	0.003	1.160	0.003
Family history allergic rhinitis	-0.033	0.436	-0.187	0.426
Family history atopic dermatitis	0.039	0.384	0.342	0.161
Aspirin use	-0.049	0.218	**-0.627**	**0.010**
School stress	0.038	0.429	0.011	0.966
Child playing	0.204	0.000	0.65	0.000
Cold sore	**-0.309**	**0.000**	-20.571	0.996
Menses irregularities	0.187	0.000	1.107	0.000
Hirsutism	0.048	0.494	**0.930**	**0.004**
Anxiety	0.053	0.053	**0.660**	**0.004**
Depression	0.130	0.000	0.828	0.001
Psychological problem	0.312	0.000	-21.671	0.998
Social problem	0.064	0.200	0.876	0.061
Food allergy	0.758	0.000	5.396	0.000
Heart burn	0.241	0.000	2.426	0.000
Irritable	0.001	0.965	0.007	0.985
IBS	0.275	0.000	2.325	0.019
Stress	0.383	0.000	3.655	0.000
House animal	**0.138**	**0.001**	0.160	0.644
House cockroach	-0.009	0.807	-0.829	0.061

Variable	Regression		Logistic regression	
	B	P value	B	P value
House wool	0.195	0.000	1.144	0.000
House spider	0.063	0.102	**0.803**	**0.001**
House grass	0.126	0.000	0.864	0.000
House tree	0.220	0.000	1.496	0.000
Family history of atopy	0.150	0.000	0.812	0.001
Water cycle	0.201	0.000	0.871	0.000
Breast feeding	**-0.129**	**0.008**	-0.371	0.122
Illiterate father	-0.032	0.508	-0.199	0.462
Illiterate mother	-0.028	0.543	-0.058	0.816
House painting	-0.004	0.911	-0.126	0.568

Table 1. Comparison between regression and logistic regression for study population in relation to asthma.

3.2. Allergy for whole study population

For allergy development (any allergy) in study population, both models demonstrated agreement of significant positive association with risk factors such as: animal exposure; family history of allergic rhinitis and atopic dermatitis; school stress; child playing; anxiety; depression; psychological problem; irritable personality; house presence of animal, wool, spider and grass; family history of atopy and presence of water cycle within house. However, both models agreed as that allergy development was with negative significant association with BMI; crowding index; house ownership; breast feeding and mother illiteracy. Table 2

Variable	Regression		Logistic regression	
	B	P value	B	P value
Oil drinking	**0.456**	**0.000**	21.851	0.996
BMI	-0.030	0.000	-0.248	0.000
Crowding index	-0.008	0.455	**-0.151**	**0.043**
House ownership	-0.322	0.000	-2.763	0.000
Oil heating	0.042	0.382	**0.741**	**0.009**
Gas heating	**0.301**	**0.000**	21.136	0.997
Air condition heating	0.066	0.124	**0.925**	**0.001**
Electricity heating	-0.054	0.194	**-0.937**	**0.001**
Fan cooling	**0.184**	**0.001**	0.428	0.114
Air condition cooling	0.060	0.153	**0.451**	**0.047**

Variable	Regression		Logistic regression	
	B	P value	B	P value
Water cooling	0.007	0.880	-0.148	0.558
Animal exposure	0.293	0.000	1.734	0.000
Child exposure to smoking	**0.100**	**0.042**	0.414	0.190
Child respiratory tract infection	**0.330**	**0.000**	20.361	0.996
Child exposure to cockroach	**0.107**	**0.005**	0.123	0.512
Child residence	-0.039	0.415	-0.334	0.176
Child hitting	0.034	0.434	0.119	0.606
Child exposure agriculture dust	-0.047	0.370	-0.060	0.823
Child agriculture work	-0.059	0.224	-0.215	0.398
Child physical activity	-0.052	0.162	0.006	0.975
Family history of asthma	0.031	0.571	0.554	0.177
Family history allergic rhinitis	0.291	0.000	2.208	0.000
Family history atopic dermatitis	0.126	0.004	0.675	0.023
Aspirin use	**0.103**	**0.014**	0.402	0.092
School stress	0.209	0.000	1.594	0.000
Child playing	0.223	0.000	1.792	0.000
Cold sore	0.056	0.356	1.097	0.015
Menses irregularities	0.057	0.204	-0.320	0.233
Hirsutism	-0.102	0.166	-0.288	0.370
Anxiety	0.137	0.000	1.586	0.000
Depression	0.228	0.000	3.121	0.000
Psychological problem	0.220	0.002	3.176	0.000
Social problem	-0.078	0.261	0.867	0.188
Food allergy	0.268	0.000	20.296	0.995
Heart burn	**0.223**	**0.000**	19.711	0.996
Irritable	0.162	0.000	1.849	0.000
IBS	-0.073	0.367	17.829	0.998
Stress	**0.217**	**0.007**	18.841	0.998
House animal	0.121	0.002	0.576	0.036
House cockroach	**0.074**	**0.048**	0.485	0.066
House wool	0.129	0.000	0.905	0.000
House spider	0.194	0.000	1.780	0.000

Variable	Regression		Logistic regression	
	B	P value	B	P value
House tree	0.312	0.000	1.727	0.000
Family history of atopy	0.298	0.000	1.626	0.000
Water cycle	0.083	0.145	0.060	0.816
Breast feeding	**-0.151**	**0.012**	-0.297	0.264
Illiterate father	**-0.165**	**0.026**	-0.619	0.083
Illiterate mother	-0.049	0.466	-0.076	0.806
House painting	-0.066	0.278	-0.400	0.152

Table 3. Comparison between regression and logistic regression for urban population in relation to asthma.

3.4. Allergy for urban study population

The two models agreement on positive significant association was achieved between allergy development in urban population and risk factors such as: oil heating; animal exposure; child exposure to cockroach; irritable personality; presence of house grass and family history of atopy. However, agreement between the two models was achieved on significant negative association between allergy development and risk factors such as: house ownership; electricity heating; and child residence. Table 4

Variable	Regression		Logistic regression	
	B	P value	B	P value
Oil drinking	**0.323**	**0.000**	20.752	0.997
BMI	-0.010	0.105	-0.142	0.014
Crowding index	**0.054**	**0.001**	0.160	0.402
House ownership	-0.218	0.000	-2.452	0.000
Oil heating	0.192	0.000	1.265	0.000
Gas heating	**0.185**	**0.019**	18.463	0.998
Air condition heating	0.085	0.265	**0.986**	**0.006**
Electricity heating	-0.132	0.002	-1.312	0.000
Fan cooling	-0.222	0.095	-18.883	0.999
Air condition cooling	-0.084	0.302	-0.139	0.659
Water cooling	**0.111**	**0.023**	-0.506	0.167
Animal exposure	0.180	0.001	0.850	0.042
Child exposure to smoking	-0.033	0.475	-0.557	0.154

Variable	Regression		Logistic regression	
	B	P value	B	P value
Child respiratory tract infection	**0.289**	**0.000**	20.430	0.996
Child exposure to cockroach	0.139	0.000	1.0656	0.001
Child residence	-0.226	0.000	-0.851	0.005
Child hitting	**-0.073**	**0.116**	2.545	0.000
Child exposure agriculture dust	-0.055	0.495	22.336	0.997
Child agriculture work	0.074	0.442	21.654	0.998
Child physical activity	**-0.161**	**0.000**	-0.274	0.433
Family history of asthma	0.067	0.247	15.993	0.996
Family history allergic rhinitis	0.131	0.212	**1.345**	**0.003**
Family history atopic dermatitis	0.196	0.288	20.620	0.995
Aspirin use	0.025	0.577	**1.439**	**0.000**
School stress	-0.008	0.874	0.805	0.097
Child playing	**0.230**	**0.000**	19.881	0.996
Cold sore	0.093	0.236	-0.267	1.000
Menses irregularities	-0.029	0.485	-0.322	0.240
Hirsutism	**0.463**	**0.000**	19.847	0.998
Anxiety	-0.018	0.666	**1.342**	**0.002**
Depression	**0.172**	**0.000**	36.112	0.992
Psychological problem	**-0.273**	**0.000**	-19.861	0.995
Social problem	**-0.296**	**0.000**	-18.040	0.994
Food allergy	**0.193**	**0.000**	20.454	0.996
Heart burn	**0.258**	**0.000**	34.915	0.993
Irritable	0.162	0.002	2.428	0.000
IBS	0.039	0.677	17.404	0.998
Stress	0.011	0.906	-1.902	1.000
House animal	0.091	0.054	**2.067**	**0.002**
House cockroach	0.008	0.839	**-1.249**	**0.003**
House wool	0.032	0.439	-0.663	0.202
House spider	**0.243**	**0.000**	21.189	0.995
House grass	0.183	0.000	2.041	0.000
House tree	0.006	0.875	0.210	0.540
Family history of atopy	0.194	0.000	1.506	0.000

Variable	Regression		Logistic regression	
	B	P value	B	P value
Water cycle	-0.040	0.399	-0.195	0.599
Breast feeding	-0.066	0.187	**-0.931**	**0.030**
Illiterate father	-0.046	0.455	-0.285	0.517
Illiterate mother	0.003	0.964	-0.300	0.482
House painting	-0.007	0.897	0.488	0.209

Table 4. Comparison between regression and logistic regression for urban population in relation to allergy.

3.5. Asthma for rural study population

In rural population, the two models demonstrated agreement on significant negative association between asthma and risk factors such as: BMI; and crowding index. Table 123. In addition, agreement on significant association was achieved between asthma development and hirsutism. Table 5

Variable	Regression		Logistic regression	
	B	P value	B	P value
Oil drinking	-0.064	0.265	-19.440	0.998
BMI	-0.021	0.003	-0.881	0.011
Crowding index	-0.037	0.001	-1.118	0.002
Oil heating	**0.786**	**0.000**	-60.025	0.997
Gas heating	-0.143	0.107	-19.411	0.999
Air condition heating	-0.286	0.082	-38.822	0.999
Electricity heating	**-0.143**	**0.013**	-19.411	0.998
Fan cooling	**0.143**	**0.002**	19.411	0.997
Air condition cooling	0.143	0.273	19.431	0.999
Water cooling	**0.143**	**0.032**	19.411	0.998
Animal exposure	**1.154**	**0.000**	42.406	0.998
Child exposure to smoking	-0.032	0.486	-17.840	0.998
Child respiratory tract infection	**1.082**	**0.000**	-41.887	0.998
Child exposure to cockroach	**0.142**	**0.000**	-18.718	0.998
Child hitting	**0.222**	**0.000**	0.908	0.151
Child exposure agriculture dust	**0.064**	**0.033**	17.147	0.996
Child agriculture work	0.052	0.116	5.250	1.000

Variable	Regression		Logistic regression	
	B	P value	B	P value
Child physical activity	**-0.184**	**0.000**	12.134	1.000
Family history of asthma	-0.094	0.211	-1.864	1.000
Family history allergic rhinitis	-0.054	0.394	-23.981	1.000
Family history atopic dermatitis	**0.107**	**0.044**	-7.652	1.000
Aspirin use	**0.472**	**0.000**	13.042	1.000
School stress	**0.218**	**0.000**	-18.989	0.998
Child playing	-0.017	0.776	-0.163	1.000
Cold sore	**-0.248**	**0.000**	-19.438	0.998
Hirsutism	0.367	0.000	2.794	0.000
Anxiety	-0.036	0.351	54.328	0.991
Depression	**0.179**	**0.000**	-17.328	0.995
Food allergy	**0.786**	**0.000**	41.324	0.996
Heart burn	**0.250**	**0.000**	20.121	0.999
Irritable	**-0.214**	**0.000**	-20.211	0.998
IBS	**0.393**	**0.000**	-20.211	0.999
Stress	**0.250**	**0.000**	ND	
House animal	0.003	0.940	-37.041	0.997
House cockroach	-0.052	0.389	-19.617	0.996
House wool	**0.238**	**0.000**	0.368	1.000
House spider	**0.497**	**0.000**	58.734	0.994
House grass	**0.389**	**0.000**	58.715	0.995
House tree	**0.176**	**0.000**	-1.643	1.000
Family history of atopy	**0.172**	**0.000**	18.587	0.994
Breast feeding	**0.208**	**0.002**	57.968	0.995
Illiterate father	**0.280**	**0.000**	56.884	0.993
Illiterate mother	-0.078	0.097	-53.158	0.998
House painting	**0.108**	**0.001**	14.570	0.993

Table 5. Comparison between regression and logistic regression for rural population in relation to asthma.

3.6. Allergy for rural study population

Agreement on significant negative association was achieved between allergy development and BMI. However, agreement between the two models on significant association between allergy development and risk factors such as: family history of asthma; aspirin use; anxiety; presence of house wool and spider. Table 6

Variable	Regression		Logistic regression	
	B	P value	B	P value
Oil drinking	0.631	0.000	23.963	0.997
BMI	-0.051	0.000	-0.485	0.000
Crowding index	-0.039	0.029	-0.155	0.097
Oil heating	0.476	0.047	-1.598	0.085
Gas heating	0.429	0.007	21.141	0.999
Air condition heating	-0.476	0.106	-0.528	1.000
Electricity heating	0.095	0.353	0.944	0.028
Fan cooling	0.071	0.388	-0.069	0.834
Air condition cooling	-0.095	0.684	-0.944	1.000
Water cooling	0.571	0.000	21.264	0.998
Animal exposure	0.580	0.002	21.608	0.999
Child exposure to smoking	0.292	0.017	20.680	0.998
Child respiratory tract infection	-0.110	0.555	-0.592	1.000
Child exposure to cockroach	-0.009	0.915	0.065	0.857
Child hitting	0.154	0.049	0.446	0.212
Child exposure agriculture dust	0.057	0.469	-0.613	0.163
Child agriculture work	0.058	0.511	1.488	0.001
Child physical activity	0.001	0.984	0.680	0.045
Family history of asthma	0.326	0.009	1.535	0.018
Family history allergic rhinitis	0.671	0.000	38.009	0.997
Family history atopic dermatitis	-0.158	0.072	-0.066	0.905
Aspirin use	0.470	0.000	1.298	0.006
School stress	0.548	0.000	21.173	0.998
Child playing	-0.072	0.499	-19.038	0.998
Cold sore	-0.308	0.003	-0.238	0.695
Hirsutism	-0.062	0.486		
Anxiety	0.305	0.001	2.397	0.000
Depression	0.321	0.001	37.191	0.996
Food allergy	0.214	0.035	20.571	0.998
Heart burn	0.250	0.115	1.421	1.000
Irritable	0.214	0.035	20.571	0.998
IBS	-0.107	0.616	20.571	0.999

Variable	Regression		Logistic regression	
	B	P value	B	P value
Stress	0.150	0.115	1.421	1.000
House animal	-0.074	0.430	0.560	0.207
House cockroach	0.175	0.200	20.656	0.998
House wool	0.425	0.000	1.907	0.000
House spider	0.314	0.013	1.132	0.040
House grass	-0.017	0.901	-0.367	0.541
House tree	-0.064	0.355	-0.452	0.159
Family history of atopy	0.070	0.474	**0.868**	**0.021**
Breast feeding	**-0.309**	**0.037**	-20.495	0.998
Illiterate father	0.269	0.004		
Illiterate mother	**-0.269**	**0.012**	-0.267	0.424
House painting	0.045	0.552	-0.119	0.717

Table 6. Comparison between regression and logistic regression for rural population in relation to allergy

4. Discussion

Rates of asthma morbidity and mortality are increasing [4] and this increase contributed to environmental exposure. Asthma is a complex multifactorial disease in which allergic factors and non-allergic triggers interact, resulting in bronchial obstruction and inflammation [19]. Asthma is the leading chronic disease of children in industrial countries; however, the disease is also common in children in developing countries [19], and may be extended to involve adolescent. The pathogenesis and underlying causes of childhood asthma is not fully understood, however, early life environmental exposure and life style may be implicated in the etiology of asthma [20,21]. Sensitization induced by allergens is essential step for the development of asthma, however, asthma exacerbation correlated to outdoor and indoor allergens, while indoor allergens influence disease prevalence and severity [22] However, timing of such environmental exposure during early development may also be important in allergic sensitization and later asthma development [23]. Early exposure to endotoxin from farm environments has been associated with reduced childhood asthma risk [24], however, endotoxin exposure later in life may increase asthma occurrence especially in agricultural settings [25].

In the present study, influenza and common cold cause allergic disease exacerbation in 46.8% of secondary school girls. In addition, stress was the predominant (66%) factor that exacerbates allergy in secondary school girls, followed by outdoor air pollution (55.3%), animal exposure (36.2%) and house dust (34%). This finding agreed with literature that implicate viral infections, rather than bacterial infections as exacerbating factor for asthma [26,27]. However, with increasing age asthma exacerbation was mainly associated with other factors such as exercise due to decline in trigger role of respiratory infections with age in children [28].

Exposure to various constituents including tobacco smoke, wood smoke, air-born allergens, dust mites, mould, and other indoor pollutants is known or suspected to trigger wheezing or exacerbate asthma in children [27]. The level of exposure to these compounds differs in regional Iraq from the situation in developed societies, as children spend more time outdoors with increasing age. Despite the increased exposure to asthma triggers, there are few population-based data examining whether exposure to environmental factors may be associated with asthma in Iraqi adolescent.

Exposure to chemical substances and pesticides exacerbate asthma attack in 53.2% of cases with allergy. Taking these together with air pollution suggest that allergy exacerbated in all cases with these factors, indicated the importance of pollution in the control of allergic diseases. Furthermore, these findings clarify that Kirkuk governorate is an area with high pollution, which warranted application of pollution control program. There is no population based study for adolescent girls in Iraq to compare with. However, there was a population based study in children [4].

Alsamarai et al [4] found that exposure to wood, oil smoke, cats, dogs, herbicides or pesticides, and animal and farm environments were associated with an increased risk of asthma among children in Samara city, Iraq. The findings suggest that the aetiology of childhood asthma is complex and may include both early life environmental exposure and early allergic sensitization. Combustion of wood liberates nitrogen dioxide, carbon monoxide, sulfur dioxide and particulate matter, all of which have been associated with increased respiratory illness [29].

Exposure to oil smoke has been shown to significantly increase the risk of asthma [30], while particles from wood combustion significantly reduced lung function in elementary school children [31]. The present study indicated that oil heating was a significant risk factor for asthma development in adolescent girls. In contrast, both air condition and electricity heating were with negative impact on asthma development in adolescent girls. The results of this study are consistent with previous observations showing that early transient wheezing and/or increased airway reactivity in children and exposure to products of combustion may be important in the pathophysiology of asthma [20,32,33]. The girls exposure to animal exacerbate allergic diseases. However, animal exposure was not shows a significant association with asthma development for whole data and when sub divided into urban and rural community. Although, animal exposure was an important risk factors for allergy development in urban, rural and whole study population. Alsamarai et al [4] observed associations between exposure to cats and dogs and childhood asthma which are consistent with other studies [20,34-37], but contrast with other studies which found pets were protective [38,39]. Presence of cats, dogs, sheep and / or cattle with the house were with significant association with asthma development in secondary school girls in Kirkuk. A review of 32 articles suggested anon-significant increase in asthma risk of 11% was associated with the presence of pets in the first two years of life [40]. However, it is difficult to explore the association between exposure to pets and childhood asthma, even in prospective studies, because of issues of temporality and possible confounders associated with keeping pets [20].

A positive association has been reported between asthma among adults and the use of herbicides and pesticides [41,42], although data on pesticide exposure and childhood asthma are limited [20]. In the present study, exposure to either pesticides or herbicides was associated with an increased risk of asthma in adolescent girls. These results are consistent with report concerning primary school children in Iraq [4] and other geographical areas [20,43]. Several studies have suggested a reduced risk of asthma with exposure to a farming environment in early life [44]. It has been suggested that exposure to a farming environment causes higher levels of exposure to bacterial endotoxin, eventually leading to the production of several cytokines that shift the balance towards the Th1- over Th2- mediated immunity, thereby reducing asthma risk [24]. In the present study and previously reported one in Iraq [4], such an inverse association with farm exposure was not evident, as there was a significantly increased risk of asthma in adolescent girls and children with farm-related exposure. In contrast, previous studies have reported that growing up in a farming environment is associated with an increased risk of asthma and that endotoxin exposure may increase asthma risk [20]. The discrepancy between studies may be due to differences in farming practice, crops, lifestyle and other "rural" factors that differ between this Iraqi environment and that in Europe and other regions from which previous reports originated. A further difference in Iraq may be the proximity of stables to the home and time spent in stables [24]; in this population stables were mostly attached to the family home and sometimes located within the house.

The protective effect of breastfeeding on the development of asthma has raised substantial interest, but the scientific evidence relating to the effect of breastfeeding is controversial [45]. The epidemiological studies have provided controversial results showing negative association consistent with a protective effect, whereas some studies have reported either no association or a positive association between the duration of breast-feeding and the risk of asthma [46-48]. The present study indicated that breastfeeding is with a protective effect on development of asthma and allergy in secondary school girls. In contrast, breastfeeding is a risk factor for asthma development in Iraqi children [4]. Both methodological issues and the complexity of the phenomenon may be responsible for these contrasting results [49]. Differences in several factors, including; the age at which various diseases were experienced, hereditary factors as well as environmental factors may influence the association between breast-feeding and the development of asthma, thus explaining the conflicting results reported to date. The finding of the present study may differ from that reported for developed countries because of variations in the duration of breast-feeding; generally about two years in Iraq. In addition, there is the potential for incorporation of local environmental pollutants into breast milk.

The duration of breast-feeding varies substantially in the reported studies, which becomes critical when fitting the variable if the relation is non-linear as previously suggested [49]. The duration of follow up and the age of onset of asthma are also important, as if breast-feeding could delay the onset of asthma, the prevalence of current asthma would be lower among breast-fed than non-breastfed young children, but similar in later life [19]. There is evidence that hereditary asthma or atopic disease [49] and exposure to environmental factors can modify the relation between the duration of breast-feeding and the risk of asthma. [4]. The controversial results referred to above may relate to the non-linear relation between the duration of breastfeeding and the risk of asthma [49].

The finding in this study is of a significant association between food allergy and asthma in adolescent girls is consistent with that reported by others in children [50]. Similarly, the association between a family history of atopy and asthma and developing asthma, with the association higher for asthma than for atopy was consistent with findings of others [4,51,52]. These study findings strengthen earlier reports suggesting that genetics might play an important role in the development of asthma in childhood [53], with parental asthma being the strongest determinant of asthma. The current study also adds to the literature suggesting that exposure to environmental tobacco smoke increases the risk of adolescent and childhood asthma [4,53].

Reported studies suggest that home environment may act as a risk factor for triggering of asthmatic attach and/or asthma development [54-56], in addition violence may be an asthma attack risk factor [57]. The present study indicated that child hitting by their parents was a significant risk factor for asthma development in urban and rural population when analyzed separately. In addition, stress was a significant risk factor for asthma development in Kirkuk adolescent girls.

Inflammatory mediators released as an outcome of stress and subsequently potentiate allergen induced responses [57,58]. Asthma may be prevented by primary and secondary approaches, however, the physicians mostly relies on performing secondary prevention approach. Our present study indicated that the predominant exacerbating factors are stress, pollution and animal exposure, all can be controlled through a healthcare and social programs and health education.

Studies in literature indicated an association between indoor and outdoor air pollutants and the evidences of such association were variable between the studies [59-66].

The present study indicated that smoking was responsible for exacerbation of allergic diseases in 19.1% of adolescent girls. However, child exposure to tobacco smoke is not a significant risk factor for development of asthma and other allergic diseases in adolescent girls. But when the data is collected together, linear regression analyses and not logistic regression analyses, shows a significant association between tobacco smoke exposure during childhood and development of allergic diseases [any one] in adolescent girls. In a previous study reported for Iraq, family history of smoking was associated with asthma (OR=1.52, 95% CI 1.17-1.97; P=0.001) [4].

Other studies suggested the association between asthma development and exacerbation and exposure to tobacco smoke [67-86].

The Institute of Medicine concluded that cockroach allergens are causally related to asthma attacks. [63] Our present study indicated that exposure to cockroach form 12.8% as exacerbating factor of asthma in adolescent girls. In addition, cockroach exposure during childhood was with significant association to development of allergy in Kirkuk population (Linear regression), urban population (Linear and Logistic regression), and rural community (Linear regression). Furthermore, present house presence of cockroach was significant risk factor for development of allergy in Kirkuk population (Linear regression), urban community (Logistic regression), but not for rural community. This could be explained on the basis that the density of cockroach is more in urban than in rural communities. In Kirkuk urban community, present house presence of cockroach was with highly significant association with asthma development (Linear and Logistic regression) in adolescent girls.

Our present study indicated that mold was responsible for 17% as exacerbating factor for asthma in adolescent girls a finding that was consistent to that reported by others [63,66]. By using both Linear regression and Logistic regression models, asthma development in adolescent girls in Kirkuk, Iraq, was with positive association with risk factors that include: oil drinking during childhood, oil heating, fan cooling, child respiratory tract infection, child exposure to agricultural dust and work, family history of asthma, child activity, depression, food allergy, heartburn, IBS, stress, presence of house wool, presence of grass and tree within house, family history of atopy, and presence of water cycle within house. However, when the data of urban and rural communities were analyzed separately, asthma development in urban community was associated with risk factors such as child respiratory tract infections, child hitting by his parents, child exposure to agriculture dust and work, child activity, aspirin use, heart burn, house presence of animal and cockroach, family history of atopy, and ho, family history of atopy, and house presence of wool and tree. The pattern for risk factors for asthma development in adolescent girls rural community was different, indicating that there are differences in risk factors influence between urban and rural population.

Several risk factors have been identified as protective against asthma. The present study indicated an inverse association between crowding index and development of asthma in adolescent girls (Linear regression), urban population (Logistic regression), and rural population (Linear and logistic regression). The same pattern was demonstrated for allergic diseases pooled together. *Ball et al* [56] *showed that exposure of young children to older children at home or to other children in child care settings protects against the development of asthma and frequent wheezing later in childhood. They hypothesized that within the first 6 months of an infant's life, the immune response of children without atopy shifts from one associated predominantly with type 2 helper T cells, such as that in adults with atopic illnesses, toward one based more on cytokines derived from type 1 helper T cells, such as that in adults without atopy.* [56,87] This could explain the prominent association between crowding index and asthma development in rural community in our study, since early exposure of young children to old one are more common in rural community. Riedler et al [88] study suggest that early-life long time exposure to stables and farm milk induces a strong protective effect against development of asthma, hay fever, and atopic sensitization. An interesting findings of this study was that house ownership, air condition heating, child residence in rural area, electricity heating, and breast feeding were acting as protective factors for development of asthma and allergic diseases in adolescent girls living.

The present study findings and the reported studies have documented that a decrease in allergic impact of environmental exposure can be achieved by application of specific interventions and subsequently may control asthma attack. However, many children and their families, particularly children who live in poverty and rely on emergency departments as their primary source of health care, and the decline in healthcare delivery in Iraq after the American invasion, may not be receiving adequate counseling about how to avoid environmental exposures. Furthermore, performing a campaigns of educational programs for parents and individual with asthma about environmental controls may play an important role in asthma prevention, control and management [89-91].

To prevent unnecessary exposures to outdoor air pollution, clinicians may provide appropriate guidance to asthmatic subjects and their parents regarding exercise during periods of high pollution. With proper management, many environmental exposures can be decreased. [92]

Some researchers have shown links between exposure to allergens, pollutants and respiratory symptoms, while in contrast some other researchers have demonstrated that better hygiene and clean indoor environment may contribute to the increased prevalence of allergic diseases and respiratory symptoms. The present study will enhance our understanding and knowledge with regard to the two different hypotheses related to asthma and respiratory symptoms.

The study is significant for several reasons: (1)- Address the influence of different variables on prevalence of respiratory symptoms among secondary school students in Iraq. (2)- Assess the extent to which personal, environmental, socio-economic factors and indoor air pollution will affect the prevalence of respiratory symptoms in school students. (3)- Enhance our knowledge and understanding about the two contrasting theories; the hygiene theory and the theory that higher exposure to air pollutants and allergens is related to asthma and respiratory symptoms. (4)- Summarize the preventive measures to reduce exposure to air pollution and allergens in school environments located in different and also efforts in improving indoor air quality of schools thus reducing the absenteeism and respiratory symptoms in students.(5). Clarify the air pollution impact on health of Kirkuk community.

Author details

Ramla Hamed Ahmed Alobaidi[1], Amina Hamed Ahmed Alobaidi[2] and Abdulghani M. Alsamarai[3*]

*Address all correspondence to: galsamarrai@yahoo.com

1 Al Mansour Constructive Company, Kirkuk, Iraq

2 Tikrit University College of Medicine, Tikrit, Iraq

3 Tikrit Teaching Hospital, Tikrit, Iraq

References

[1] Bernstein, JA, Neil Alexis, Hyacinth Bacchus, Leonard Bernstein, Pat Fritz, Elliot Horner, Ning Li, Stephany Mason, Andre Nel, John Oullette, Kari Reijula, Tina Repo-

nen, James Seltzer, Alisa Smith, Susan M. Tarlo. The health effects of nonindustrial indoor air pollution. J Allergy Clin Immunol 2008;121:585-91.

[2] Khare M. Air pollution, monitoring, modeling and health. InTech Janeza Trdine 9, 51000 Rijeka, Croatia. 2012

[3] Alsamarai AGM, Alwan AM, Ahmad AH, Salih MA, Salih JA, Aldabagh MA, Alturaihi S, Abdulaziz ZH, Salih AA, Salih SK and Murbat MM. The relationship between asthma and allergic rhinitis in the Iraqi population. Allergology International 2009;58: 549-555.

[4] Alsamarai AGM, Salih MA, Alobaidi AHA, Alwan AM, Abdulaziz ZH. Risk factors for asthma in Iraqi children. Jour Rural Tropical Public Health 2009; 8:45-52.

[5] Alsamarai AGM. Infectious diseses fellowship program: proposed model for establishment in Iraqi Universities. Ann Iraqi Sci 2008;1:319-324.

[6] Mendell MJ, Heath GA. Do indoor pollutants and thermal conditions in schools influence student performance? A critical review of the literature. Indoor Air 2005;15:27-52.

[7] Rumchev, K., J. Spickett, et al. Association of domestic exposure to volatile organic compounds with asthma in young children. Thorax. 2004;59: 746-751

[8] Zhao Z, Zhang Z, Wang Z, Ferm M, Liang Y, Norbck D. Asthmatic symptoms among pupils in relation to winter indoor and outdoor air pollution in schools in Taiyuan, China. Environ Health Perspect 2008;116:90–97.

[9] McGwin G, Lienert J, Kennedy JR. Formaldehyde exposure and asthma in children: a systematic review. 2009. http://www.scielosp.org/pdf/csc/v16n9/a20v16n9.pdf

[10] Parker, J. Reducing asthma triggers in schools: Recommendations for Effective Policies, Regulations, and Legislation. NEW SOLUTIONS: A Journal of Environmental and Occupational Health Policy 2006;16(1): 87 - 105.

[11] Basagaña, X., J. Sunyer, Manolis Kogevinas, Jan-Paul Zock, Enric Duran-Tauleria, Deborah Jarvis, Peter Burney, and Josep Maria Anto on Behalf of the European Community Respiratory Health Survey. Socioeconomic Status and Asthma Prevalence in Young Adults. American Journal of Epidemiology 2004;160:178-188.

[12] Rona, R. J. Asthma and poverty. Thorax 2000;55: 239-244

[13] Weitzman, M., A. Sobol, et al. Racial, social, and environmental risks for childhood asthma. Am J Dis Child 1990;144(11): 1189-1194.

[14] Ring J. Davos Decleration: Allergy as a global problem. Allergy 2012;67:141143.

[15] Bousquet J, Anto J, Auffray C, Akdis M, Cambon-Thomsen A, Keil T, et al. MeDALL (Mechanisms of the Development of ALLergy): an integrated approach from phenotypes to systems medicine. Allergy 2011;66:596–604.

[16] Pawankar R, Canonica GW, Holgate ST, Lockey RF eds. World Allergy Organization (WAO) White Book on Allergy. WAO, Milwaukee, 2011; 1–216.

[17] Heinzerling L, Burbach G, van Cauwenberge P, Papageorgiou P, Carlsen KH, Lødrup Carlsen KC et al. Establishing a standardized quality management system for the European Health Network GA2LEN. Allergy 2010;65:743–752.

[18] Alsamarai AGM, et al. Development of air pollution index for Kirkuk Governorate. Ann Iraqi Sci 2008;1:231-235

[19] Busse WW, Holgate ST. Asthma and Rhinitis. 2nd ed., Vol: 1; Oxford, Blackwell Science 245-841.2003.

[20] Salam MT, Li Yu-Fen, Langholz B, Gilliland FD. Early life environmental risk factors for asthma: findings from children's health study. Environmental Health Perspective 2004;112: 760-5.

[21] Johnson CC, Ownby DR, Zoratti EM, Alford SH, Williams LK, Joseph CL. Environmental epidemiology of pediatric asthma and allergy. Epidemiology Review 2002; 24:154-75.

[22] Adkinson NF, Yunginger JW, Busse WW, Bochner BS, Holgate ST, Simon FE. Middletons Allergy: Principles and Practice. 6th ed. Vol: Two, USA, Mosby; 1175-208.2000.

[23] Melen E, Wickman M, Nordvall SL, van Hage-Hamsten M, Lindfors A. Influence of early and current environmental exposure factors on sensitization and outcome of asthma in pre-school children. Allergy 2001;56: 646-52.

[24] Braun-Fahrlander C. The role of the farm environment and animal contact for the development of asthma and allergies. Clinical Experimental Allergy 2001;31:1799-803.

[25] Schwartz DA. Does inhalation of endotoxin cause asthma? American Journal Respiratory Critical Care Medicine 2001;163: 305-6.

[26] Johnston SL. Mechanisms of asthma exacerbation. Clinical Experimental Allergy 1998;28(suppl): 181-6.

[27] Weiss ST. Environmental risk factors in childhood asthma. Clinical Experimental Allergy 1998;28(suppl): 29-34.

[28] Sarafino EP, Pterson ME, Murphy EL. Age and impacts of triggers in childhood asthma. Journal Asthma 1998;35: 213-7.

[29] Larson TV, Koenig JQ. Wood smoke: emissions and no cancer respiratory effects. Annals Review Public Health 1994;15:133-56.

[30] Chen P, Yu R, Hou X, Tan P, Xie H, Kong L, et al. Epidemiological survey on bronchial asthma in Liaoning province. ZhoghuaJie He Hu Xi ZaZhi 2002;25: 603-6.

[31] Koenig JQ, Larson TV, Hanley QS, Rebolledo V, Dumler K, Checkoway H, et al. Pulmonary function changes in children associated with fine particulate matter. Environmental Research 1993;63: 26-38.

[32] Belanger K, Beckett W, Triche E, Bracken MB, Holford T, Ren P, et al. Symptoms of wheeze and persistent cough in the first year of life: associations with indoor allergens, air contaminants, and maternal history of asthma. American Journal of Epidemiology 2003;158: 195-202.

[33] Sotir M, Yeatts K, Shy C. Presence of asthma risk factors and environmental exposures related to upper respiratory infection- triggered wheezing in middle school age children. Environmental Health Perspectives 2003;111:657-62.

[34] Nafstad P, Magnus P, Gaarder Pl, Jaakkola JJ. Exposure to pets and atopy-related diseases in the first 4 years of life. Allergy 2001;56: 307-12.

[35] Ronmark E, Perzanowski M, Platts-Mills T, lundback B. Incidence rates and risk factors for asthma among schoolchildren: a 2-years follow-up report from the obstructive lung diseases in Northern Sweden (OLIN) studies. Respiratory Medicine 2002;96: 1006-13.

[36] McConnell R, Berhane K, Gilliland F, Islam T, Gauderman WJ, London SJ, et al. Indoor risk factors for asthma in a prospective study of adolescents. Epidemiology 2002;13: 288-95.

[37] Zheng T, Niu S, Lu B, Fan X, Sun F, Wang J, et al. Childhood asthma in Beijing, China: a population-based case-control study. American Journal Epidemiology 2002;156: 977-83.

[38] Hesselmar B, Aberg N, Aberg B, Eriksson B, Bjorksten B. Does early exposure to cat or dog protect against later allergy development? Clinical Experimental Allergy 1999;29: 611-7.

[39] Remes ST, Castro-Rodriguez JA, Holberg CJ, Martinez FD, Wright AL. Dog exposure in infancy decreases the subsequent risk of frequent wheeze but not of atopy. Journal of Allergy Clinical Immunology 2001;108: 509-15.

[40] Apelberg BJ, Aoki Y, Jaakkola JJ. Systematic review: exposure to pets and risk of asthma and asthmalike symptoms. Journal of Allergy and Clinical Immunology 2001;107:455-60.

[41] . Bener A, Lestringant GG, Beshwari MM, Pasha MA. Respiratory symptoms, skin disorders and serum IgE levels in farm workers. Allergy Immunology (Paris) 2001;31: 52-6.

[42] Hoppin JA, Umbach DM, London SJ, Alavanja MC, Sandler DP. Chemicals predictors of wheeze among farmer pesticide applicators in the Agricultural Health Study. American Journal Respiratory Critical Care Medicine 2002;165: 683-9.

[43] Karmaus W, Kuehr J, Kruse H. Infections and atopic disorders in childhood and organochlorine exposure. Archives of Environmental Health 2001;56: 485-92.

[44] Von Ehrenstein OS, Von Mutius E, Illi S, Baunmann L, Bohm O, Von Kries R. Reduced risk of hay fever and asthma among children of farmers. Clinical Experimental Allergy 2000;30: 187-93.

[45] Friedman NJ. Zeiger RS. The role of breastfeeding in development of allergies and asthma. Journal of Allergy Clinical Immunology 2005;115: 1238-48.

[46] Chulada PC, Arbes SJ, Dunson D, Zeldin DC. Breastfeeding and the prevalence of asthma and wheezing in children: analysis from the third national health and nutrition examination survey, 1988-1994. Journal of Allergy Clinical Immunology 2003;111: 328-36.

[47] Nafstad P, Jaakola JJK. Breast feeding, passive smoking and asthma and wheeze in children. Journal of Allergy Clinical Immunology 2003;112: 807-8.

[48] Oddy WH, Sherriff JL, DE Klerk NH, et al.The relation of breastfeeding and body mass index to asthma and atopy in children: a prospective cohort study to age 6 years. American Journal of Public Health 2004; 94: 1531-7.

[49] Fredriksson P, Jaakola N, Jaakola JJK. Breastfeeding and childhood asthma: a six year population based cohort study. B M C Pediatrics 2007; 7:39-46.

[50] Simpson AB, Glutting J, Yousef E. Food allergy and asthma morbidity in children. Pediatric Pulmonology 2007;42: 489-95.

[51] Bjerg A, Hedman L, Perzanowski MS, Platt-Mills T, Lundback B, Ronmark E. Family history of asthma and atopy: in depth analyses of the impact on asthma and wheeze in 7 to 8 year old children. Pediatrics 2007;120:741-8.

[52] Palvo F, Toledo EC, Menin AMCR, Jorge PPO, Godoy MF, Sole D. Risk factors of childhood asthma in Sao Jose do Rio Preto, Sao Paulo, Brazil. Journal Tropical Pediatrics 2008;54: 253-7.

[53] Jaakola JJK, Nfstad P, Magnus P. Environmental tobacco smoke, parental atopy and childhood asthma. Environmental Health Perspective2001; 109: 579-82.

[54] Cullinan P, Taylor AJ. Asthma in children: environmental factors. BMJ. 1994;308:1585–1586

[55] Holt PG, Macaubas C, Stumbles PA, Sly PD. The role of allergy in the development of asthma. Nature. 1999;42(6760 suppl):B12–B17

[56] Ball TM, Castro-Rodriguez JA, Griffith KA, Holberg CJ, Martinez FD, Wright AL. Siblings, day-care attendance, and the risk of asthma and wheezing during childhood. N Engl J Med. 2000;343:538–543

[57] Wright RJ, Steinbach SF. Violence: an unrecognized environmental exposure that may contribute to greater asthma morbidity in high risk inner-city populations. Environ Health Perspect. 2001;109:1085–1089

[58] Wright RJ, Rodriguez M, Cohen S. Review of psychosocial stress and asthma: an integrated biopsychosocial approach. Thorax. 1998;53:1066–1074

[59] Figley KD, Elrod RH. Endemic asthma due to castor bean dust. JAMA. 1928;90:79–82

[60] Sunyer J, Anto JM, Rodrigo MJ, Morrell F. Case-control study of serum immunoglobulin-E antibodies reactive with soybean in epidemic asthma. Lancet. 1989;1:179–182

[61] Anto JM, Sunyer J, Rodriguez-Roisin R, Suarez-Cervera M, Vazquez L. Community outbreaks of asthma associated with inhalation of soybean dust. N Engl J Med. 1989;320:1097–1102

[62] Anto JM, Sunyer J, Reed CE, et al. Preventing asthma epidemics due to soybeans by dust-control measures. N Engl J Med. 1993;329:1760–1763

[63] Institute of Medicine, Committee on the Assessment of Asthma and Indoor Air. Clearing the Air: Asthma and Indoor Air Exposures. Washington, DC: National Academy Press; 2000

[64] Etzel RA. Indoor air pollution and childhood asthma: effective environmental interventions. Environ Health Perspect. 1995;103(suppl 6): 55–58

[65] Platts-Mills TA. Allergen-specific treatment for asthma: III. Am Rev Respir Dis. 1993;148:553–555

[66] Pope AM, Patterson R, Burge H, et al, eds. Indoor Allergens: Assessing and Controlling Adverse Health Effects. Institute of Medicine, Committee on the Health Effects of Indoor Allergens. Washington, DC: National Academy Press; 1993

[67] Matthews TJ. Smoking during pregnancy in the 1990s. Natl Vital Stat Rep. 2001;49:1–14

[68] Tager IB, Hanrahan JP, Tosteson TD, et al. Lung function, pre- and post-natal smoke exposure, and wheezing in the first year of life. Am Rev Respir Dis. 1993;147:811–817

[69] Pirkle JL, Flegal KM, Bernert JT, Brady DJ, Etzel RA, Maurer KR. Exposure of the U.S. population to environmental tobacco smoke: the Third National Health and Nutrition Examination Survey, 1988–1991. JAMA. 1996;275:1233–1240

[70] American Academy of Pediatrics, Committee on Environmental Hazards. Involuntary smoking—a hazard to children. Pediatrics. 1986;77: 755–757

[71] Murray AB, Morrison BJ. The effect of cigarette smoke from the mother on bronchial responsiveness and severity of symptoms in children with asthma. J Allergy Clin Immunol. 1986;77:575–581

[72] Evans D, Levison J, Feldman CH, et al. The impact of passive smoking on emergency room visits of urban children with asthma. Am Rev Respir Dis. 1987;135:567–572

[73] Burchfiel CM, Higgins MW, Keller JB, Howatt WF, Butler WJ, Higgins IT. Passive smoking in childhood: respiratory conditions and pulmonary function in Tecumseh, Michigan. Am Rev Respir Dis. 1986;133:966–973

[74] Chilmonczyk BA, Salmun LM, Megathlin KN, et al. Association between exposure to environmental tobacco smoke and exacerbations of asthma in children. N Engl J Med. 1993;328:1665–1669

[75] Ehrlich R, Kattan M, Godbold J, et al. Childhood asthma and passive smoking. Urinary cotinine as a biomarker of exposure. Am Rev Respir Dis. 1992;145:594–599

[76] Holberg CJ, Wright AL, Martinez FD, Morgan WJ, Taussig LM. Child day care, smoking by caregivers, and lower respiratory tract illness in the first 3 years of life. Group Health Medical Associates. Pediatrics. 1993;91:885–892

[77] Krzyzanowski M, Quackenboss JJ, Lebowitz MD. Chronic respiratory effects of indoor formaldehyde exposure. Environ Res. 1990;52:117–125

[78] Martinez FD, Cline M, Burrows B. Increased incidence of asthma in children of smoking mothers. Pediatrics. 1992;89:21–26

[79] Murray AB, Morrison BJ. Passive smoking by asthmatics: its greater effect on boys than girls and on older than on younger children. Pediatrics. 1989;84:451–459

[80] O'Connor GT, Weiss ST, Tager IB, Speizer FE. The effect of passive smoking on pulmonary function and nonspecific bronchial responsiveness in a population-based sample of children and young adults. Am Rev Respir Dis. 1987;135:800–804

[81] Oldigs M, Jorres R, Magnussen H. Acute effects of passive smoking on lung function and airway responsiveness in asthmatic children. Pediatr Pulmonol. 1991;10:123–131

[82] Rylander E, Pershagen G, Eriksson M, Bermann G. Parental smoking, urinary cotinine, and wheezing bronchitis in children. Epidemiology.1995;6:289–293

[83] Sherman CB, Tosteson TD, Tager IB, Speizer FE, Weiss ST. Early childhood predictors of asthma. Am J Epidemiol. 1990;132:83–95

[84] Weitzman M, Gortmaker S, Walker DK, Sobol A. Maternal smoking and childhood asthma. Pediatrics. 1990;85:505–511

[85] Murray AB, Morrison BJ. The decrease in severity of asthma in children of parents who smoke since the parents have been exposing them to less cigarette smoke. J Allergy Clin Immunol. 1993;91:102–110

[86] Centers for Disease Control and Prevention. Strategies for reducing exposure to environmental tobacco smoke, increasing tobacco-use cessation, and reducing initiation

in communities and health-care systems.MMWR Morb Mortal Wkly Rep. 2000;49(RR-12):1

[87] Prescott SL, Macaubas C, Smallcombe T, Holt BJ, Sly PD, Holt PG. Development of allergen-specific T-cell memory in atopic and normal children. Lancet. 1999;353:196–200

[88] Riedler J, Braun-Fahrlander C, Eder W, et al. Exposure to farming in early life and development of asthma and allergy: a cross-sectional survey. Lancet. 2001;358:1129–1133

[89] Jones AP. Asthma and the home environment. J Asthma. 2000;37:103–124

[90] Environmental controls and lung disease. Report of the ATS Workshop on Environmental Controls and Lung Disease. Santa Fe, New Mexico, March 24–25, 1988. Am Rev Respir Dis. 1990;142:915–939

[91] Ingram JM, Heymann PW. Environmental controls in the management of asthma. Immunol Allergy Clin North Am. 1993;13:785–801

[92] Etzel RA. Environmental Exposures Influence the Development and Exacerbation of Asthma. Pediatrics 2003;112:233–239.

7

A Disintegrin and Metalloproteinase (ADAM) 10 and 17 in Th2 Mediated Responses

Lauren Folgosa Cooley, Rebecca K. Martin and
Daniel H. Conrad

1. Introduction

Asthma is a chronic airway disease characterized by wheezing, cough, shortness of breath, chest tightness, and "asthma attacks" caused by obstruction in airflow. In the United States, prevalence has increased since 2001 with children and African Americans having the highest incidence [1]. Asthma-related medical costs are \$3,300 per diagnosed individual including missed school and work days and asthma-related deaths totaled 3,404 in 2010 [2;3]. Worldwide, 300 million people are diagnosed with asthma and 70% of those suffer from other allergies as well [4]. Helminth infection, however, is considered a disease of developing countries and is rarely concomitant with allergies [5]. The World Health Organization estimates that 1.5 billion people, or 24% of the world's population, is infected by soil transmitted helminthes, with the majority of cases occurring in east Asia, China, and Sub-Saharan Africa [6]. Allergy, asthma, and helminth infection are considered classic Th2 diseases with immunoglobulin E (IgE) as the predominant antibody class coordinating the response. IgE levels are tightly regulated, being the antibody with the lowest levels *in vivo* [7]. Interestingly, very small amounts of antigen are detected by IgE, making it a "gatekeeper", as it is first to detect foreign particles in areas of interface with the environment. When these foreign particles are innocuous, such as pollen, cat dander or peanut proteins, IgE moves from beneficial to potentially life threatening. IgE mediates allergic responses from mild reactions to severe, such as allergic rhinitis, atopic dermatitis, urticaria, asthma, and anaphylactic shock [8].

IgE regulates the immune response in one of three ways. First, antigen specific IgE binds the high affinity IgE receptor, FcεRI, on mast cells (MCs) or basophils where it can persist for up to 21 days waiting to bind to antigen, cross-link the FcεRI and degranulate the cell [9]. Degranulation results in release of vasoactive mediators such as histamine, leukotrienes, prostaglandins, and other biologically active products, inducing the classic symptoms of allergic diseases (e.g. wheal and flare or urticaria) depending upon the location of the reaction, while additionally activating the MC or basophil to induce late stage cytokine production [8]. Second, circulating IgE can bind to its antigen creating an IgE-immune complex. IgE immune complexes are picked up by circulating follicular (FO) B cells by binding to CD23, the low affinity IgE receptor (FcεRII). These CD23+B cells then traffic to the splenic follicles where antigen transfer occurs followed by rapid increases in antigen-specific CD4+T cell proliferation and IgG responses [10]. Third, circulating IgE can bind to CD23 on B cells, inducing a negative regulatory response to shut down and control excessive IgE synthesis [11].

Enzymatic regulation of CD23 and downstream IgE synthesis was initially how a disintegrin and metalloproteinase (ADAM) 10 (ADAM10) became an important topic in Th2 mediated disease responses [12]. ADAMs are a family of zinc dependent proteases involved in ectodomain cleavage of transmembrane proteins and regulated intramembrane proteolysis. Of all the ADAMs, ADAM10 and ADAM17, also known as tumor necrosis factor alpha (TNF) converting enzyme (TACE), are most closely related with regards to structure and share many overlapping substrates [13;14]. Structurally, they contain a zinc dependent metalloproteinase domain, disintegrin and cysteine rich ligand binding domain, transmembrane domain, and cytoplasmic domain [15]. ADAM10 is widely expressed in many cells types and is a highly investigated target in disease processes ranging from cancer and Alzheimer's disease to asthma [15]. Since its discovery, many ADAM10 substrates have been identified including CD23, Notch1, TNF, amyloid precursor protein (APP) and epidermal growth factor (EGF), further supporting its ability to participate in an array of pathologic processes [16]. ADAM10 has been of much interest in allergic and other Th2 mediated diseases as it is the principle sheddase of the low affinity IgE receptor, CD23. Through an unknown mechanism, soluble CD23 (sCD23) negatively regulates IgE production, meaning increased ADAM10 and thus sCD23 production leads to enhanced IgE production [12;17]. Furthermore, increased sCD23 is seen in sera of allergic patients in active allergy season, which corresponds with increased circulating IgE [18]. Increased cleavage of CD23 leaves less membrane bound CD23 (mCD23) to negatively regulate IgE production as well as increased sCD23 to interact with other pro-inflammatory receptors such as CD11b-CD18 on monocytes [19;20]. Therefore, blocking cleavage of CD23 could be an important target in regulating IgE synthesis and thus the first step in the allergic cascade.

ADAM17, the principal protease of membrane TNF (mTNF), epidermal growth factor receptor (EGFR) ligands, and other vasoactive mediators, has been classically studied in inflammatory syndromes and cancer, with less emphasis on its role in allergy [14]. While ADAM17 is the principle sheddase of mTNF, ADAM10 can cleave TNF albeit to a lesser extent [21]. Dysregulation of TNF is critical for the pathologic characteristics underlying many disease states including cancer, type 2 diabetes, and rheumatoid arthritis [22]. Furthermore, increased TNF production is a key factor implicated in B cell aging, which ultimately curtails class-switched antibody production [23]. B cell TNF is, further, required for maintaining proper secondary lymphoid tissue architecture and antibody production and in its absence severe defects are seen [24;25]. ADAM17 is potentially a new target for diagnostic and/or therapeutic intervention in Th2 mediated diseases, as it and TNF are reduced in B cells of allergic patients [23;26;27].

Herein, the role of ADAM10 and ADAM17 in B cell responses, maintenance of secondary lymphoid tissue architecture, and Th2 mediated diseases, such as allergic rhinitis, asthma, and helminth infection is explored.

2. ADAM10 in B cell development and function

Through their cleaved substrates, members of the ADAM family regulate a wide range of functions, including cell migration, proliferation, and adhesion [28]. With regards to B cell development and function, ADAM10 and ADAM17 have both been extensively studied with respect to lymphocyte development through initiation of the canonical Notch signaling pathway, germinal center responses, and plasma cell function [17;23;26;29;30]. Four Notch receptors exist in humans and rodents, which can interact with five different ligands [31]. Upon ligand-receptor interaction, ADAM10 initiates S2 cleavage followed by S3 cleavage by y secretase, effectively releasing the Notch intracellular domain (NICD), which translocates to the nucleus leading to altered gene expression [32;33]. The role of ADAM10 in Notch signaling has been extensively studied as ADAM10 deficient embryos are similar to those of Notch 1-4 deficient embryos [34] and Notch 1 signaling is impaired in ADAM10 deficient thymocytes [30]. Furthermore, ADAM10 but not ADAM17 is required for Notch 1 rate-limiting, S2 cleavage, which has important implications in novel approaches to targeting Notch 1 signaling in cancer [35]. B lymphocytes, however, preferentially express Notch 2 [32] and Notch 2 signaling is noted in pre, pro, immature, follicular and marginal zone (MZ) B cells. MZBs are unique B cells, which behave in a T independent manner and are critical for early antibody production against blood borne pathogens [36]. Interestingly, their development is dependent on ADAM10 as it is critical for initiation of Notch 2 signaling [17]. B cell ADAM10, furthermore, has been shown to be critical for antibody production by follicular B2 cells. While the role of ADAM10 in IgE production is discussed below, *Chaimowitz et al.* described that in the absence of B cell ADAM10, germinal center formation is impaired and antigen specific IgM and IgG1 production is reduced 14 days post immunization with NP-KLH, a T dependent antigen [29]. These mice, additionally, lack a normal number of antigen specific plasma cells and remaining plasma cells are abnormal in function. Specifically, Bcl6, a transcriptional repressor, which must be downregulated during plasma cell differentiation, was increased in plasma cells from which ADAM10 is deleted after class switching to IgG1 [37].

3. ADAM10 and ADAM17 in germinal center formation and secondary lymphoid tissue architecture

TNF and its closely related family members have been extensively studied in the development and maintenance of secondary lymphoid tissue architecture. Because ADAM10 and ADAM17 are closely related ADAMs, many questions have been raised about their functional redundancy under physiologic as well as in various genetically manipulated animal models. While ADAM17 is the principle sheddase of TNF, ADAM10 is known to cleave TNF, especially in the absence of ADAM17 [38]. In addition to TNF, *Le Gall et al.* described that in the absence of ADAM17, ADAM10 cleaves epidermal growth factor receptor (EGFR) ligands, which are classically considered ADAM17 substrates. However, under physiologic conditions, ADAM17 dominates as the principal sheddase [38]. *Mezyk-Kopec et al.* further demonstrated that in ADAM17 deficient mouse embryonic fibroblasts, ADAM10 increases and ADAM10 dependent cleavage of TNF is seen [39]. *Folgosa et al.* described a compensatory relationship between ADAM10 and ADAM17 in B cells. In C57Bl/6 B cell specific ADAM10 deficient mice, B cell ADAM17 expression and activity increased resulting in excessive cleavage of TNF [26]. Excessive B cell TNF production has been implicated in B cell aging and reduced antibody production, which may help to explain the reduction in antibody production by B cell specific ADAM10 deficient mice [23]. Furthermore, the direct contribution of *B cell* TNF to maintenance of secondary lymphoid tissue architecture has been widely studied. Specifically, failure to produce B cell sTNF, as seen in mutated B cells with an un-cleavable form of mTNF, and excessive B cell sTNF production, as in ADAM10 deficient B cells, both result in dramatic alterations in secondary lymphoid tissue architecture [25;26]. Both aberrant B cell TNF conditions result in abnormal B cell/T cell localization with loss of a proper cortico-medullary junction, reduced germinal center formation, and impaired follicular dendritic cell (FDC) network development. Furthermore, naïve and draining lymph nodes (post-immunization) of B cell ADAM10 deficient mice, which exhibit excessive B cell TNF production, have increased angiogenesis and collagen deposition [26]. Therefore, secondary lymphoid architecture is highly sensitive to B cell TNF levels, which is maintained by a proper ratio of ADAM10 to ADAM17 expression and function. Interestingly, however, these differences are not noted in ADAM10$^{B-/-}$mice on a Th2-biased background, Balb/c [27]. Th2 prone strains were shown to have enhanced ADAM10 but reduced ADAM17 and TNF relative to Th1 prone strains and are less adept at increasing ADAM17 expression in the absence of B cell ADAM10 [27]. These findings suggest that the B cell and its ADAM10/ADAM17 profile plays a role in the classic Th1/Th2 paradigm rendering the B cell more than a passive participant waiting for a T cell signal.

4. ADAM10 and ADAM17 in murine and human allergic airway disease

4.1. ADAM10 is the principle sheddase of CD23

CD23 is a unique Fc receptor as it is a type 2 transmembrane protein and a member of the calcium dependent (C type) lectin family. It exists in two isoforms, CD23a and CD23b, and has three domains: (1) IgE interacting carboxy terminal domain, (2) stalk regions, and (3) a short cytoplasmic tail [11]. Surface CD23 levels can be increased in an IL-4 or IL-13 dependent manner [11]. In humans, peripheral blood mononuclear cells stimulated with IL-4 exhibit increased CD23 shedding and IgE production whereas treatment with anti-CD23, which prevents its cleavage, inhibits IgE production [40]. Several enzymes have been implicated in the cleavage of CD23 including ADAM8 [41] and other hydroxymate sensitive metalloproteinases [42], but ADAM10 was determined by *Weskamp et al.* in a series of loss and gain of ADAM protease function experiments to be the principle sheddase of CD23 in B cells [12]. Once cleaved from the surface, sCD23 negatively regulates IgE production by an unknown mechanism. Several models exist that attempt to explain this relationship including: (1) High levels of IgE stabilize mCD23 and reduce further IgE production while allergen proteases and anti-CD23 stalk monoclonal antibodies destabilize CD23, increase its proteolysis, and increase IgE production [11]; and, (2) sCD23 crosslinks membrane IgE and CD21 resulting in increased IgE production [43]. This relationship between ADAM10, CD23, and IgE has since ignited much interest in the asthma and allergy fields regarding the use of ADAM10 or CD23 cleavage inhibitors as a mechanism to prevent IgE synthesis.

4.2. ADAM10, ADAM17, and their substrates in murine and human airway hypersensitivity

Mouse models of airway hypersensitivity are classically used to model asthma in humans. The role of ADAM10 and ADAM17 and their substrates has been widely studied in lung inflammation models used to simulate upper and lower airway disease. First, as described herein, ADAM10 is critical in the regulation of IgE production through its substrate, CD23. Transgenic mice overexpressing CD23 (CD23Tg) had been shown previously to have reduced IgE and lung inflammation [44;45]. In a OVA-induced lung inflammation model, *Mathews et al.*, using C57Bl/6 CD23Tg and B cell specific ADAM10 deficient (ADAM10$^{B-/-}$) mice, demonstrated that when mCD23 is increased, symptoms and features of IgE-dependent experimental asthma are reduced (17). Specifically, airway cellular infiltration, eosinophilia, airway resistance, and OVA-specific IgE production were reduced in mice lacking B cell-ADAM10 [46]. Furthermore, treatment with an ADAM10 inhibitor decreased antigen-specific IgE, Th2 cytokines in the lung, AHR, lung inflammation, and infiltration of eosinophils. Additionally, ADAM10 inhibitor therapy resulted in reduction of the Th2 transcription factor, GATA3, expression but had no effect on Th1 transcription factor, Tbet [46]. Interestingly, recent evidence has shown that ADAM10 and ADAM17 regulation in B cells is highly strain dependent. Classic Th1 (including C57Bl/6, SJL/J) and Th2-prone strains (including Balb/c, A/J) strains were characterized as high (SJL/J), intermediate (C57Bl/6), and low (Balb/c, A/J) IgE responders based on *in vivo* IgE production post immunization [47]. Furthermore, B cells from Th2 prone mouse strains (Balb/c, A/J), which are more susceptible to allergic airway disease induction and exhibit increased IgE synthesis have increased ADAM10 and reduced ADAM17 and TNF compared to those from Th1 prone mouse strains (C57Bl/6, SJL/J). In a house-dust mite (HDM) airway hypersensitivity model, Balb/c WT, which exhibit increased B cell ADAM10, experience more severe disease induction than C57Bl/6 WT including HDM specific IgE production, goblet cell metaplasia, mucus production, and airway cellular infiltration. Furthermore, Balb/c B cell specific ADAM10 deficient mice fail to reduce antigen specific IgE, cellular infiltration, mucus production, or goblet cell metaplasia to the extent of C57Bl/6 B cell specific ADAM10 deficient mice [27]. This evidence is further substantiated by B cell ADAM10, ADAM17, and TNF differences in Th2 prone allergic patients compared to non-allergic controls (Th1-prone). In human patients with allergic disease or asthma, increased circulating IgE is a diagnostic criteria, and has been correlated with increased circulating sCD23[18], implicating ADAM10 in the disease cascade. Recent evidence has shown that patients with actively symptomatic allergic rhinitis exhibit increased B cell ADAM10 supporting these findings. Furthermore, allergic patient B cells were described as having reduced ADAM17 and TNF, suggesting that these are protective against an allergic phenotype [27]. However, there is also evidence suggesting TNF inhibition would be beneficial in reducing asthma symptoms and disease manifestations. TNF can amplify inflammation by recruiting neutrophils, eosinophils, and monocytes as well as aiding in T cell activation. Furthermore, TNF can enhance airway remodeling by causing fibroblast proliferation and also contributes to enhanced airway resistance [48]. Therefore, while reduced B cell TNF may be more indicative of Th2-prone B cells, TNF produced by other cells can cause detrimental airway symptoms. Overall, Figure 1 demonstrates the novel model synthesizing evidence for ADAM10 and ADAM17 regulation in B cells from Th1 and Th2 prone mouse strains and humans. Th2 prone mouse strains and humans exhibit reduced ADAM10 and increased ADAM17 relative to Th1 counterparts resulting in increased sCD23 and IgE and decreased TNF and cell proliferation, as suggested by *Folgosa Cooley et al.* [27] and *Frasca et al.*[23;49]

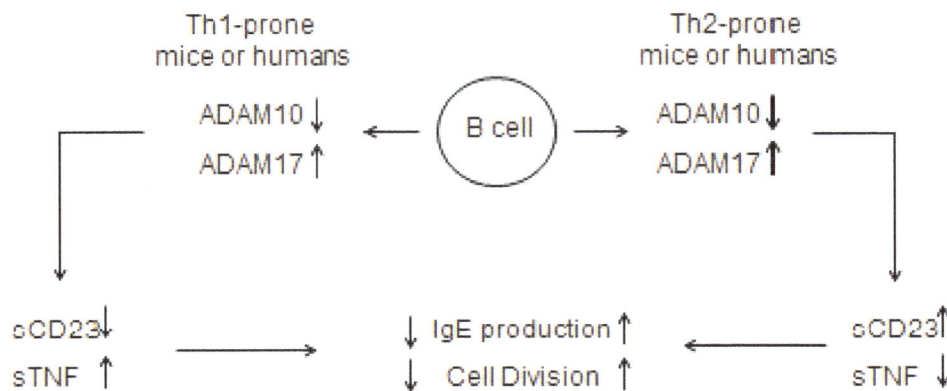

Figure 1. Novel model for regulation of ADAM10 and ADAM17 in B cells of Th1-prone compared to Th2-prone mice or humans.

Lastly, while glutamate is classically known for its role as an excitatory neurotransmitter, glutamate receptors have been found on T cells [50], macrophages [51], and human B cells [52]. The kainate receptor is a multi-subunit, ionotropic glutamate receptor. *Sturgill et al.* was first to describe the presence of the kainate receptor on B cells and demonstrated that kainate receptor activation increases ADAM10 expression, CD23 cleavage, and B cell proliferation [52]. Therefore, localized kainite receptor inhibition could be a unique approach to treating allergic airway disease as it could reduce CD23 cleavage, rounds of B cell proliferation, and thus IgE synthesis. Overall, there is substantial evidence advocating for the therapeutic benefit of ADAM10 or CD23 cleavage inhibitors in the treatment of allergic airway disease.

In addition to B cells, neutrophils or leukocytes and their respective ADAM10 and ADAM17 levels have also been described in lung inflammation models. Neutrophils recruitment occurs early during inflammation and their mediators affect the activity and recruitment of many other immune cells. The number of neutrophils in sputum was seen to be elevated in patients with both acute and chronic asthma and especially those with lower eosinophil numbers and those unresponsive to corticosteroid treatment [53-55]. Both ADAM10 and ADAM17, with some conflicting reports, have been described to be important for leukocyte migration to the airway in lung inflammation models. In leukocyte specific ADAM17 deficient mice, *Arndt et al.* described a decrease in alveolar leukocyte recruitment following aerosolized LPS induction of acute airway inflammation. Furthermore, there was reduction in alveolar levels of CXCL1 and CXCL5, both neutrophil chemokines [56]. *Pruessmeyer et al.*, however, in leukocytes isolated from either hematopoietic cell specific ADAM10 or ADAM17 deficient mice showed that ADAM10 and not ADAM17 is required for leukocyte migration to the alveoli following LPS induced acute lung inflammation [57]. Therefore, ADAM10 inhibition could lead to reduced neutrophil infiltration.

Epidermal growth factor receptor (EGFR) signaling is reported to be integral in tissue repair, airway remodeling in asthma, and MUC5AC mucin production in lung inflammation models [58-60]. ADAM17 is responsible for the processing of epidermal growth factor receptor ligands including transforming growth factor alpha (TGFα) [14]. In normal human bronchial epithelial (NHBE) cells, *Booth et al.* demonstrated that ADAM17 induced TGFα cleavage as well as IL13 mediated proliferation. Furthermore, IL13, a key Th2 cytokine, was noted to redistribute TGFα to apical regions of NHBE for ADAM17 cleavage resulting in epithelial hypertrophy [61]. Therefore, further exploration of the IL13/ADAM17/TGFα axis is integral in better understanding methods to curb airway remodeling in chronic asthma. *Shiomi et al.* additionally described the importance of the ADAM17 on compressive stress to airway epithelial cells or bronchoconstriction, which is mediated through ERK and AKT phosphorylation. In this study, conditional deletion of ADAM17 from murine tracheal epithelial cells reduced ERK and AKT phosphorylation and thus attenuated compressive stress gene regulation [62]. Furthermore, ADAM17 is known to regulate transforming growth factor beta (TGFβ) through cleavage of vasorin, a TGFβ trap. Therefore, when ADAM17 is inhibited, less vasorin is cleaved, and TGFβ signaling is increased [63]. In asthma patients, TGFβ1 is increased in bronchoalveolar lavage samples as well as in lung biopsy samples. Furthermore, TGFβ1 was found predominately in inflammatory cells beneath the basement membrane in bronchial biopsy samples and may be important for collagen deposition and thus airway remodeling [64]. Taken together, this evidence suggests that reduced ADAM17 levels as seen in human patients' B cells (discussed above) could lend to increased TGFβ1 and thus enhanced asthma symptoms compared to control patients, who exhibited higher ADAM17 levels.

5. ADAM10, CD23 and MDSCs in helminth infection

In industrialized countries, incidence of helminth infection is greatly reduced and when observed it is commonly associated with a reduced parasite burden [65]. Worldwide, over one billion individuals are heavily infected with helminth and are rarely affected by allergic disease [5], a correlation demonstrated by many epidemiological studies [65;66]. Allergic diseases share many factors with helminth infections, including a similar cytokine milieu (e.g. IL-13, IL-4, IL-5) and most importantly up-regulation of IgE [65;66]. These factors contribute to the symptomology of allergic disease, yet in helminth infected individuals, are protective [65;66]. This is despite helminth being the strongest natural promoter of IgE synthesis [67]. It is well established that parasite-specific IgE is important for anti-helminth immunity, but helminthes are also known to elicit large amounts of polyclonal or non-specific IgE in the sera of infected individuals. This finding has been thought to be a protective response by the parasite [67]. Helminth evolution has selected for this trait that benefits parasite life and reproduction, assisting the helminth in immune evasion [67].

In both allergy and helminth infection, IgE responses have been associated with CD23 expression and thus ADAM10 enzymatic activity [68-70]. The product, sCD23, has been a diagnostic indicator in many different diseases [69;71]. In an epidemiological study of individuals infected with the helminth *Schistosoma haematobium*, increased sCD23 levels correlated with infection intensity, but were inversely correlated with helminth-specific IgE [69]. Though ADAM10 activity was not measured in this study, increased ADAM10 mediated CD23 cleavage during helminth infection may be inducing this correlation.

Mast cells (MCs), which are important in mediating response to helminth infection, have been shown to express ADAM10 [72]. ADAM10 deletion results in reduced proliferation and migration of bone marrow derived masts cells *in vitro* (BMMC) [72]. Furthermore, loss of ADAM10 has been shown to regulate the MC response to stem cell factor (SCF), which binds to c-kit on MCs to induce proper migration and distribution of tissue mast cells in mice [72]. Currently, the substrate ADAM10 cleaves in this scenario is unknown. It has been hypothesized that Notch 1 may be involved, as Notch 1 promotes IgE-mediated cytokine production in mast cells, but other substrates such as Notch 2 and CD44 have also been considered [73-75].

ADAM10Tg mice, generated by injection of ADAM10 cDNA under control of the H-2Kb promoter and the IgH enhancer, overexpress murine ADAM10 and were initially made to study the role of ADAM10 in lymphocyte development [76-78]. Inclusion of the IgH enhancer results in preferential expression on B lineage cells. This overexpression of ADAM10 was observed on bone marrow (BM) cells and markedly reduced the numbers of pro, pre, and immature B cells in the BM resulting in an almost complete loss of peripheral B2 B cells due to improper Notch cleavage and signaling [17]. The only B cell population unaltered by ADAM10 overexpression was B1a and B1b cells, which typically reside in the peritoneal and pleural cavities [17]. ADAM10Tg animals also exhibit significant myeloid accumulation. In the BM of these mice, CD11b+Gr-1+cells constitute over 90% of total BM cells. These cells leave the BM and migrate to all secondary lymphoid organs, where they are defined as myeloid derived suppressor cells (MDSCs). Recent work has shown a similar scenario exists in human disease, with defects in Notch signaling driving MDSC accumulation [79].

MDSCs accumulate in a spectrum of disease states including cancer, the natural aging process, solid organ transplantation, parasitic infections, sepsis, autoimmune disease, trauma, and burns [80-83]. MDSCs are classified as either monocytic (CD11b+Ly6C+Ly6G-) or granulocytic (CD11b+Ly6C^{int}Ly6G+) subsets [84]. This heterogeneous population was observed within the MDSCs in the ADAM10Tg [17]. Although MDSC accumulation is a byproduct of ADAM10 overexpression in early hematopoietic progenitors, ADAM10 expression is not altered in these cells. ADAM10Tg mice, therefore, could be exploited to study MDSC-mediated immune regulation in an environment devoid of confounding factors.

While MDSCs are most well-defined for their immunosuppressive role in cancer, a new role for accumulation of MDSCs in Th2-driven parasitic infection, such as *Nippostrongylus brasiliensis*, shows they play an immunosupportive role [80;85;86]. ADAM10Tg mice infected with *N. brasiliensis* have significantly reduced L4 lung worms, L5 adult worms and fecal egg burden [87]. These findings directly correlated with MDSC levels, as depletion of MDSCs reversed these findings.

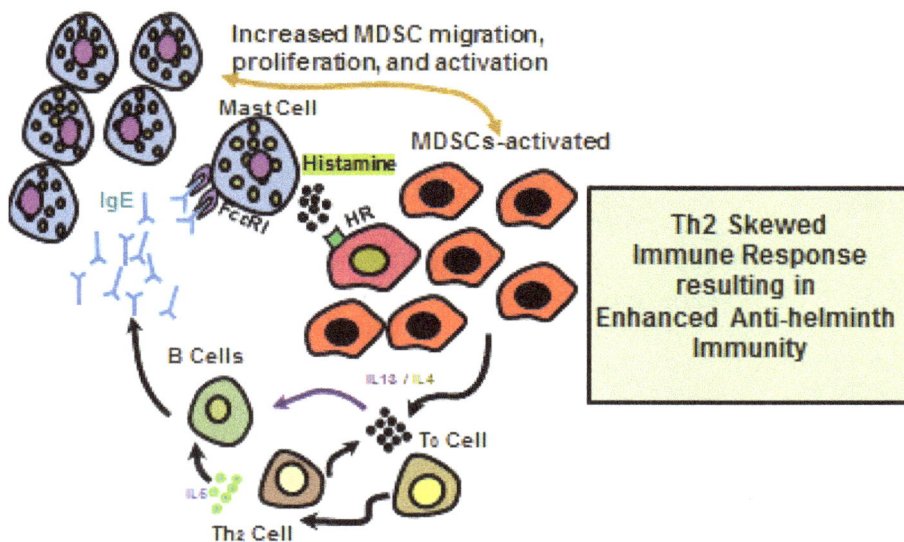

Figure 2. Model of MDSC/MC interaction. MCs are required for MDSC activity. MCs in the liver release mediators, wich create a chemokine gradient that increases migration of MDSCs, resulting in accumulation in the liver. MCs release mediators, such as histamine, that induce MDSC activation, proliferation and Th2-skewed immune responses that promote allergy and parasitic clearance and diminish antitumor responses.

Recent evidence is beginning to suggest that mast cells (MCs) contribute to the recruitment and activity of these MDSCs [86;88;89]. While MCs have been well documented to mediate allergic inflammation, new evidence is emerging to define the novel interaction between the MDSC and the MC. In MC-deficient mice, MDSC enhanced parasitic clearance is completely reversed. Additionally, co-culture of MCs and MDSCs results in enhanced IgE-mediated cytokine production by the MC [90]. Without MCs, MDSCs fail to migrate to the liver. This is thought to be through MC mediators such as histamine and IL-13 [86;87]. Histamine has been shown to induce MDSC proliferation, migration and activation (Figure 2) [87]. This is reflected in humans as reported by *Martin et al.* that patients with symptomatic allergic inflammation and increased ADAM10 have increased circulating MDSCs [27;87]. Figure 2 demonstrates the proposed model for MDSC/Mast Cell interaction, with MCs in the liver releasing histamine, which induces MDSC activation, proliferation, and release of Th2 cytokines such as IL13 and IL4, which in turn skews the immune response Th2. Therefore, while this model is favorable for elimination of helminth infection, it would diminish antitumor responses.

6. ADAM10, CD23 and IgE immune complexes

Antibody, in complex with its antigen, provides the immune system with a feedback response against the complexed antigen. This feedback mechanism results in immune stimulation or suppression depending upon the antibody class [91]. IgE, complexed with antigen, has long been shown to induce a significantly increased immune response over antigen alone. This response results in increased antigen specific T cell proliferation and antigen specific IgG *in vivo* [92]. ADAM10 may additionally play a role in this up regulation as ADAM10 B$^{-/-}$mice show significantly increased T cell proliferation over WT mice [93]. This may be due to the increased CD23 found on the surface of ADAM10 B$^{-/-}$mice, but may additionally be related to a not previously described ADAM10 effect. The low affinity receptor for IgE, CD23 has been known to internalize IgE antigen complexes and promote antigen presentation. Extensive studies using CD23$^{-/-}$animals proved CD23 to be essential to the immunostimulatory properties of IgE antigen complexes [92]. Recent findings show that CD23$^+$B cells rapidly transfer the antigen to the spleen [94] and were dispensable after 4 hours post IgE antigen complex injection. After that period, DCs were required [95]. These findings suggested that IgE antigen complexes or fragments thereof were being carried to the secondary lymphoid system, in this case the spleen, by CD23$^+$B cells and then were being transferred to DCs.

Exosomes are defined as tiny membrane bound particles ranging from 30-150nm. Although originally discovered in the 1980s and thought to be primarily for cellular waste [96], exosomal research has undergone a resurgence given the protein and micro-RNA cargo that is packed into these particles [97]. In a previous publication, *Mathews et al.* demonstrated that CD23 and its protease, ADAM10 were found in B cell derived exosomes (bexosomes) from both mouse and human B cells [98]. Additionally, β2-adrenergic stimulation of B cells further increased both CD23 and ADAM10 levels in bexosomes [99]. *Martin et al.* showed that B cells stimulated with anti-CD40 and IL-4, in the presence of IgE antigen complexes, release bexosomes that contain both CD23 and IgE. In agreement with earlier studies [100], these bexosomes were capable of directly stimulating antigen specific T cells *in vitro*, presumably via the MHC peptide complexes found on these bexosomes [93]. Culture of these bexosomes with bone marrow derived DCs (BMDC), followed by isolation and injection of DCs additionally enhanced *in vivo* antigen specific T cell proliferation. Overall, *Martin et al.* shows that bexosomes are responsible for antigen transfer from B cells to DCs, thus, providing a mechanism and suggesting a model to explain the importance of DCs in the immunostimulatory activity of IgE complexes [93].

7. Conclusion

ADAM 10 and 17 proteases have been widely studied in Th2 mediated disease responses including allergic rhinitis, asthma, and helminth infection. Enzymatic regulation of ADAM10 and 17 substrates as well as the relative amount of ADAM10 and 17 on immune cells is critical for preventing Th2 mediated disease as well as maintenance of normal antibody production, germinal center formation, and secondary lymphoid tissue architecture. While the role of ADAM10 in Th2 diseases is classically recognized for its regulation of IgE synthesis by CD23 cleavage, predisposition to asthma as well as severity of disease appears to be in part controlled by a tight regulation of ADAM10 and ADAM17 proteolytic activity, which in turn controls the cleavage of key substrates such as CD23, TNF, TGFα, and TGFβ1. These substrates ultimately effect IgE production, airway remodeling, inflammatory cell infiltration, and airway responsiveness.

Attenuation of MC degranulation and neutralization of MC mediators such as histamine and leukotrienes are common targets of therapeutic interventions used in asthma and allergic airway disease. MC histamine release is critical, however, for function, migration, and activation of MDSCs, which have been shown to alleviate helminth infection by decreasing parasite burden. This finding was studied using a unique model of MDSC accumulation in a mouse model that overexpresses ADAM10. Therefore, while MDSCs is could be considered harmful in severe allergy, they may also be essential for protection against helminth infection.

This review has demonstrated the essential role of ADAM10 and 17 and their substrates in Th2 mediated disease and provided a review of evidence supporting the continued exploration of ADAM10 and ADAM17 as potential therapeutic and diagnostic targets.

Acknowledgements

Work discussed in this review, which is from the author's laboratory is supported by grant RO1AI18697 from NIAID/NIH, American Asthma Foundation 11-0094 AAF, and a bridge grant from the VCU School of Medicine.

Author details

Lauren Folgosa Cooley[1,2,3], Rebecca K. Martin[2,3] and Daniel H. Conrad[2*]

*Address all correspondence to: dconrad@vcu.edu

1 Center for Clinical and Translational Research (CCTR), Virginia Commonwealth University, Richmond, VA, USA

2 Department of Microbiology and Immunology, Virginia Commonwealth University, Richmond, VA, USA

3 Lauren Folgosa Cooley and Rebecca K. Martin equally contributed to the writing of this review

References

[1] Akinbami LJ, Moorman JE, Bailey C, Zahran HS, King M, Johnson CA, et al. Trends in asthma prevalence, health care use, and mortality in the United States, 2001-2010. NCHS Data Brief 2012;(94):1-8.

[2] Centers for Disease Control and Prevention. Vital Signs: Asthma in the US, May 2011. http://www.cdc.gov/vitalsigns/pdf/2011-05-vitalsigns.pdf (accessed 29 September 2014).

[3] Murphy SL, Xu JQ, Kochanek KD. Deaths: Final data for 2010. National vital statistics reports; vol 61 no 4. Hyattsville, MD: National Center for Health Statistics. 2013.

[4] World Health Organization. Global surveillance, prevention and control of chronic respiratory diseases: a comprehensive approach, 2007. http://www.who.int/gard/publications/GARD20Book202007.pdf?ua=1 (accessed 29 September 2014).

[5] Weissman IL, Anderson DJ, Gage F. Stem and progenitor cells: origins, phenotypes, lineage commitments, and transdifferentiations. Annu Rev Cell Dev Biol 2001;17:387-403.

[6] World Health Organization. Soil-transmitted helminth infections, 2014. http://www.who.int/mediacentre/factsheets/fs366/en/ (accessed 29 September 2014).

[7] Wu LC, Zarrin AA. The production and regulation of IgE by the immune system. Nat Rev Immunol 2014;14(4):247-59.

[8] Larche M, Akdis CA, Valenta R. Immunological mechanisms of allergen-specific immunotherapy. Nat Rev Immunol 2006;6(10):761-71.

[9] Zheng Y, Shopes B, Holowka D, Baird B. Conformations of IgE bound to its receptor Fc epsilon RI and in solution. Biochemistry 1991;30(38):9125-32.

[10] Gustavsson S, Hjulstrom S, Liu T, Heyman B. CD23/IgE-mediated regulation of the specific antibody response in vivo. J Immunol 1994;152(10):4793-800.

[11] Conrad DH, Ford JW, Sturgill JL, Gibb DR. CD23: an overlooked regulator of allergic disease. Curr Allergy Asthma Rep 2007;7(5):331-7.

[12] Weskamp G, Ford JW, Sturgill J, Martin S, Docherty AJ, Swendeman S, et al. ADAM10 is a principal 'sheddase' of the low-affinity immunoglobulin E receptor CD23. Nat Immunol 2006;7(12):1293-8.

[13] Edwards DR, Handsley MM, Pennington CJ. The ADAM metalloproteinases. Mol Aspects Med 2008;29(5):258-89.

[14] Le Gall SM, Bobe P, Reiss K, Horiuchi K, Niu XD, Lundell D, et al. ADAMs 10 and 17 represent differentially regulated components of a general shedding machinery for

membrane proteins such as transforming growth factor alpha, L-selectin, and tumor necrosis factor alpha. Mol Biol Cell 2009;20(6):1785-94.

[15]   Klein T, Bischoff R. Active metalloproteases of the A Disintegrin and Metalloprotease (ADAM) family: biological function and structure. J Proteome Res 2011;10(1):17-33.

[16]   Seals DF, Courtneidge SA. The ADAMs family of metalloproteases: multidomain proteins with multiple functions. Genes Dev 2003;17(1):7-30.

[17]   Gibb DR, El SM, Kang DJ, Rowe WJ, El SR, Cichy J, et al. ADAM10 is essential for Notch2-dependent marginal zone B cell development and CD23 cleavage in vivo. J Exp Med 2010;207(3):623-35.

[18]   Di LG, Drago A, Pellitteri ME, Candore G, Colombo A, Potestio M, et al. Serum levels of soluble CD23 in patients with asthma or rhinitis monosensitive to Parietaria. Its relation to total serum IgE levels and eosinophil cationic protein during and out of the pollen season. Allergy Asthma Proc 1999;20(2):119-25.

[19]   Lecoanet-Henchoz S, Gauchat JF, Aubry JP, Graber P, Life P, Paul-Eugene N, et al. CD23 regulates monocyte activation through a novel interaction with the adhesion molecules CD11b-CD18 and CD11c-CD18. Immunity 1995;3(1):119-25.

[20]   Lecoanet-Henchoz S, Plater-Zyberk C, Graber P, Gretener D, Aubry JP, Conrad DH, et al. Mouse CD23 regulates monocyte activation through an interaction with the adhesion molecule CD11b/CD18. Eur J Immunol 1997;27(9):2290-4.

[21]   Hikita A, Tanaka N, Yamane S, Ikeda Y, Furukawa H, Tohma S, et al. Involvement of a disintegrin and metalloproteinase 10 and 17 in shedding of tumor necrosis factor-alpha. Biochem Cell Biol 2009;87(4):581-93.

[22]   Tracey KJ, Cerami A. Tumor necrosis factor, other cytokines and disease. Annu Rev Cell Biol 1993;9:317-43.

[23]   Frasca D, Romero M, Diaz A, Alter-Wolf S, Ratliff M, Landin AM, et al. A molecular mechanism for TNF-alpha-mediated downregulation of B cell responses. J Immunol 2012;188(1):279-86.

[24]   Tumanov AV, Kuprash DV, Mach JA, Nedospasov SA, Chervonsky AV. Lymphotoxin and TNF produced by B cells are dispensable for maintenance of the follicle-associated epithelium but are required for development of lymphoid follicles in the Peyer's patches. J Immunol 2004;173(1):86-91.

[25]   Tumanov AV, Grivennikov SI, Kruglov AA, Shebzukhov YV, Koroleva EP, Piao Y, et al. Cellular source and molecular form of TNF specify its distinct functions in organization of secondary lymphoid organs. Blood 2010;116(18):3456-64.

[26]   Folgosa L, Zellner HB, El Shikh ME, Conrad DH. Disturbed follicular architecture in B cell A disintegrin and metalloproteinase (ADAM)10 knockouts is mediated by

compensatory increases in ADAM17 and TNF-alpha shedding. J Immunol 2013;191(12):5951-8.

[27] Folgosa Cooley L, Martin RK, Zellner HB, Irani AM, El Shikh ME, Conrad DH. Increased B cell ADAM10 in allergic patients and Th2 prone mice. Submitted for publication.

[28] Overall CM, Blobel CP. In search of partners: linking extracellular proteases to substrates. Nat Rev Mol Cell Biol 2007;8(3):245-57.

[29] Chaimowitz NS, Martin RK, Cichy J, Gibb DR, Patil P, Kang DJ, et al. A disintegrin and metalloproteinase 10 regulates antibody production and maintenance of lymphoid architecture. J Immunol 2011;187(10):5114-22.

[30] Tian L, Wu X, Chi C, Han M, Xu T, Zhuang Y. ADAM10 is essential for proteolytic activation of Notch during thymocyte development. Int Immunol 2008;20(9):1181-7.

[31] Kopan R, Ilagan MX. The canonical Notch signaling pathway: unfolding the activation mechanism. Cell 2009;137(2):216-33.

[32] Saito T, Chiba S, Ichikawa M, Kunisato A, Asai T, Shimizu K, et al. Notch2 is preferentially expressed in mature B cells and indispensable for marginal zone B lineage development. Immunity 2003;18(5):675-85.

[33] Kopan R. Notch signaling. Cold Spring Harb Perspect Biol 2012;4(10).

[34] Hartmann D, de SB, Serneels L, Craessaerts K, Herreman A, Annaert W, et al. The disintegrin/metalloprotease ADAM 10 is essential for Notch signalling but not for alpha-secretase activity in fibroblasts. Hum Mol Genet 2002;11(21):2615-24.

[35] van TG, van DP, Verlaan I, van der Wall E, Kopan R, Vooijs M. Metalloprotease ADAM10 is required for Notch1 site 2 cleavage. J Biol Chem 2009;284(45):31018-27.

[36] Lopes-Carvalho T, Foote J, Kearney JF. Marginal zone B cells in lymphocyte activation and regulation. Curr Opin Immunol 2005;17(3):244-50.

[37] Chaimowitz NS, Kang DJ, Dean LM, Conrad DH. ADAM10 regulates transcription factor expression required for plasma cell function. PLoS One 2012;7(8):e42694.

[38] Le Gall SM, Bobe P, Reiss K, Horiuchi K, Niu XD, Lundell D, et al. ADAMs 10 and 17 represent differentially regulated components of a general shedding machinery for membrane proteins such as transforming growth factor alpha, L-selectin, and tumor necrosis factor alpha. Mol Biol Cell 2009;20(6):1785-94.

[39] Mezyk-Kopec R, Bzowska M, Stalinska K, Chelmicki T, Podkalicki M, Jucha J, et al. Identification of ADAM10 as a major TNF sheddase in ADAM17-deficient fibroblasts. Cytokine 2009;46(3):309-15.

[40] Pene J, Rousset F, Briere F, Chretien I, Wideman J, Bonnefoy JY, et al. Interleukin 5 enhances interleukin 4-induced IgE production by normal human B cells. The role of soluble CD23 antigen. Eur J Immunol 1988;18(6):929-35.

[41] Kelly K, Hutchinson G, Nebenius-Oosthuizen D, Smith AJ, Bartsch JW, Horiuchi K, et al. Metalloprotease-disintegrin ADAM8: expression analysis and targeted deletion in mice. Dev Dyn 2005;232(1):221-31.

[42] Marolewski AE, Buckle DR, Christie G, Earnshaw DL, Flamberg PL, Marshall LA, et al. CD23 (FcepsilonRII) release from cell membranes is mediated by a membrane-bound metalloprotease. Biochem J 1998;333 (Pt 3):573-9.

[43] Hibbert RG, Teriete P, Grundy GJ, Beavil RL, Reljic R, Holers VM, et al. The structure of human CD23 and its interactions with IgE and CD21. J Exp Med 2005;202(6): 751-60.

[44] Haczku A, Takeda K, Hamelmann E, Loader J, Joetham A, Redai I, et al. CD23 exhibits negative regulatory effects on allergic sensitization and airway hyperresponsiveness. Am J Respir Crit Care Med 2000;161(3 Pt 1):952-60.

[45] Payet-Jamroz M, Helm SL, Wu J, Kilmon M, Fakher M, Basalp A, et al. Suppression of IgE responses in CD23-transgenic animals is due to expression of CD23 on non-lymphoid cells. J Immunol 2001;166(8):4863-9.

[46] Mathews JA, Ford J, Norton S, Kang D, Dellinger A, Gibb DR, et al. A potential new target for asthma therapy: a disintegrin and metalloprotease 10 (ADAM10) involvement in murine experimental asthma. Allergy 201;66(9):1193-200.

[47] Watanabe N, Kobayashi A. Regulation of immunoglobulin E production in mice immunized with an extract of Toxoplasma gondii. Infect Immun 1989;57(5):1405-8.

[48] Babu KS, Davies DE, Holgate ST. Role of tumor necrosis factor alpha in asthma. Immunol Allergy Clin North Am 2004;24(4):583-vi.

[49] Frasca D, Landin AM, Alvarez JP, Blackshear PJ, Riley RL, Blomberg BB. Tristetraprolin, a negative regulator of mRNA stability, is increased in old B cells and is involved in the degradation of E47 mRNA. J Immunol 2007;179(2):918-27.

[50] Ganor Y, Besser M, Ben-Zakay N, Unger T, Levite M. Human T cells express a functional ionotropic glutamate receptor GluR3, and glutamate by itself triggers integrin-mediated adhesion to laminin and fibronectin and chemotactic migration. J Immunol 2003;170(8):4362-72.

[51] Boldyrev AA, Kazey VI, Leinsoo TA, Mashkina AP, Tyulina OV, Johnson P, et al. Rodent lymphocytes express functionally active glutamate receptors. Biochem Biophys Res Commun 2004;324(1):133-9.

[52] Sturgill JL, Mathews J, Scherle P, Conrad DH. Glutamate signaling through the kainate receptor enhances human immunoglobulin production. J Neuroimmunol 2011;233(1-2):80-9.

[53] Fahy JV, Kim KW, Liu J, Boushey HA. Prominent neutrophilic inflammation in sputum from subjects with asthma exacerbation. J Allergy Clin Immunol 1995;95(4): 843-52.

[54] Green RH, Brightling CE, Woltmann G, Parker D, Wardlaw AJ, Pavord ID. Analysis of induced sputum in adults with asthma: identification of subgroup with isolated sputum neutrophilia and poor response to inhaled corticosteroids. Thorax 2002;57(10):875-9.

[55] Jatakanon A, Uasuf C, Maziak W, Lim S, Chung KF, Barnes PJ. Neutrophilic inflammation in severe persistent asthma. Am J Respir Crit Care Med 1999;160(5 Pt 1): 1532-9.

[56] Arndt PG, Strahan B, Wang Y, Long C, Horiuchi K, Walcheck B. Leukocyte ADAM17 regulates acute pulmonary inflammation. PLoS One 2011;6(5):e19938.

[57] Pruessmeyer J, Hess FM, Alert H, Groth E, Pasqualon T, Schwarz N, et al. Leukocytes require ADAM10 but not ADAM17 for their migration and inflammatory recruitment into the alveolar space. Blood 2014;123(26):4077-88.

[58] Le Cras TD, Acciani TH, Mushaben EM, Kramer EL, Pastura PA, Hardie WD, et al. Epithelial EGF receptor signaling mediates airway hyperreactivity and remodeling in a mouse model of chronic asthma. Am J Physiol Lung Cell Mol Physiol 2011;300(3):L414-L421.

[59] Tamaoka M, Hassan M, McGovern T, Ramos-Barbon D, Jo T, Yoshizawa Y, et al. The epidermal growth factor receptor mediates allergic airway remodelling in the rat. Eur Respir J 2008;32(5):1213-23.

[60] Shao MX, Ueki IF, Nadel JA. Tumor necrosis factor alpha-converting enzyme mediates MUC5AC mucin expression in cultured human airway epithelial cells. Proc Natl Acad Sci U S A 2003;100(20):11618-23.

[61] Booth BW, Sandifer T, Martin EL, Martin LD. IL-13-induced proliferation of airway epithelial cells: mediation by intracellular growth factor mobilization and ADAM17. Respir Res 2007;8:51.

[62] Shiomi T, Tschumperlin DJ, Park JA, Sunnarborg SW, Horiuchi K, Blobel CP, et al. TNF-alpha-converting enzyme/a disintegrin and metalloprotease-17 mediates mechanotransduction in murine tracheal epithelial cells. Am J Respir Cell Mol Biol 2011;45(2):376-85.

[63] Malapeira J, Esselens C, Bech-Serra JJ, Canals F, Arribas J. ADAM17 (TACE) regulates TGFbeta signaling through the cleavage of vasorin. Oncogene 2011;30(16): 1912-22.

[64]   Duvernelle C, Freund V, Frossard N. Transforming growth factor-beta and its role in asthma. Pulm Pharmacol Ther 2003;16(4):181-96.

[65]   Flohr C, Quinnell RJ, Britton J. Do helminth parasites protect against atopy and allergic disease? Clin Exp Allergy 2009;39(1):20-32.

[66]   Yazdanbakhsh M, Kremsner PG, van RR. Allergy, parasites, and the hygiene hypothesis. Science 2002;296(5567):490-4.

[67]   Mingomataj EC, Xhixha F, Gjata E. Helminths can protect themselves against rejection inhibiting hostile respiratory allergy symptoms. Allergy 2006;61(4):400-6.

[68]   Aberle N, Gagro A, Rabatic S, Reiner-Banovac Z, Dekaris D. Expression of CD23 antigen and its ligands in children with intrinsic and extrinsic asthma. Allergy 1997;52(12):1238-42.

[69]   Black CL, Muok EM, Mwinzi PN, Carter JM, Karanja DM, Secor WE, et al. Increases in levels of schistosome-specific immunoglobulin E and CD23(+) B cells in a cohort of Kenyan children undergoing repeated treatment and reinfection with Schistosoma mansoni. J Infect Dis 2010;202(3):399-405.

[70]   Mwinzi PN, Ganley-Leal L, Black CL, Secor WE, Karanja DM, Colley DG. Circulating CD23+B cell subset correlates with the development of resistance to Schistosoma mansoni reinfection in occupationally exposed adults who have undergone multiple treatments. J Infect Dis 2009;199(2):272-9.

[71]   Acharya M, Borland G, Edkins AL, Maclellan LM, Matheson J, Ozanne BW, et al. CD23/FcepsilonRII: molecular multi-tasking. Clin Exp Immunol 2010;162(1):12-23.

[72]   Faber TW, Pullen NA, Fernando JF, Kolawole EM, McLeod JJ, Taruselli M, et al. ADAM10 is required for SCF-induced mast cell migration. Cell Immunol 2014 Jul; 290(1):80-8.

[73]   Nakano K, Siar CH, Tsujigiwa H, Nagatsuka H, Nagai N, Kawakami T. Notch signaling in benign and malignant ameloblastic neoplasms. Eur J Med Res 2008;13(10): 476-80.

[74]   Nakano N, Nishiyama C, Yagita H, Koyanagi A, Akiba H, Chiba S, et al. Notch signaling confers antigen-presenting cell functions on mast cells. J Allergy Clin Immunol 2009;123(1):74-81.

[75]   Nakano N, Nishiyama C, Yagita H, Koyanagi A, Ogawa H, Okumura K. Notch1-mediated signaling induces MHC class II expression through activation of class II transactivator promoter III in mast cells. J Biol Chem 201;286(14):12042-8.

[76]   Malek SN, Dordai DI, Reim J, Dintzis H, Desiderio S. Malignant transformation of early lymphoid progenitors in mice expressing an activated Blk tyrosine kinase. Proc Natl Acad Sci U S A 1998;95(13):7351-6.

[77] Payet ME, Woodward EC, Conrad DH. Humoral response suppression observed with CD23 transgenics. J Immunol 1999;163(1):217-23.

[78] Pircher H, Mak TW, Lang R, Ballhausen W, Ruedi E, Hengartner H, et al. T cell tolerance to Mlsa encoded antigens in T cell receptor V beta 8.1 chain transgenic mice. EMBO J 1989 Mar;8(3):719-27.

[79] Cheng P, Kumar V, Liu H, Youn JI, Fishman M, Sherman S, et al. Effects of notch signaling on regulation of myeloid cell differentiation in cancer. Cancer Res 2014;74(1): 141-52.

[80] Cuenca AG, Delano MJ, Kelly-Scumpia KM, Moreno C, Scumpia PO, Laface DM, et al. A paradoxical role for myeloid-derived suppressor cells in sepsis and trauma. Mol Med 2011;17(3-4):281-92.

[81] Dilek N, van RN, Le MA, Vanhove B. Myeloid-derived suppressor cells in transplantation. Curr Opin Organ Transplant 2010;15(6):765-8.

[82] Gomez CR, Boehmer ED, Kovacs EJ. The aging innate immune system. Curr Opin Immunol 2005;17(5):457-62.

[83] Highfill SL, Rodriguez PC, Zhou Q, Goetz CA, Koehn BH, Veenstra R, et al. Bone marrow myeloid-derived suppressor cells (MDSCs) inhibit graft-versus-host disease (GVHD) via an arginase-1-dependent mechanism that is up-regulated by interleukin-13. Blood 2010;116(25):5738-47.

[84] Movahedi K, Guilliams M, Van den Bossche J, Van den Bergh R, Gysemans C, Beschin A, et al. Identification of discrete tumor-induced myeloid-derived suppressor cell subpopulations with distinct T cell-suppressive activity. Blood 2008;111(8): 4233-44.

[85] Pastula A, Marcinkiewicz J. Myeloid-derived suppressor cells: a double-edged sword? Int J Exp Pathol 2011;92(2):73-8.

[86] Saleem SJ, Martin RK, Morales JK, Sturgill JL, Gibb DR, Graham L, et al. Cutting edge: mast cells critically augment myeloid-derived suppressor cell activity. J Immunol 2012;189(2):511-5.

[87] Martin RK, Saleem SJ, Folgosa L, Zellner HB, Damle SR, Nguyen GK, et al. Mast cell histamine promotes the immunoregulatory activity of myeloid-derived suppressor cells. J Leukoc Biol 2014;96(1):151-9.

[88] Cheon EC, Khazaie K, Khan MW, Strouch MJ, Krantz SB, Phillips J, et al. Mast cell 5-lipoxygenase activity promotes intestinal polyposis in APCDelta468 mice. Cancer Res 2011;71(5):1627-36.

[89] Yang Z, Zhang B, Li D, Lv M, Huang C, Shen GX, et al. Mast cells mobilize myeloid-derived suppressor cells and Treg cells in tumor microenvironment via IL-17 pathway in murine hepatocarcinoma model. PLoS One 2010;5(1):e8922.

[90] Morales JK, Saleem SJ, Martin RK, Saunders BL, Barnstein BO, Faber TW, et al. Myeloid-derived suppressor cells enhance IgE-mediated mast cell responses. J Leukoc Biol 2014;95(4):643-50.

[91] Hjelm F, Carlsson F, Getahun A, Heyman B. Antibody-mediated regulation of the immune response. Scand J Immunol 2006;64(3):177-84.

[92] Getahun A, Hjelm F, Heyman B. IgE enhances antibody and T cell responses in vivo via CD23+B cells. J Immunol 2005;175(3):1473-82.

[93] Martin RK, Brooks KB, Henningsson, F, Heyman, B, and Conrad DH. Antigen transfer from exosomes to dendritic cells as an explanation for the immune enhancement seen by IgE immune complexes. PLOS One 2014;9(11):e110609.

[94] Hjelm F, Karlsson MC, Heyman B. A novel B cell-mediated transport of IgE-immune complexes to the follicle of the spleen. J Immunol 2008;180(10):6604-10.

[95] Henningsson F, Ding Z, Dahlin JS, Linkevicius M, Carlsson F, Gronvik KO, et al. IgE-mediated enhancement of CD4+T cell responses in mice requires antigen presentation by CD11c+cells and not by B cells. PLoS One 2011;6(7):e21760.

[96] Trams EG, Lauter CJ, Salem N, Jr., Heine U. Exfoliation of membrane ecto-enzymes in the form of micro-vesicles. Biochim Biophys Acta 1981;645(1):63-70.

[97] Bobrie A, Colombo M, Raposo G, Thery C. Exosome secretion: molecular mechanisms and roles in immune responses. Traffic 2011;12(12):1659-68.

[98] Mathews JA, Gibb DR, Chen BH, Scherle P, Conrad DH. CD23 Sheddase A disintegrin and metalloproteinase 10 (ADAM10) is also required for CD23 sorting into B cell-derived exosomes. J Biol Chem 2010;285(48):37531-41.

[99] Padro CJ, Shawler TM, Gormley MG, Sanders VM. Adrenergic regulation of IgE involves modulation of CD23 and ADAM10 expression on exosomes. J Immunol 2013;191(11):5383-97.

[100] Qazi KR, Gehrmann U, Domange JE, Karlsson MC, Gabrielsson S. Antigen-loaded exosomes alone induce Th1-type memory through a B-cell-dependent mechanism. Blood 2009;113(12):2673-83.

8

Specific Immunotherapy in Food Allergy — Towards a Change in the Management Paradigm

José Manuel Lucas, Ana Moreno-Salvador and
Luis García-Marcos

1. Introduction

Food allergy is one of the leading causes of allergic disease and the main cause of anaphylactic reactions and mortality due to allergic problems, producing important economic problems and social restrictions for the affected patients and their families.

The increase in the prevalence and persistence of food allergy throughout the world has a significant impact not only upon patient safety but also on quality of life and healthcare expenditure. Indeed, food allergy constitutes a major public health problem.

The attitude or approach to food allergy has always been to avoid the cause and adopt measures against adverse reactions in the event of accidental intake. However, in the last few years a new management strategy has been explored: the active induction of food tolerance.

One of the most promising therapies is desensitization to specific food allergens through oral or sublingual immunotherapy, and research in this field is advancing quickly for some established allergens. In this respect, the technique has demonstrated its effectiveness, and its transfer to clinical practice is presently undergoing evaluation.

This chapter addresses the epidemiology and natural history of food allergy, the mechanisms of immune tolerance to foods, the forms of desensitization and induction of tolerance to allergens with applications to foods, and affords an update on the experience gained with the induction of tolerance to different foods, the respective protocols and guides, efficacy and safety considerations, and adverse reaction risk factors. An evaluation is also made of the current state of biological therapy utilization in conjunction with specific immunotherapy for food allergens.

Lastly, a discussion is made of the opportunities and limitations facing the clinical use of the specific immunotherapy in food allergy, and of the areas of future research.

2. Epidemiology of food allergy

Food allergy is a worldwide problem, affecting at least 1-2% of all adults and between 6-8% of the pediatric population [1–3]. The reported prevalences are conditioned by the diagnostic methods used, the patient ages considered, and also by genetic, ethnic, geographic and cultural factors. Consequently, the published data differ greatly from one country to another [4].

The diagnostic methodology used exerts a great influence. In this respect, a recent metaanalysis [5] found the self-reported incidence of allergy to cow's milk (CM), egg, peanut or crustaceans to be 12%-a figure that dropped to 3% when the diagnosis was established from double-blind, placebo-controlled food challenge(DBPCFC) or provocation testing. In the case of cow's milk, between 1.2% and 17% of those surveyed claimed to be allergic, depending on the study. In this regard, if the diagnosis was established by prick testing or the determination of specific IgE, the frequency was found to be 2-9%, versus a prevalence of 0-3% when DBPCFC was the selected diagnostic technique.

In the United States [6] it is estimated that 8% of all children will suffer food allergy, and that 40% of these patients will experience severe reactions, while 30% will be allergic to several foods – peanut, cow's milk and crustaceans being the most commonly implicated foods. In a one-year of age Australian population, the prevalence of allergic individuals as established by provocation testing (i.e., challenge-proven allergy) reached 10% [7].

The prevalence of food allergy appears to be increasing rapidly, particularly in the industrialized world [8–10] and in widely different regions such as the United Kingdom [11], the United States [12], Australia [13], Sweden [9] or China [14].

2.1. The most frequently implicated foods

The age of the studied population and the geographical setting exert a key influence upon the types of foods that cause allergy. The most common cause of food allergy in pediatric patients is cow's milk, followed by egg (and peanut in the United States). In turn, crustaceans, nuts and peanut become the most common causes of more serious allergic reactions among adults, since allergy to cow's milk and egg disappears in approximately three out of every four patients, while the opposite is observed for the rest of foods.

2.2. Cow's milk

Allergy to cow's milk is the most common type of food allergy in children, affecting 2-3% of all individuals in this age group. Approximately one-half of all cases are mediated by IgE, with the development of immediate allergic reactions which in some cases may prove systemic and serious (e.g., anaphylaxis). The rest of the cases are not mediated by IgE, and are characterized by generally less serious gastrointestinal problems-with the exception of FPIES (food protein-induced enterocolitis syndrome).

Most patients show a favorable course, with disappearance of the allergy in up to 83% of all subjects by 5 years of age. The specific IgE levels are a good predictor of tolerance, though recent publications indicate that longer periods of time are currently needed to acquire natural tolerance, and that tolerance now develops in adolescence and not in the early schooling period as was common in the past [15,16]. Despite measures of caution, accidental intake still occurs, often on a day to day basis in the home [17], with the description of even fatal anaphylactic reactions [18].

2.3. Egg

Allergy to chicken egg (usually to egg white) is the second most common form of food allergy in pediatric patients, being observed in 1-3% of all children [19]. The underlying pathogenesis is mainly IgE-mediated. Approximately two-thirds of all patients acquire natural tolerance [13,20,21], though a recent study has evidenced the persistence of egg allergy in 42% of the patients upon reaching adolescence [22]. This change in tendency may contribute to increase the number of adults with allergy to egg. In this regard, it has been estimated that 0.2% of all adults are allergic to egg [23], so this figure is likely to increase.

2.4. Peanut

Allergy to peanut is one of the most frequent forms of food allergy in western countries, and can give rise to serious IgE-mediated reactions in response to even small intakes or exposure levels. The condition is found in up to 1.8% of all children in the United Kingdom [24] and in 1.3% of the adult population in the United States [23]. When diagnosed by provocation or challenge testing, the prevalence reaches 3% of all children in Australia [7]. The prevalence of peanut allergy appears to be increasing, and most individuals continue to suffer allergy to this food in adult life [25]. Indeed, only 20% of the affected patients overcome peanut allergy [26], and the percentage of tolerant subjects is related to the degree of sensitization [27]. Over 15% of all affected patients suffer accidental exposure on a yearly basis [28,29].

2.5. Multiple foods

Allergy to multiple foods is important, since up to 30% of all allergic children suffer allergy to more than one food [6,30] – the magnitude of the condition increasing with the degree of atopy of the patient. These patients have poorer quality of life than those with allergy to a single food [31], and are at an increased risk of suffering nutritional deficiencies [32]. Likewise, patients with allergy to multiple foods have lesser chances of acquiring natural tolerance to the implicated foods [22].

3. Current treatment of food allergy

The traditionally recommended approach to the management of food allergy consisted of strict avoidance of the causal allergen; early recognition of the allergic reaction; and the availability of adrenalin to deal with serious reactions. However it is known that strict avoidance is very difficult to achieve, and is limited by difficulty in interpreting food labels [33] and by the existence of hidden allergens in commercial foods [34]. Accidental intake is therefore common, and can be expected to occur in up to 50% of all patients in the course of a two-year period, even in very cautious patients. Undertreatment is moreover a common problem [35].

3.1. Management of anaphylaxis

The main risk posed by food allergy is the induction of IgE-mediated systemic reactions. In this regard, food allergy is the leading cause of both anaphylaxis and mortality due to anaphylaxis. Between 40-100% of all deaths attributable to anaphylaxis in patients with food allergy are due to commercial foods or foods prepared outside the home [18,36,37]

Management includes teaching the patients and caregivers to quickly recognize the symptoms of anaphylaxis and promptly self-inject insulin and notify the emergency care services [38].

However, difficulties are found regarding correct use on the part of the caregivers [39], and in assuming the responsibility of care on the part of the patients [40] – particularly in the case of adolescents [41,42]. In such patients, one-fourth of all anaphylactic episodes occur outside the home. It is therefore necessary to instruct the caretakers in school on how to handle anaphylaxis, and to reinforce self-care instructions among these adolescents [43].

4. Quality of life

The need for a strict avoidance diet, the high probability of accidental exposure, and the risk of anaphylaxis in food allergies alters the life of the patients and their families, and generates anxiety and psychosocial stress, with a negative impact upon quality of life [44–46], to an extent greater than that observed with other chronic disorders of childhood [47,48].

This loss of quality of life affects even the daily relations of the patient, with an increased frequency of bullying in such children [49]. Allergic children are also at an increased risk of suffering abuse.

5. Economic costs

Food allergy implies an important economic cost [50], reaching an estimated 25 billion USD each year in the United States – the largest part of this sum (approximately 20 billion USD) being assumed by the families as direct costs, working hours lost, visits to the emergency service, etc. [51]. The generated costs are not only of a personal nature but moreover also affect the healthcare services, the food industry, the caregivers, and society as a whole [52].

6. Immunology of food tolerance

The gastrointestinal tract (GIT) is constantly exposed to an enormous number of exogenous antigens, including commensal bacteria and ingested proteins. In this respect, the GIT is the most relevant site of exposure to antigens in the entire body, and therefore of antigen absorption and presentation to the host.

An epithelial layer separates the allergens from the lymphocyte population, antigen-presenting cells (APCs) and other immune cells of the *lamina propria* that globally conform the so-called mucosa-associated lymphatic tissue (MALT). Within the latter, the dendritic cells (DCs) interact with the food allergens, determining the outcome of the adaptive response (immunity versus tolerance)[53]. In this respect, immune tolerance is defined as suppression of the antigen-specific cellular or humoral immune response.

Following the intake of proteins with the diet, enzyme-mediated digestion reduces their immunogenicity, probably through destruction of the conformational epitopes. However, other foods sharing common characteristics (molecular weight < 70 kDa, linear epitopes, water solubility) are resistant to both physical and chemical degradation, and thus maintain their allergenicity upon reaching the small intestine. Under normal conditions, the intact macromolecules are taken up by a transcellular transport mechanism, and the antigenic material is deposited through the basolateral surface of the epithelial cell layer; as a result, a significant amount of food allergens reach the systemic circulation following a meal.

Another antigen uptake mechanism consists of direct antigen presentation to the CD11c +dendritic cell population. The function of these cells is related to macrophage activity, and there is evidence that the CD11+macrophage population plays an important role in the T cell-mediated antigen-specific response during the development of immune tolerance to food antigens.

More recent evidence supports that impairment in regulatory T cell (Treg) induction and innate immunity might also contribute to Th2 polarization in early life. Prospective birth cohort studies have shown that IgE production in response to egg, milk, and peanut commonly occurs even in healthy infants. In non-allergic subjects, this Th2 bias appears to be transient, and IgE levels decrease, possibly through a counterbalancing induction of antigen-specific Th1 responses (i.e., IFN-γ); in contrast, these Th2 responses consolidate and strengthen in allergic children, perhaps through the induction of IL-4 signaling [54].

A full 80% of all plasmatic cells are located in the intestine. The small bowel contains cell generating pIgA (polymeric IgA)(80%), followed in order of prevalence by secretory pIgM (polymeric IgM)(15-20%) and secretory IgG (3-4%). IgA deficiency in children has been reported to be associated with an elevated frequency of food allergy. In this context, it has been postulated that IgA plays a protective role in the context of food allergy [55].

The presence of antigen-specific IgG in the intestinal lumen can exert a significant influence upon immunity to food and flora. IgG-mediated antigen uptake through FcRn in the neonatal intestine is tolerogenic, and suggests that antigen exposure through breast milk would be a helpful preventative strategy, particularly when the mother has existing IgG antibodies to that antigen. Once allergic sensitization has been established, it is not clear whether IgG-facilitated antigen uptake through FcRn would amplify existing proallergic adaptive immune responses or promote active immune tolerance. Studies are needed to address the influence of FcRn on responses to food antigens [55].

Immunoglobulin E can be found in secreted form under the conditions of allergy and helminth infection-this being associated with an epithelial receptor for IgE. IgE-facilitated antigen uptake results in increased delivery of antigen to allergic effector cells, activates proinflammatory pathways in intestinal epithelial cells, and enhances antigen delivery to dendritic cells. IgE-facilitated antigen uptake by B cells can also have an adjuvant-like effect on the resulting adaptive immune response.

This complex interaction among physical factors, antigen characteristics and timing, together with the effects of innate immune stimulation, condition the development of oral tolerance through a common pathway directly or indirectly influenced by APCs. It recently has been shown that mucosal dendritic cells are probably the key element in determining allergic sensitization versus tolerance in naïve subjects.

Multiple tolerance mechanisms probably intervene, and may include anergy or deletion of T cells. There is evidence relating oral tolerance with the capacity of the mucosal dendritic cells to induce positive forkhead box protein [Foxp3]+Treg cells in MLNs (mesenteric lymph nodes). CD103, retinoic acid (RA), indoleamine-2,3-dioxygenase, co-stimulator molecules of the B7 family and TGF-β appear to act by allowing dendritic cells to induce such conversion. In contrast, the dendritic cells of the *lamina propria* do not express CD103, and are proinflammatory. This suggests that tolerogenic dendritic cells could inhibit site-specific signaling of the intestinal epithelium through interaction with E-cadherin (a CD103 ligand). This is probably the microenvironment provided by the mucosa to allow antigen presentation resulting in either inflammatory response or tolerance within the MLNs. Antigen-presenting cells other than conventional dendritic cells might also participate in oral tolerance induction.

Oral tolerance might be operative through multiple mechanisms in multiple tissue compartments. For example, intestinal macrophages can also efficiently induce Foxp3+Treg cells in an IL-10-, RA-and TGF-β-dependent fashion. Plasmacytoid dendritic cells, a specialized dendritic cell subset known for their ability to produce vast quantities of type I interferons, can also activate inducible Foxp3+IL-10. Integration of environmental information by dendritic cells results in specific activation and differentiation of T cell subsets, including the Foxp3+Treg cells, as the primary effectors of oral tolerance.

Repeated exposures to low doses of antigen are thought to be the optimal stimulus for the development of Treg cells, which suppress immune responses through soluble or cell-bound regulatory cytokines such as IL-10 and TGF-β. Natural CD4+CD25+Treg cells develop in the thymus and express the specific transcription factor Foxp3+, which confers regulatory function to these cells to block both Th1 and Th2 responses. Inducible regulatory T cells (iTreg) are CD4+cells that can differentiate from naïve precursors, acquiring regulatory properties in the periphery after exposure to antigen. In many cases these cells acquire the expression of Foxp3, and they exist in at least two forms distinguished by the antiinflammatory cytokines produced: IL-10 (Tr1 cells) and TGF-β (Th3 cells). Whereas natural CD4+CD25+Treg cells are thought to primarily govern peripheral tolerance to self-antigens, Treg cells are more likely responsible for tolerance to exogenous substances, such as allergens [56].

Mechanistically, functional allergen-specific Treg cells can attenuate allergic responses through: 1.-the suppression of mast cells, basophils, and eosinophils; 2.-the suppression of inflammatory dendritic cells and induction of tolerogenic dendritic cells; 3.-the suppression of allergen-specific Th2 cells, hence contributing to T cell anergy; and 4.-the early induction of IgG4 and late reduction of IgE production. All of these mechanisms can be mediated through the secretion of IL-10 and TGF-beta, or through cell contact-dependent suppression. The Treg cells therefore appear to play an important role in tolerance following immunotherapy in food allergy [57,58].

7. Active therapy against food allergy

Between 15-20% of all patients with allergy to cow's milk and egg will remain allergic, while those who acquire tolerance will take years to become tolerant. In contrast, most patients with allergy to fish, crustaceans, peanut or nuts will remain allergic to these foods for life [59].

The health risks for such patients, the alterations in their diet, social discrimination, impaired quality of life, and the costs generated by such illnesses have led to re-evaluation of the passive management strategies with a view to establishing active treatment options – replacing the management through avoidance paradigm with an active intervention approach based on specific desensitization and tolerance of the causal food.

In this context, active intervention has been considered for years with the purpose of solving this health problem, particularly in patients with a high risk of anaphylaxis and in those who will not benefit from natural resolution of the problem. Such intervention involves nonspecific therapeutic measures and, more recently, specific treatments for each type of food.

Immunotherapy would be a plausible option in view of its demonstrated efficacy in patients with allergy to aeroallergens and stinging insect venom [60]. For this reason, the use of immunotherapy in application to food allergens has been postulated for over two decades – giving rise to a series of experiments and producing a body of knowledge over the last decade, referred particularly to the oral route, which we will try to explain in this chapter.

Considering that non-IgE mediated allergy does not appear amenable to such treatment strategies, we will only deal with IgE-mediated food allergy.

8. Immunotherapy in application to foods

The site of antigen administration and contact is important for the efficacy and safety of specific food immunotherapy. According to the administration route involved, we can distinguish among four different types of specific food immunotherapy: subcutaneous immunotherapy (SCIT), epicutaneous immunotherapy (EPIT), sublingual immunotherapy (SLIT) and oral immunotherapy or specific oral tolerance induction (SOTI)[61].

8.1. Specific Subcutaneous Immunotherapy (SCIT)

There is extensive experience with the use of subcutaneous immunotherapy in application to aeroallergens and insect venom – more than 100 years having gone by since the technique was first developed – though very little experience has been gained to date with its use in application to food allergy. In patients with pollen-fruit syndrome [62], immunotherapy has been found to be effective against aeroallergens that share antigenicity with certain plant foods [63–65], securing desensitization to such allergens and foods. However, the utilization of specific food allergens via the subcutaneous route (e.g., peanut), produced important [66] and serious adverse reactions, with the death of one patient following error in the composition of the placebo dose containing allergen. As a result, and despite evidence of a certain degree of efficacy, these problems caused the early evaluation attempts to be suspended [67]. In effect, since then, this specific immunotherapy administration route to treating food allergy has been discontinued. However, the introduction of recombinant allergens, the elimination of epitopes for IgE with the maintenance of T cell-recognized epitopes [68], immunotherapy with peptides, DNA immunotherapy, and other advances that are currently in the preclinical investigation phase, will make it possible to resume studies with this administration route.

8.2. Specific Epicutaneous Immunotherapy (EPIT)

Specific epicutaneous immunotherapy (EPIT) is based on the capacity of the Langerhans cells of the epidermal basal layer to migrate and reach the lymph nodes, where they regulate the cells implicated in allergic inflammation [69,70]. A pilot study in patients with allergy to cow's milk [71] demonstrated a modest increase in the amount of milk tolerated, with only local symptoms, none of which proved serious. A recent phase IIa double-blind, placebo-controlled (DBPC) efficacy study in patients with allergy to peanut (ARACHILD) [72] was able to secure a more than 10-fold increase versus baseline in the tolerated levels after 18 months of treatment in 67% of the patients. The study has currently been extended to 36 months, with good safety results. Other studies involving this same administration route for the induction of peanut desensitization are currently also in course.

8.3. Specific Sublingual Immunotherapy (SLIT)

Specific sublingual immunotherapy (SLIT), which makes use of the capacity of the Langerhans cells of the oral mucosa to suppress allergic cell response [69,73,74], has been successfully applied against aeroallergens in rhinitis and asthma [75,76]. In the same way as SCIT, the technique has afforded improvement in patients with plant allergy exhibiting cross-allergenicity with certain pollens. In this regard, SLIT has been used against the latter [77] and against latex – avoiding the increase in foods to which reactions occurred [78].

Use has been made of SLIT with specific food allergens such as kiwi [79]. One case report documented persistent tolerance after 5 years [80]. DBPC studies have been made with hazelnut [81], with the maintenance of protection over the long term [82], and with peach [83], in which tolerance could be increased 3-to 9-fold. At present, an observational study is underway to evaluate the efficacy and safety of SLIT with Pru p3 extract in pediatric patients. A pilot study with cow's milk [84] was able to increase the tolerated amount of milk three-fold in a group of 8 children. A placebo-controlled SLIT study with peanut [85] in turn secured a 10-fold increase in the amount of peanut that could be ingested without symptoms after 44 weeks of therapy in the active treatment group. A more recent placebo-controlled SLIT study with peanut [86] found 70% of the patients to be able to ingest 5 g of peanut or increase the tolerated amount up to 10-fold versus the amounts tolerated at baseline, after 44 weeks of treatment.

8.4. Specific Oral Immunotherapy / Specific Oral Tolerance Induction (SOTI)

Specific oral tolerance induction (SOTI) is currently the most widely evaluated approach, having exhibited effectiveness over the short and long term, though with limitations in relation to its safety profile. Tolerance is taken to represent non-reactivity to the allergen even after a period of time without contact with the allergen. In this regard, desensitization constitutes a prior step, but does not guarantee lasting tolerance. SOTI is able to achieve desensitization in a large percentage of patients – this being enough to avoid reactions secondary to accidental ingestion and incorporation of the food to the diet. Such desensitization is possibly the most important objective of the technique, since the number of patients that are able to achieve permanent tolerance is considerably smaller. As a result, it has been proposed that SOTI should actually be referred to as specific oral desensitization induction.

A prospective comparison of SOTI versus SLIT [87] has confirmed greater efficacy if SLIT is followed by a SOTI phase involving high maintenance doses. The retrospective comparison of SLIT and SOTI in application to peanut allergy [88] has shown greater efficacy with the latter technique, though with more adverse effects. In this respect, it seems that SLIT is comparatively safer but less effective than SOTI in application to foods.

Since SOTI is the most widely investigated type of specific immunotherapy in food allergy, we will address the technique a little more in depth.

8.4.1. Mechanism of immune tolerance in SOTI

SOTI acts at intestinal dendritic cell level [89,56], lowering the specific IgE levels and increasing the specific IgG4 titers, with an increase in IL-10, IL-5, IFN-γ, TNF-α and Foxp3 cells. Studies involving T cell microarrays have shown inhibition oriented towards apoptosis at genetic level [90]. The technique also reduces basophil IgE receptor production [91].

8.4.2. Regimens and phases in SOTI

The technique aims to induce desensitization and subsequent tolerance by administering small amounts of allergens that cause no clinical manifestations or only mild manifestations. The amounts are gradually increased over time until the ingested allergen level reached is considered to protect against adverse reactions and secure tolerance after ingestion of the food over the following months.

Three phases can be distinguished during this process. On the first day an initial rush-type **rapid desensitization phase** is established, followed by an **escalation or up-dosing phase** involving daily administration of the tolerated dose in the home of the patient, with controlled periodic up-dosing (usually on a weekly basis) until the maintenance or desensitization dose is reached. This represents the start of the **maintenance phase**, in which the maximum dose reached is ingested either daily or on alternating days over the subsequent months in order to maintain desensitization and protection against accidental exposure, and to secure full tolerance in at least some of the patients. This in turn must be confirmed through provocation testing after an exclusion period or treatment cessation period of one or more months.

The different management protocols use these phases in different ways as regards the doses and times. Some protocols prolong the initial rush phase to reach maintenance dosing within about 5 days [92–94], avoiding the weekly up-dosing phase which usually covers 2-4 months. This practice typically implies more adverse effects. In contrast, the initial protocols used by Patriarca et al. did not use the rush phase and prolonged the escalation phase for more months, with increments in the home of the patient introduced on a daily basis or every few days in the form of very small amounts, until the full desensitization dose was reached [95]. The mentioned group continues to maintain this protocol in modified form [96,97]. There is also some experience with the use of a SLIT desensitization phase followed by SOTI [87] – this being an option in those patients who fail to tolerate the initial rush phase. In other studies the rush phase is prolonged to two days and the up-dosing or dose escalation phase to 16 weeks [98,99]. The authors use a one-day rush phase and a 10-week dose escalation phase.

The most recent protocols typically contemplate all three phases, and follow-up evaluation after the last phase, which is essential in order to confirm tolerance.

8.4.3. Experiences and clinical trials with SOTI

8.4.3.1. Peanut

In a non-controlled SOTI study, 28 children between 1-16 years of age with peanut allergy were randomized 2:1 to active treatment or placebo. Three patients in the active treatment group abandoned the study due to adverse effects, while the rest reached the 4000 mg dose, and after 12 months were able to tolerate 5000 mg (20 peanuts), versus 280 mg in the control group (p<0.001). Significant reductions were observed in the size of the prick test and in the specific IgE and Th2 cytokine levels – with a significant increase in specific IgG4 titers and Treg cell count [100].

In another study, 29 patients completed the protocol and were able to consume 3.9 g of peanut protein, with a significant decrease in the size of the prick test and in basophil activation after 6 months of maintenance dosing. Specific IgE was seen to decrease, with a significant increase in specific IgG4 between months 12-18 of this treatment phase, together with elevations in the levels of IL-10, IL-5, IFN-γ, TNF-α and Foxp3 T cells, with demonstration of inhibition oriented towards apoptosis at genetic level [90].

In another non-controlled study, 23 patients with anaphylaxis due to peanut allergy diagnosed by DBPCFC received SOTI in the form of a rush protocol during 7 days until a dose of 0.5 g was reached. After 8 weeks of daily intake and a two-week avoidance phase, DBPCFC was repeated, with tolerance of only 0.15 g of peanut. Twenty-two patients continued with the maintenance phase, and after an average of 7 months, 13 of them (60%) reached the protective dose, with a final tolerance of 0.25-4 g of peanut (initial tolerance being 0.02-1 g). Three of the 22 patients suspended intake during this phase. A significant increase was recorded in specific IgG4, with a decrease in Th2 cytokine levels [101].

8.4.3.2. Cow's Milk (CM)

A total of 22 children with allergy to cow's milk were randomized 2:1 to SOTI with 500 mg of CM protein (15 ml CM) daily during four months, or to placebo. At final challenge testing, the active treatment group tolerated 5140 mg, versus 40 mg in the control group. The IgE levels did not vary, though the IgG4 levels increased significantly in the SOTI group [102].

Another study selected 97 children with DBPCFC-diagnosed allergy to CM with serious reactions and very high anti-CM IgE titers. Sixty patients reacted to very low doses. The subjects were randomized 1:1 to SOTI or an exclusion diet. After one year of treatment, 36% of the patients in the SOTI group were fully tolerant (> 150 ml), 54% were able to consume limited amounts of milk (5-150 ml), and 10% were unable to complete the protocol because of persistent respiratory or digestive problems. None of the control subjects passed the final DBPCFC test. [103]

A case series has described CM desensitization as a result of a rush-type SOTI protocol in four patients, with long-term desensitization being achieved in all cases [93].

A multicenter study involving 60 pediatric patients with a mean age of two years (range 24-36 months) randomized the subjects 1:1 to an exclusion diet or SOTI (2-day rush phase followed by a 16-week escalation phase until reaching a maintenance dose of 200 ml of CM). After one year, 90% of the patients in the SOTI group were fully tolerant, versus 23% of the patients in the exclusion diet group [98].

Another study randomized 30 patients diagnosed with CM allergy by DBPCFC to SOTI or placebo (soya milk), with an 18-week up-dosing phase and no prior rush period. Thirteen patients were maintained in the SOTI group, of which 10 reached the final dose of 200 ml (77%). None of the control subjects passed the DBPCFC test [104].

Thirteen patients with CM allergy were subjected to SOTI with no initial rush phase and with an 18-week escalation period until a dose of 200 ml of CM was reached. The three controls received soya milk. Tolerance was achieved in 8 of the patients in the SOTI group (7 cases of full tolerance and one partial tolerance), while the controls maintained DBPCFC positivity [105].

In another study, 28 children between 6-14 years of age with CM allergy (36% of an anaphylactic type) were recruited after oral provocation testing and randomized in a double-blind, placebo-controlled SOTI study. Sixteen out of 18 patients in the active treatment group and 8 out of 10 in the placebo series completed the study. After one year of SOTI, 81% of the children consumed 200 ml of CM or equivalent products. After confirming the absence of tolerance among the controls, the latter were enrolled in a similar protocol and were seen to tolerate 200 ml of CM after 6 months. After 3.5 years, tolerance was maintained in 79% [106].

Lastly, in another study, 60 children aged between 13 months and 6.5 years were randomized to SOTI or an exclusion diet. After 6 months, 89% of the patients in the active treatment group tolerated 200 ml of CM, versus 60% of the controls (p<0.025). A decrease in the size of the prick test was recorded in the active treatment group, while the size was seen to increase among the controls [107].

8.4.3.3. Egg

A total of 55 patients with egg allergy were included in a randomized, double-blind, placebo-controlled trial. Forty patients received SOTI. Of these, 55% passed a 5 g oral egg white powder provocation test after 10 months, versus none of the individuals in the control group. In turn, 75% of the subjects in the active treatment group passed a 10 g oral provocation test after 22 months. Desensitization was associated to a decrease in specific IgE, an increase in IgG4 after 10 months, a reduction in basophil activation, and a decrease in the size of the prick test after 22 months [108].

Eighty-four patients with egg allergy that tolerated up to 1 g of raw egg white were randomized to SOTI or an avoidance diet. After 6 months, 69% of the patients in the active treatment group and 51% of the controls passed a oral provocation test, and the mean size prick test size and specific IgE titers decreased significantly in the active treatment group. Furthermore, the patients subjected to SOTI who failed to pass the provocation test had comparatively greater tolerance and lesser severity of symptoms [107].

Of 19 patients between 4-14 years of age who started SOTI for egg allergy, 16 achieved full tolerance (85%), being able to consume a 10 g dose of powdered pasteurized egg (equivalent to one egg). In addition, a decrease was recorded in the population of effector-memory CD4+T cells, with an increase in a subclass of CD4+T cells with a hypo-proliferative and non-reactive phenotype [109]. These authors also recorded an increase in Treg cell count in those individuals who reached tolerance [110].

In a study comprising 72 patients between 5-15 years of age, the presence of egg allergy was confirmed by open oral challenge testing. Forty subjects were randomized to SOTI with powdered pasteurized egg – tolerance being achieved in 92.5% of them, and in 21.8% of the controls [111].

Another study involving 8 patients documented desensitization in 6 subjects (75%) [112].

In a retrospective review of 43 children with egg allergy, 30 were found to be willing to participate in a SOTI study with egg, involving maintenance of the maximum tolerated dose two or three times a week. The 13 patients who declined to participate conformed the control group. Nine of the 30 children in the active treatment group reached tolerance of one egg after one year of SOTI – a figure that was seen to increase to 17 out of 30 subjects after two years of treatment. In comparison, none of the controls achieved tolerance. Of the 14 desensitized patients that could be followed-up on, 11 reached full tolerance [113].

A randomized and controlled study recorded partial tolerance (10-40 ml of raw hen's egg emulsion) in 90% of the patients (n=9) subjected to SOTI with egg during 6 months, versus none of the controls [114].

8.4.3.4. Metaanalyses

A metaanalysis of SOTI with cow's milk included 5 randomized controlled trials (RCTs) and 5 observational studies that met the inclusion criteria. The RCTs comprised 218 patients and showed that oral immunotherapy versus an elimination diet increased the probability of acquiring full tolerance to cow's milk [relative risk: 10.0 (95%CI: 4.1-24.2)]. The adverse effects of immunotherapy included frequent local symptoms (16% of the doses), mild laryngeal spasm [relative risk: 12.9 (1.7-98.6)], mild asthma [rate ratio: 3.8 (95%CI: 2.9-5.0)] and reactions requiring oral corticosteroids [relative risk: 11.3 (95%CI: 2.7-46.5)] or intramuscular adrenalin [relative risk: 5.8 (95%CI: 1.6-21.9)]. The findings of the observational studies were consistent with those of the RCTs. The metaanalysis concluded that larger RCTs are needed [115].

Another metaanalysis of SOTI with cow's milk selected 16 publications, of which 5 were clinical trials. The studies were generally small and presented methodological inconsistencies, with low quality evidence. Each study used a different SOTI protocol. A total of 196 pediatric patients were studied (106 subjected to SOTI and 90 controls). Sixty-two percent of the patients in the SOTI group and 8% of the controls reached tolerance of about 200 ml of cow's milk [relative risk 6.61 (95%CI: 3.51-12.44)]. In addition, another 25% of the subjects in the SOTI group achieved partial tolerance (10-184 ml), versus none of the controls [relative risk 9.34 (95%CI: 2.72-32.09)]. None of the studies evaluated the patients some time after immunotherapy suspension. Adverse reactions were common, affecting 92% of the patients, though most were mild and of a local nature. One out of every 11 patients receiving SOTI required intramuscular adrenalin. The studies conducted to date have involved small numbers of patients, and the quality of the evidence is generally low. The current data show that SOTI can lead to desensitization in the majority of individuals with cow's milk allergy, though the development of long-term tolerance has not been established. A major drawback of such therapy is the frequency of adverse effects, although most are mild and self-limited. The use of parenteral epinephrine is not infrequent [116].

Regarding SOTI for allergy to cow's milk, achieving desensitization or even tolerance to cow's milk does not imply desensitization to milk from other mammalian species to which the patient may be sensitized [117,118] – a circumstance observed in 25% of the cases in one study [119]. Consequently, the exclusion of milk and milk products from other species must be maintained if exposure testing does not confirm the existence of tolerance to such foods.

8.4.3.5. Other foods

Individual SOTI studies have yielded positive results in reference to other foods such as tomato [94], celery [120], apple [121] or wheat [122,123].

8.4.3.6. Multiple foods

A field of great interest refers to the study of simultaneous allergy to multiple foods (up to 5), since one-third of all patients with food allergy are allergic to two or more different foods. In this respect, a trial has been carried out in 40 patients [124], of which 15 were allergic only to peanut, while 25 were allergic to more foods. The patients received up to 4 g of each food during the maintenance phase, and tolerance was seen to increase 10-fold versus the initial DBPCFC dose. The same authors have conducted a study of desensitization to multiple foods with omalizumab therapy, which allowed a shortening of the dose escalation phase [125].

8.4.3.7. Global metaanalyses

A metaanalysis of 33 case reports and 21 trials (18 RCTs and 3 controlled clinical trials) revealed a substantially lesser risk of allergic food reactions in those individuals subjected to SOTI [relative risk 0.21 (95%CI: 0.12-0.38)]. The immunological data showed a significant decrease in prick test size and an increase in the specific IgG4 titers. The risk of local reactions was seen to increase (in the form of mild oropharyngeal and gastrointestinal manifestations)[relative risk 1.47 (95%CI: 1.11-1.95)], though no significant increase in systemic reactions was observed [relative risk 1.08 (95%CI: 0.97-1.19)]. The authors concluded that there is strong evidence that oral immunotherapy is able to induce immune changes and promote desensitization to different foods. However, oral immunotherapy should not be used outside the defined experimental conditions [126].

9. Safety

The side effects associated to SOTI are generally mild or moderate, with a predominance of oropharyngeal manifestations that are easy to deal with [100–102,127,128]. However, more serious reactions have also been reported, such as generalized urticaria / angioedema, wheezing and dyspnea, laryngeal edema, intense abdominal pain and recurrent vomiting. This latter adverse effect is the most limiting problem, preventing the continuation of SOTI in 10-15% of the patients [129].

There have been reports of eosinophilic esophagitis during the maintenance phase in patients who did not have this problem before SOTI [130]. Although large series report a low incidence (2%), in our experience the problem may be more frequent (10% in a small series of patients). In this respect, the suspicion of eosinophilic esophagitis should be reinforced in cases with classic symptoms of retroesternal pain, dysphagia, or less specific like recurrent cough or digestive discomfort.

In a study of SOTI with peanut [100], most patients suffered some symptoms. During the first day of the up-dosing phase, two subjects abandoned the study, another two made use of adrenalin, and 47% developed symptoms requiring antihistamines. Symptoms were observed in 1.2% of the 407 doses during the escalation phase. Despite this observation, however, 16 of the 19 patients subjected to SOTI were able to tolerate 4000 mg with only minimal adverse effects. Likewise, in SOTI with cow's milk, 45% of the doses produced symptoms, versus 11% in the placebo group – most manifestations being mild and of an oropharyngeal nature [102]. During the first year of SOTI with egg, 25% of the 11,860 active treatment doses were associated with symptoms, versus 4% of the 4018 placebo doses [127].

The frequency of adverse reactions is 10 times greater if the patient is moreover asthmatic [17].

9.1. Triggering factors

Viral infections, menstruation and physical exercise have been associated with reductions in the tolerance threshold among patients who are already receiving SOTI maintenance doses [131]. The development of other acute disease conditions may also require temporary SOTI dose adjustment [101]. In a long-term SOTI follow-up study, 22% of the patients with allergy to cow's milk who had previously completed SOTI and had passed provocation testing with the food reported limitations in milk intake due to symptoms often associated with physical exercise (25%) and disease processes (6%) [132].

Rush-type SOTI protocols designed to shorten the interval required to reach maintenance therapy have been associated to an increase in the incidence of undesired symptoms and adrenalin use [103,101, 133, 134].

9.2. Prevention

It is advisable to avoid physical exercise in the hours before and after administration of the dose, and to temporarily reduce the amount ingested by 50% in the case of viral disease or respiratory symptoms. It is also advisable to administer the dose with other foods in order to avoid gastrointestinal adverse effects.

Antihistamines have been used as premedication, and a study has used antileukotrienes to control the gastrointestinal manifestations [135].

Thus, SOTI appears to be effective in securing desensitization, but it is not without risks. Different metaanalyses indicate that the existing body of information is still insufficient to guarantee the efficacy of the technique, and concern is still expressed about the safety of SOTI. In this respect, further studies are recommended before considering transfer of the technique from the experimental setting to clinical practice [115,116,126,136–138].

10. Long-term outcome

Does desensitization to a food imply long-term tolerance or only temporary tolerance?

Although a considerable number of years have gone by since the first inductions of oral tolerance to food were performed, few controlled studies have examined what happens after several years of SOTI. Such information is crucial in order to define the frequency with which full tolerance is achieved, as well as to identify the underlying patient-related factors involved, and characterize the different desensitization options.

A communication published in 2005 [139] reported the loss of tolerance in two patients after a two-month exclusion period following tolerance of the allergen maintenance dose during several months (cow's milk allergy with 27 weeks of tolerance of the 100 ml dose in one case, and egg allergy with 39 weeks of tolerance of half an egg in the other). In turn, a third patient who took 52 weeks in reaching the maximum dose again developed symptoms after four weeks of exclusion. In these individuals the specific IgE titers did not exceed class IV. The authors postulated that tolerance is dependent upon a series of variables such as the baseline tolerance level, the duration of SOTI, the elimination diet involved, and the course of the illness at individual level. Patients with a low probability of natural remission of their allergy may require long-term maintenance therapy. There is little information on the interval between the doses in the maintenance phase needed in order to preserve the acquired tolerance, though for safety reasons, daily intake should be recommended.

A study published in 2007 [140] reported the follow-up data corresponding to four patients who had undergone desensitization to cow's milk three years earlier. Three of them were found to have no detectable levels of specific IgE against casein, and presented no symptoms during intake – though no exclusion period followed by reintroduction of the allergen had been applied to ensure definitive tolerance.

The first long-term follow-up study on patients with cow's milk allergy [141] revealed that 86% of the individuals reached desensitization (18 out of 21 patients), and tolerance persisted in 14 out of 20 individuals (70%) upon evaluation an average of four years and 8 months after the start of desensitization [142]. In addition, none of the patients needed to use adrenalin.

Since no control groups were established, these studies could not rule out the possibility that tolerance in some of these individuals may have been attributable to natural mechanisms, and were unable to establish whether tolerance persisted after the cessation of daily allergen intake.

In another study [143], 15 patients with successful induction of desensitization to cow's milk were subjected to oral provocation after 13 to 75 weeks with doses of 16 g. This dose was tolerated by 6 of the patients, though here again there was no prior exclusion period. During the follow-up period, adverse reactions were recorded that required adrenalin injection on 6 occasions (0.2% of the doses).

In a much larger patient sample [144], 66 subjects were diagnosed with allergy to cow's milk by DBPCFC (including 44 anaphylactic cases). Initial tolerance was achieved in 64 patients (97%) – complete in 51 (> 150 ml) and partial in 13 (5-150 ml) – and was seen to persist after one year of follow-up, with significant reduction of the specific IgE titers and of the size of the prick test. As in the above studies, tolerance was not evaluated after an exclusion period.

In another study [145], following SOTI with egg or milk during a mean period of 21 months, tolerance as demonstrated by DBPCFC was recorded in 36% of the patients two months after suspending SOTI. Surprisingly, tolerance in the control group reached 35%, indicating a lack of efficacy of SOTI in achieving tolerance. In another non-controlled study, 7 patients received SOTI with egg [146], and four of them passed DBPCFC testing after 24 months. In turn, two of these four individuals passed a second DBPCFC test three months after suspending SOTI.

The commented relatively low yet promising success rates in inducing tolerance were improved upon in a follow-up study [112] involving a SOTI dosing regimen in which the maintenance dosage was increased stepwise until the levels of specific IgE against egg were < 2 kU/l. At this point DBPCFC was performed, and those patients who passed the test again underwent DBPCFC one month after suspending SOTI. The 6 patients that passed the first test also passed the second test.

Another study [87] first administered sublingual immunotherapy (SLIT) with milk, followed by patient randomization to either continuation with SLIT or conversion to SOTI with two different maintenance doses during 80 weeks. Six weeks after the end of immunotherapy, one of the 10 patients in the SLIT group (maintenance dose 7 mg/day) was found to be tolerant, versus three of the 10 patients administered 1000 mg of milk as maintenance in SOTI, and 5 of the 10 patients administered 2000 mg of milk as maintenance in SOTI. Although this was a non-controlled study with few patients, the results obtained support the idea that higher doses and longer durations of immunotherapy can afford a sustained lack of allergic responses after the end of therapy, or tolerance of the allergen.

A placebo-controlled study of SOTI with egg [127], involving 40 children in the active treatment group and 15 in the placebo group, recorded desensitization in 75% of the patients after 22 months, with a 28% tolerance rate after 24 months as established by DBPCFC performed two months after the end of SOTI. None of the controls passed the provocation test after 10 months, though they were not again subjected to oral challenge after 22 or 24 months – except one subject with specific IgE levels of < 2 kU/l, who failed to pass the test. After 30 to 36 months of follow-up, those patients who had acquired tolerance were seen to retain tolerance. This study suggests that approximately one-quarter of all children with egg allergy achieve tolerance after two years of SOTI – though the absence of provocation testing after two years in the control group may complicate interpretation of the data – particularly in view of the high degree of spontaneous tolerance registered among the controls [147].

In another study, after SOTI and 5 years of maintenance therapy with 4000 mg of peanut, 50% of the patients passed oral provocation testing and were able to incorporate peanut to their diet without restrictions [148].

11. Biological therapies associated to SOTI

In the course of the induction of oral tolerance to foods, patients may experience serious adverse effects (e.g., anaphylaxis) or problems of lesser magnitude but which preclude desensitization in 10-20% of the cases. This raises doubts not only about the safety of such techniques but also as regards their efficacy in application to patients with antecedents of food-induced anaphylactic reactions, which are precisely the individuals that could benefit most from desensitization or even tolerance.

For these reasons, different authors have recommended the use of a protective "umbrella" during the initial phases, in which IgE-mediated allergic reactions are most frequent, with a view to avoiding at least the most serious incidents.

11.1. Omalizumab

The availability of a humanized anti-IgE monoclonal antibody marked as omalizumab (Xolair®, Genentech / Novartis) has allowed its use to prevent adverse effects – particularly anaphylaxis – in those patients who because of their degree of sensitization or seriousness of previous adverse reactions are at particularly high risk. In addition to improving patient safety, such preventive treatment would result in improved efficacy, since it would allow us to reach doses sufficient to ensure complete desensitization and possible subsequent tolerance [149].

On the other hand, under this type of protection against anaphylaxis, we could shorten the escalation or up-dosing period and even reach doses higher than those previously used.

Omalizumab is a recombinant anti-IgE monoclonal antibody (anti-IgE mAb) with a molecular weight of 150 kDa; 95% of the antibody is derived from human kappa IgG1, to which certain murine complementary determinant regions are coupled. These in turn bind selectively and with high affinity to the CHε3 domain of the Fc of IgE, preventing binding of this domain to the high-affinity IgE receptors (Fc$_\varepsilon$RI) of mast cells and basophils – thus inhibiting the release of mediators by these cells through Fab binding to the antigen. Binding to the low-affinity receptors (Fc$_\varepsilon$RII) of dendritic cells, T cells, eosinophils and other cells related to allergic inflammation is also inhibited.

The absence of binding to these receptors also down-regulates the expression of IgE receptors (Fc$_\varepsilon$RI) on the part of mast cells and basophils, which is dependent upon the levels of IgE. On the other hand, the antigen-presenting cells (APCs), i.e., dendritic cells, also reduce their activity [150], and the formation of Th2 lymphocytes is consequently not stimulated. The basophils also experience a change in activity, paradoxically increasing their sensitivity to the allergen, but maintaining lowered activity in the presence of a specific IgE / total IgE ratio of < 4% [151,152].

The circulating anti-IgE/IgE complexes do not activate complement, and by keeping the antigen-binding fraction free, are able to capture antigens from the bloodstream – preventing them from reaching the specific IgE already bound to the cells.

One week after the start of treatment with anti-IgE mAb, basophil FcεRI expression is strongly suppressed, while mast cell FcεRI expression is suppressed after 10 weeks [153]. This rapid basophil suppression, together with the clinical improvement, reflects the importance of these cells [154,155].

After the first hour of treatment with omalizumab, the free IgE titers in blood decrease linearly with respect to the dose, a maximum effect being observed within 6 days, when more than 96% of the IgE levels are cleared from plasma – though total IgE increases because the half-life of the IgE-Anti-IgE complex is longer than that of IgE. The half-life of omalizumab is about 3-4 weeks [156].

11.2. Administration regimen and dose

The dose is established according to the instructions of the manufacturer in relation to the total IgE titers and patient body weight. In this regard, the minimum dose is 0.016 IU/kg/IgE (IU/ml)/4 weeks, in fractionated subcutaneous doses if needed [157].

It is estimated that 9 weeks are needed to reach the maximum effect, reduction of IgE and a decrease in the expression of its receptors. A clinical trial involving asthmatic patients found the clinical response to manifest after 16 weeks of therapy in most patients (158], though a study in children and adolescents found the maximum effect to manifest after four weeks of treatment (159,160]. Differences in criterion and patient population may account for this discrepancy. Most studies establish a minimum treatment period of 8 weeks prior to the start of induction therapy. The posterior coverage period varies, but corresponds at least to the interval required to reach the maximum maintenance dose. Treatment cessation has been abrupt, and the protective activity is known to cease completely within about three half-lives (some 9-12 weeks). Stepwise cessation over time and/or dose could result in a prolongation of the protective action without incurring in major costs increments.

11.3. Clinical applications

Soon after the marketing of omalizumab, the use of these anti-IgE antibodies in food allergy was considered [161]. Data evidencing its benefit referred to food tolerance were obtained in patients who received the drug for asthma control, and who were seen to be able to consume a larger amount of foods to which they were known to be allergic. Indeed, the patients were able to start consuming some foods which they were previously unable to consume even in very small amounts.

The usefulness of omalizumab in avoiding IgE-mediated allergic reactions other than allergic asthma, such as for example food allergy, has been evidenced in different studies [162,163]. The drug has been shown to be effective in raising the oral provocation sensitivity threshold among patients with peanut allergy, when used in monotherapy [155,164,165].

The protective activity of omalizumab has been confirmed in immunotherapy for allergic rhinitis [166,167] and asthma [168]. Its utilization in rush immunotherapy [169], involving an increased frequency of systemic adverse reactions, afforded increased protection, including protection against anaphylaxis, when administered during the 9 weeks prior to immunotherapy and then for 12 months concomitant to immunotherapy. In this respect, omalizumab was seen to be superior to the use of antihistamines as premedication. Likewise, increased efficacy of immunotherapy has been documented in patients receiving anti-IgE mAb.

11.4. Clinical trials with omalizumab and SOTI

The above considerations have led to the use of omalizumab pretreatment in food tolerance induction protocols [170]. To date, only non-controlled double-blind pilot studies involving few patients are available, though several randomized, double-blind, placebo-controlled trials are currently underway.

The first published study to report a possible role for omalizumab administered together with oral immunotherapy in allergic patients [171] assessed the usefulness of the drug in inducing tolerance to cow's milk in the context of a phase I pilot trial involving a small patient sample. Evaluation of the immunological changes revealed the inhibition of cutaneous mast cells and peripheral blood basophils in a non-specific allergen manner during therapy with omalizumab, and in an antigen-specific manner after completing the milk desensitization protocol [172].

Thirteen patients with peanut allergy confirmed by DBPCFC participated in a pilot trial involving pretreatment with omalizumab during 12 weeks, after which the drug was continued in combination with the immunotherapy up-dosing phase for another 8 weeks [173]. This made it possible to increase the initial peanut dose without major side effects, and to shorten the weekly up-dosing phase. With the dose of the first day (992 mg of peanut flour, equivalent to about 2 peanuts), the patients could be protected against anaphylactic reactions caused by accidental ingestion of the allergen. Within 8 weeks, the maintenance dose of 4000 mg was reached in 12 out of 13 patients, with tolerance after 30-32 weeks of 8000 mg as evidenced by DBPCFC – this dose being 160-400 times greater than the dose causing symptoms at first DBPCFC testing. Fifty-four percent of the patients (7 out of 13 individuals) suffered no adverse reactions during the first rush phase, while the rest experienced grade 1 effects requiring antihistamine use in only two patients. During the weekly up-dosing phase, 49 adverse effects were documented, of which 97% corresponded to grade 1 and none to grade 3. During maintenance therapy, without the administration of omalizumab, a total of 17 adverse effects were recorded, two of which corresponded to grade 3. Those patients that experienced adverse effects after suspending omalizumab had higher specific IgE titers both at the end and at the start, as well as a larger prick test size. The prolongation of omalizumab in patients of this kind was thus proposed.

Another non-controlled phase I study used omalizumab during 16 weeks, including 8 weeks as pretreatment, in the induction of tolerance to different foods in combination with oral immunotherapy [174]. This management strategy allowed rapid desensitization using higher starting doses than those used in another trial carried out by the same authors [175], involving up to 5 foods at once, and with no grade 2 (moderate) or grade 3 (severe) symptoms during the up-dosing phase. Adrenalin proved necessary in only one case, during the maintenance phase (representing 0.01% of the administered maintenance doses).

11.5. Side effects of omalizumab

These antibodies have been reported to cause side effects [156,157] – the most important being local inflammatory reactions. Anaphylaxis has been reported in 0.2% of the patients. It has been suggested that such treatment should be administered in an appropriate healthcare setting, with an adequate period of observation after administration (2 hours on the first occasion and half an hour with the subsequent doses), with the availability of preloaded adrenalin [176,177]. A recent study has observed no increased risk of tumors associated to long-term treatment [178]. In contrast, the risk of parasitic infestations appears to increase; treatment in high-prevalence areas therefore should be restricted.

Another very important aspect to be taken into account is the cost-effectiveness ratio, with a view to ascertaining whether the treatment is acceptable from the healthcare and insurance perspectives. No such data referred to the specific therapeutic indication of food allergy have yet been obtained, however.

Further clinical data are currently needed, involving double-blind, placebo-controlled trials, as well as cost-effectiveness analyses, in order to establish the recommendations for use in concrete patient groups as treatment in combination with SOTI, such as for example:

- Patients at particularly high risk due to increased sensitivity (usually associated to increased clinical reactivity) and/or who have suffered serious reactions to the food allergen

- Patients unable to reach levels considered necessary to ensure desensitization

- Protocols involving a rush phase and rapid up-dosing

- Patients undergoing desensitization to several foods at the same time

11.6. Interferon-γ and SOTI

Few data are available on the usefulness of interferon-γ in combination with SOTI, though the preliminary results are encouraging [179].

12. Conclusion

Immunoglobulin E-mediated food allergy in high risk patients or in individuals with a poor prognosis in terms of tolerance may benefit from new immunotherapeutic techniques such as SOTI. The advantages of SOTI are a great decrease in the risk of serious allergic reactions in patients with particularly severe food allergy, and the possibility of introducing such foods in the patient diet – with the resulting improvement in quality of life. Further studies are needed to better characterize those patients most amenable to effective SOTI, establish the required duration of therapy, define the immunological markers for assessing the course of treatment, the role of associated biological therapies and draft safe and effective consensus-based protocols and guides, before transferring desensitization to the general clinical practice setting.

There is evidence that this new approach is changing the management paradigm in food allergy, and in our opinion, like other authors [180], possibly it's time for the practice of SOTI in medical centers with medical staff trained and under secure supervision of his risks.

Author details

José Manuel Lucas*, Ana Moreno-Salvador and Luis García-Marcos

*Address all correspondence to: josem.lucas@carm.es

Pediatric Clinical Immunology and Allergy Unit, "Virgen de la Arrixaca" University Children's Hospital, University of Murcia, Murcia, Spain

References

[1] Sicherer SH. Epidemiology of food allergy. J Allergy Clin Immunol. 2011;127(3):594–602.

[2] Chafen JJS, Newberry SJ, Riedl MA, Bravata DM, Maglione M, Suttorp MJ, et al. Diagnosing and managing common food allergies: a systematic review. JAMA. 2010;303(18):1848–56.

[3] Sicherer SH, Sampson HA. Food allergy: Epidemiology, pathogenesis, diagnosis, and treatment. J Allergy Clin Immunol. 2014;133(2):291–307.

[4] Prescott SL, Pawankar R, Allen KJ, Campbell DE, Sinn JK, Fiocchi A, et al. A global survey of changing patterns of food allergy burden in children. World Allergy Organ J. 2013;6(1):21.

[5] Rona RJ, Keil T, Summers C, Gislason D, Zuidmeer L, Sodergren E, et al. The prevalence of food allergy: a meta-analysis. J Allergy Clin Immunol. 2007;120(3):638–46.

[6] Gupta RS, Springston EE, Warrier MR, Smith B, Kumar R, Pongracic J, et al. The prevalence, severity, and distribution of childhood food allergy in the United States. Pediatrics. 2011;128(1):e9–17. http://pediatrics.aappublications.org/content/128/1/e9.long (Accesed 02 September 2014)

[7] Osborne NJ, Koplin JJ, Martin PE, Gurrin LC, Lowe AJ, Matheson MC, et al. Prevalence of challenge-proven IgE-mediated food allergy using population-based sampling and predetermined challenge criteria in infants. J Allergy Clin Immunol. 2011;127:668–76.

[8] Prescott S, Allen KJ. Food allergy: riding the second wave of the allergy epidemic. Pediatr Allergy Immunol. 2011;22(2):155–60.

[9] Johnson J, Malinovschi A, Alving K. Ten year review reveals changing trends and severity of allergic reactions to nuts and other foods. Acta Paediatr. 2014;103(8):862–7.

[10] Berin M, Sampson H. Food allergy: an enigmatic epidemic. Trends Immunol. 2013;34(8):390–7.

[11] Venter C, Hasan Arshad S, Grundy J, Pereira B, Bernie Clayton C, Voigt K, et al. Time trends in the prevalence of peanut allergy: three cohorts of children from the same geographical location in the UK. Allergy. 2010;65(1):103–8.

[12] McGowan EC, Keet CA. Prevalence of self-reported food allergy in the National Health and Nutrition Examination Survey (NHANES) 2007-2010. J Allergy Clin Immunol. 2013;132(5):1216–9.

[13] Wood RA. The natural history of food allergy. Pediatrics. 2003;111(6 Pt 3):1631–7.

[14] Hu Y, Chen J, Li H. Comparison of food allergy prevalence among Chinese infants in Chongqing, 2009 versus 1999. Pediatr Int. 2010;52(5):820–4.

[15] Martorell A, Plaza AM, Nevot S, Echeverria L, Alonso E, Garde J. The predictive value of specific immunoglobulin E levels in serum for the outcome of the development of tolerance in cow's milk allergy. Allergol et Immunopathol (Mad). 2008;36:14–5.

[16] Skripak JM, Matsui EC, Mudd K, Wood R a. The natural history of IgE-mediated cow's milk allergy. J Allergy Clin Immunol. 2007;120(5):1172–7.

[17] Boyano-Martínez T, García-Ara C, Pedrosa M, Díaz-Pena JM, Quirce S. Accidental allergic reactions in children allergic to cow's milk proteins. J Allergy Clin Immunol. 2009;123(4):883–8.

[18] Bock SA, Muñoz-Furlong A, Sampson HA. Further fatalities caused by anaphylactic reactions to food, 2001-2006. J Allergy Clin Immunol. 2007;119(4):1016–8.

[19] Eggesbo M, Botten G, Halvorsen R, Magnus P. The prevalence of allergy to egg: a population-based study in young children. Allergy. 2001;1992(56):403–11.

[20] Boyano-Martínez T, García-Ara C, Díaz-Pena JM, Martín-Esteban M. Prediction of tolerance on the basis of quantification of egg white-specific IgE antibodies in children with egg allergy. J Allergy Clin Immunol. 2002;110(2):304–9.

[21] Martorell A, Alonso E, Boné J, Echeverría L, López MC, Martín F, et al. Position document: IgE-mediated allergy to egg protein. Allergol Immunopathol. 2013;41(5): 320–36.

[22] Savage JH, Matsui EC, Skripak JM, Wood RA. The natural history of egg allergy. J Allergy Clin Immunol. 2007;120(6):1413–7.

[23] Liu AH, Jaramillo R, Sicherer SH, Wood RA, Bock SA, Burks AW, et al. National prevalence and risk factors for food allergy and relationship to asthma: results from the National Health and Nutrition Examination Survey 2005-2006. J Allergy Clin Immunol. 2010;126(4):798–806.

[24] Hourihane JO, Aiken R, Briggs R, Gudgeon LA, Grimshaw KEC, DunnGalvin A, et al. The impact of government advice to pregnant mothers regarding peanut avoidance on the prevalence of peanut allergy in United Kingdom children at school entry. J Allergy Clin Immunol. 2007;119(5):1197–202.

[25] Sicherer SH, Sampson HA. Peanut allergy: emerging concepts and approaches for an apparent epidemic. J Allergy Clin Immunol. 2007;120(3):491–503.

[26] Skolnick HS, Conover-Walker MK, Koerner CB, Sampson HA, Burks W, Wood RA. The natural history of peanut allergy. J Allergy Clin Immunol. 2001;107(2):367–74.

[27] Fleischer DM, Conover-Walker MK, Christie L, Burks AW, Wood RA. The natural progression of peanut allergy: Resolution and the possibility of recurrence. J Allergy Clin Immunol. 2003;112(1):183–9.

[28] Clark AT, Ewan PW. Good prognosis, clinical features, and circumstances of peanut and tree nut reactions in children treated by a specialist allergy center. J Allergy Clin Immunol. 2008;122(2):286–9.

[29] Yu JW, Kagan R, Verreault N, Nicolas N, Joseph L, St Pierre Y, et al. Accidental ingestions in children with peanut allergy. J Allergy Clin Immunol. 2006;118(2):466–72.

[30] Wang J. Management of the patient with multiple food allergies. Curr Allergy Asthma Rep. 2010;10(4):271–7.

[31] Sicherer SH, Noone SA, Muñoz-Furlong A. The impact of childhood food allergy on quality of life. Ann Allergy Asthma Immunol. 2001;87(6):461–4.

[32] Sova C, Feuling MB, Baumler M, Gleason L, Tam JS, Zafra H, et al. Systematic review of nutrient intake and growth in children with multiple IgE-mediated food allergies. Nutr Clin Pract. 2013;28(6):669–75.

[33] Joshi P, Mofidi S, Sicherer SH, York N. Food and drug reactions and anaphylaxis Interpretation of commercial food ingredient labels by parents of food-allergic children. J Allergy Clin Immunol. 2002;109(6):1019–21.

[34] Altschul AS, Scherrer DL, Muñoz-Furlong A, Sicherer SH. Manufacturing and labeling issues for commercial products: relevance to food allergy. J Allergy Clin Immunol. 2001;108(3):468.

[35] Fleischer DM, Perry TT, Atkins D, Wood RA, Burks AW, Jones SM, et al. Allergic reactions to foods in preschool-aged children in a prospective observational food allergy study. Pediatrics. 2012;130(1):e25–32. http://pediatrics.aappublications.org/content/130/1/e25.long (Accesed 02 September 2014)

[36] Pumphrey RSH, Gowland MH. Further fatal allergic reactions to food in the United Kingdom, 1999-2006. J Allergy Clin Immunol. 2007;119(4):1018–9.

[37] Liew WK, Williamson E, Tang MLK. Anaphylaxis fatalities and admissions in Australia. J Allergy Clin Immunol. 2009;123(2):434–42.

[38] Simons FER, Ardusso LR, Bilò MB, Cardona V, Ebisawa M, El-Gamal YM, et al. International consensus on (ICON) anaphylaxis. World Allergy Organ J. 2014;7(1):9. http://www.waojournal.org/content/7/1/9 (Accessed 02 September 2014)

[39] Järvinen K, Celestin J. Anaphylaxis avoidance and management: educating patients and their caregivers. J Asthma Allergy. 2014;7:95–104.

[40] Simons E, Sicherer SH, Simons FER. At What Age Should Children and Teenagers Be Able To Recognize Anaphylaxis and Self-Inject Epinephrine? J Allergy Clin Immunol. 2012;129(2):AB179.

[41] Gallagher M, Worth A, Cunningham-Burley S, Sheikh A. Epinephrine auto-injector use in adolescents at risk of anaphylaxis: a qualitative study in Scotland, UK. Clin Exp Allergy. 2011;41(6):869–77.

[42] Marrs T, Lack G. Why do few food-allergic adolescents treat anaphylaxis with adrenaline?--Reviewing a pressing issue. Pediatr Allergy Immunol. 2013;24(3):222–9.

[43] Gupta RS. Anaphylaxis in the Young Adult Population. Am J Med. 2014;127(1):S17–S24.

[44] Bollinger ME, Dahlquist LM, Mudd K, Sonntag C, Dillinger L, McKenna K. The impact of food allergy on the daily activities of children and their families. Ann Allergy Asthma Immunol. 2006;96(3):415–21.

[45] Cummings AJ, Knibb RC, Erlewyn-Lajeunesse M, King RM, Roberts G, Lucas JS a. Management of nut allergy influences quality of life and anxiety in children and their mothers. Pediatr Allergy Immunol. 2010;21(4 Pt 1):586–94.

[46] Lieberman JA, Sicherer SH. Quality of life in food allergy. Curr Opin Allergy Clin Immunol. 2011;11(3):236–42.

[47] Gupta RS, Springston EE, Kim JS, Smith B, Pongracic J a, Wang X, et al. Food allergy knowledge, attitudes, and beliefs of primary care physicians. Pediatrics. 2010;125(1): 126–32. http://pediatrics.aappublications.org/content/125/1/126.long (Accesed 02 September 2014)

[48] Cummings AJ, Knibb RC, King RM, Lucas JS. The psychosocial impact of food allergy and food hypersensitivity in children, adolescents and their families: a review. Allergy. 2010 ;65(8):933–45.

[49] Lieberman JA, Weiss C, Furlong TJ, Sicherer M, Sicherer SH. Bullying among pediatric patients with food allergy. Ann Allergy Asthma Immunol. Ann. Allergy Asthma Immunol. 2010;105(4):282–6.

[50] Patel DA, Holdford DA, Edwards E, Carroll NV. Estimating the economic burden of food-induced allergic reactions and anaphylaxis in the United States. J Allergy Clin Immunol. 2011;128(1):110–5.

[51] Gupta R, Holdford D, Bilaver L, Dyer A, Holl JL, Meltzer D. The economic impact of childhood food allergy in the United States. JAMA Pediatr. 2013;167(11):1026–31.

[52] Miles S, Fordham R, Mills C, Valovirta E, Mugford M. A framework for measuring costs to society of IgE-mediated food allergy. Allergy. 2005 ;60(8):996–1003.

[53] Chehade M, Mayer L. Oral tolerance and its relation to food hypersensitivities. J Allergy Clin Immunol. 2005;115(1):3–12.

[54] Hadis U, Wahl B, Schulz O, Hardtke-Wolenski M, Schippers A, Wagner N, et al. Intestinal Tolerance Requires Gut Homing and Expansion of FoxP3+Regulatory T Cells in the Lamina Propria. Immunity. 2011;34:237–46.

[55] Berin M. Mucosal antibodies in the regulation of tolerance and allergy to foods. Semin immunopathol. 2012;34(5):633–42.

[56] Vickery B, Scurlock A, Jones S, Burks A. Mechanisms of immune tolerance relevant to food allergy. J Allergy Clin Immunol. 2011 ;127(3):576–86.

[57] Jo J, Garssen J, Knippels L, Sandalova E. Role of Cellular Immunity in Cow's Milk Allergy: Pathogenesis, Tolerance Induction, and Beyond. Mediators Inflamm. 2014;2014:249784. http://www.hindawi.com/journals/mi/2014/249784/ (Accesed 02 September 2014)

[58] Palomares O. The Role of Regulatory T Cells in IgE-Mediated Food Allergy. J Investig Allergol Clin Immunol. 2013;23(6):371–82.

[59] Boyce JA, Assa'ad A, Burks AW, Jones SM, Sampson HA, Wood RA, et al. Guidelines for the Diagnosis and Management of Food Allergy in the United States: Summary of the NIAID-Sponsored Expert Panel Report. J Allergy Clin Immunol. 2010;126(6): 1105–18.

[60] Burks AW, Calderon MA, Casale T, Cox L, Demoly P, Jutel M, et al. Update on allergy immunotherapy: American Academy of Allergy, Asthma & Immunology/European Academy of Allergy and Clinical Immunology/PRACTALL consensus report. J Allergy Clin Immunol. 2013;131(5):1288–96.

[61] Jones SM, Burks AW, Dupont C. State of the art on food allergen immunotherapy: oral, sublingual, and epicutaneous. J Allergy Clin Immunol. 2014;133(2):318–23.

[62] Scheurer D. Pollen-food allergy syndrome. Clin Exp allergy. 2000;30:905–7.

[63] Asero R. Effects of birch pollen-specific immunotherapy on apple allergy in birch pollen-hypersensitive patients. Clin Exp allergy. 1998;28(11):1368–73.

[64] Asero R. Fennel, cucumber, and melon allergy successfully treated with pollen-specific injection immunotherapy. Ann Allergy Asthma Immunol. 2000;84:460–2.

[65] Bolhaar S, Tiemessen M. Efficacy of birch-pollen immunotherapy on cross-reactive food allergy confirmed by skin tests and double-blind food challenges. Clin Exp Allergy. 2004;34:761–9. http://onlinelibrary.wiley.com/doi/10.1111/j. 1365-2222.2004.1939.x/full (Accesed 02 September 2014)

[66] Nelson HS, Lahr J, Rule R, Bock A, Leung D. Treatment of anaphylactic sensitivity to peanuts by immunotherapy with injections of aqueous peanut extract. J Allergy Clin Immunol. 1997;99(6 Pt 1):744–51.

[67] Oppenheimer JJ, Nelson HS, Bock SA, Christensen F, Leung DY. Treatment of peanut allergy with rush immunotherapy. J Allergy Clin Immunol. 1992;90:256–62.

[68] Prickett SR, Voskamp AL, Phan T, Dacumos-Hill A, Mannering SI, Rolland JM, et al. Ara h 1 CD4+T cell epitope-based peptides: candidates for a peanut allergy therapeutic. Clin Exp Allergy. 2013;43(6):684–97.

[69] Novak N, Gros E, Bieber T, Allam J-P. Human skin and oral mucosal dendritic cells as "good guys" and "bad guys" in allergic immune responses. Clin Exp Immunol. 2010;161(1):28–33.

[70] Dioszeghy V, Mondoulet L, Dhelft V, Ligouis M, Puteaux E, Benhamou P-H, et al. Epicutaneous immunotherapy results in rapid allergen uptake by dendritic cells through intact skin and downregulates the allergen-specific response in sensitized mice. J Immunol. 2011;186:5629–37.

[71] Dupont C, Kalach N, Soulaines P, Legoué-Morillon S, Piloquet H, Benhamou P-H. Cow's milk epicutaneous immunotherapy in children: A pilot trial of safety, acceptability, and impact on allergic reactivity. J Allergy Clin Immunol. 2010;125(5):1165–7.

[72] Dupont C, Bourrier T, de Blay F, Guénard-Bilbault L, Sauvage C, Cousin M-O, et al. Peanut Epicutaneous Immunotherapy (EPIT) In Peanut-Allergic Children: 18 Months Treatment In The Arachild Study. J Allergy Clin Immunol. 2014;133(2):AB102.

[73] Mousallem T, Burks AW. Immunology in the Clinic Review Series; focus on allergies: immunotherapy for food allergy. Clin Exp Immunol. 2012;167(1):26–31.

[74] Moingeon P. Update on immune mechanisms associated with sublingual immunotherapy: practical implications for the clinician. J Allergy Clin Immunol Pract. 2013;1(3):228–41.

[75] Cox LS, Larenas Linnemann D, Nolte H, Weldon D, Finegold I, Nelson HS. Sublingual immunotherapy: a comprehensive review. J Allergy Clin Immunol. 2006 ;117(5): 1021–35.

[76] Bousquet J, Casale T, Lockey RF, Baena-cagnani CE, Pawankar R, Potter PC, et al. Sub-Lingual Immunotherapy. World Allergy Organ J. 2009;2(11):233–81. http://www.waojournal.org/content/2/11/233 (Accesed 02 September 2014)

[77] Bergmann K-C, Wolf H, Schnitker J. Effect of Pollen-Specific Sublingual Immunotherapy on Oral Allergy Syndrome. World Allergy Organ J. 2008;1:79–84. http://www.waojournal.org/content/1/5/79 (Accesed 02 September 2014)

[78] Bernardini R, Campodonico P, Burastero S, Azzari C, Novembre E, Pucci N, et al. Sublingual immunotherapy with a latex extract in paediatric patients: a double-blind, placebo-controlled study. Curr Med Res Opin. 2006;22(8):1515–22.

[79] Mempel M, Rakoski J, Ring J, Ollert M. Severe anaphylaxis to kiwi fruit: Immunologic changes related to successful sublingual allergen immunotherapy. J Allergy Clin Immunol. 2003;111(6):1406–9.

[80] Kerzl R, Simonowa A, Ring J, Ollert M, Mempel M. Life-threatening anaphylaxis to kiwi fruit: protective sublingual allergen immunotherapy effect persists even after discontinuation. J Allergy Clin Immunol. 2007;119(2):507–8.

[81] Enrique E, Pineda F, Malek T, Bartra J, Basagaña M, Tella R, et al. Sublingual immunotherapy for hazelnut food allergy: a randomized, double-blind, placebo-controlled study with a standardized hazelnut extract. J Allergy Clin Immunol. 2005;116(5): 1073–9.

[82] Enrique E, Malek T, Pineda F. Sublingual immunotherapy for hazelnut food allergy: a follow-up study. Ann Allergy Asthma Immunol. 2008 ;100:283–4.

[83] Fernández-Rivas M, Garrido Fernández S, Nadal J a, Díaz de Durana MDA, García BE, González-Mancebo E, et al. Randomized double-blind, placebo-controlled trial of sublingual immunotherapy with a Pru p 3 quantified peach extract. Allergy. 2009;64(6):876–83.

[84] De Boissieu D, Dupont C. Sublingual immunotherapy for cow's milk protein allergy: a preliminary report. Allergy. 2006 ;61(10):1238–9.

[85] Kim EH, Bird JA, Kulis M, Laubach S, Pons L, Shreffler W, et al. Sublingual immunotherapy for peanut allergy: clinical and immunologic evidence of desensitization. J Allergy Clin Immunol. 2011;127(3):640–6.

[86] Fleischer D, Burks A, Vickery B. Sublingual immunotherapy for peanut allergy: a randomized, double-blind, placebo-controlled multicenter trial. J Allergy Clin Immunol. 2013;131(1):119–27.

[87] Keet C. The safety and efficacy of sublingual and oral immunotherapy for milk allergy. J Allergy Clin Immunol. 2012;129(2):448–55.

[88] Chin SJ, Vickery BP, Kulis MD, Kim EH, Varshney P, Steele P, et al. Sublingual versus oral immunotherapy for peanut-allergic children: a retrospective comparison. J Allergy Clin Immunol. 2013;132(2):476–8.

[89] Scurlock AM, Vickery BP, Hourihane JO, Burks AW. Pediatric food allergy and mucosal tolerance. Mucosal Immunol. 2010;3(4):345–54.

[90] Jones SM, Pons L, Roberts JL, Scurlock AM, Perry TT, Kulis M, et al. Clinical efficacy and immune regulation with peanut oral immunotherapy. J Allergy Clin Immunol; 2009;124(2):292–300.

[91] Thyagarajan A, Jones S. Evidence of pathway specific basophil anergy induced by peanut oral immunotherapy in peanut allergic children. Clin Exp Allergy. 2012 ;

42(8):1197–205.   http://onlinelibrary.wiley.com/doi/10.1111/j.1365-2222.2012.04028.x/ full (Acessed 02 September 2014)

[92] Bauer A, Mudiyanselage SE, Wigger-Alberti P, Elsner P. Oral rush desensitization to milk.   Allergy.   1999   ;54:894–5.   http://onlinelibrary.wiley.com/doi/10.1034/j. 1398-9995.1999.00228.x/full (Accesed 02 September 2014)

[93] Martorell A, Félix Toledo R, Cerdá Mir JC, Martorell Calatayud A. Oral rush desensitization to cow milk. Following of desensitized patients during three years. Allergol Immunopathol (Mad). 2007;35(5):174–6.

[94] Nucera E, Schiavino D, Buonomo A, Roncallo C, Pollastrini E, Lombardo C, et al. Oral rush desensitization with tomato: a case report. J Investig Allergol Clin Immunol. 2006;16(3):214–7.

[95] Patriarca G, Schiavino D, Nucera E. Food allergy in children: results of a standardized protocol for oral desensitization. Hepatogastroenterology. 1998;45:32–8. http:// www.apalweb.it/FILES/RISORSE/Full-text/Patriarca1998_oral_desensitization.pdf (Accesed 02 September 2014)

[96] Patriarca G, Nucera E, Pollastrini E, Roncallo C, Pasquale T De, Lombardo C, et al. Oral Specific Desensitization in Food-Allergic Children. Dig Dis Sci. 2007;52:1662–72.

[97] Nucera E, Aruanno A, Lombardo C, Patriarca G, Schiavino D. Apple desensitization in two patients with PR-10 proteins allergy. Allergy. 2010 ;65(8):1060–1.

[98] Martorell A, De la Hoz B, Ibáñez MD, Bone J, Terrados MS, Michavila A, et al. Oral desensitization as a useful treatment in 2-year-old children with cow's milk allergy. Clin Exp Allergy. 2011;41(9):1297–304.

[99] Alvaro M, Giner MT, Vázquez M, Lozano J, Domínguez O, Piquer M, et al. Specific oral desensitization in children with IgE-mediated cow's milk allergy. Evolution in one year. Eur J Pediatr. 2012 ;171:1389–95.

[100] Varshney P, Jones SM, Scurlock AM, Perry TT, Kemper A, Steele P, et al. A randomized controlled study of peanut oral immunotherapy: clinical desensitization and modulation of the allergic response. J Allergy Clin Immunol. 2011;127(3):654–60.

[101] Blumchen K, Ulbricht H, Staden U, Dobberstein K, Beschorner J, de Oliveira LCL, et al. Oral peanut immunotherapy in children with peanut anaphylaxis. J Allergy Clin Immunol. 2010;126(1):83–91.

[102] Skripak J, Nash S, Rowley H, Brereton N. A randomized, double-blind, placebo-controlled study of milk oral immunotherapy for cow's milk allergy. J Allergy Clin Immunol. 2008;122(6):1154–60.

[103] Longo G, Barbi E, Berti I, Meneghetti R, Pittalis A, Ronfani L, et al. Specific oral tolerance induction in children with very severe cow's milk-induced reactions. J Allergy Clin Immunol. 2008;121(2):343–7.

[104] Pajno GB, Caminiti L, Ruggeri P, De Luca R, Vita D, La Rosa M, et al. Oral immuno-therapy for cow's milk allergy with a weekly up-dosing regimen: a randomized sin-gle-blind controlled study. Ann Allergy Asthma Immunol. 2010;105(5):376–81.

[105] Caminiti L, Passalacqua G, Barberi S, Vita D, Barberio G, De Luca R, et al. A new pro-tocol for specific oral tolerance induction in children with IgE-mediated cow's milk allergy. Allergy Asthma Proc. 2014;30(4):443–8.

[106] Salmivesi S, Korppi M, Mäkelä MJ, Paassilta M. Milk oral immunotherapy is effective in school-aged children. Acta Paediatr. 2013;102(2):172–6.

[107] Morisset M, Moneret-Vautrin DA, Guenard L, Cuny JM, Frentz P, Hatahet R, et al. Oral desensitization in children with milk and egg allergies obtains recovery in a sig-nificant proportion of cases. A randomized study in 60 children with cow's milk al-lergy and 90 children with egg allergy. Eur Ann Allergy Clin Immunol. 2007;39(1): 12–9.

[108] Burks AW, Jones SM, Wood RA, Fleischer DM, Sicherer SH, Lindblad RW, et al. Oral immunotherapy for treatment of egg allergy in children. N Engl J Med. 2012;367(3): 233–43. http://www.nejm.org/doi/full/10.1056/NEJMoa1200435 (Accesed 02 Septem-ber 2014)

[109] Fuentes-Aparicio V, Alonso-Lebrero E, Zapatero L, Infante S, Lorente R, Angeles Muñoz-Fernández M, et al. Oral immunotherapy in hen's egg-allergic children in-creases a hypo-proliferative subset of CD4+T cells that could constitute a marker of tolerance achievement. Pediatr Allergy Immunol. 2012;23(7):648–53.

[110] Fuentes-Aparicio V, Alonso-Lebrero E, Zapatero L, Infante S, Lorente R, Muñoz-Fer-nández MÁ, et al. Induction of Treg cells after oral immunotherapy in hen's egg-al-lergic children. Pediatr Allergy Immunol. 2014;25(1):103–6.

[111] Fuentes-Aparicio V, Alvarez-Perea A, Infante S, Zapatero L, D'Oleo A, Alonso-Leb-rero E. Specific oral tolerance induction in paediatric patients with persistent egg al-lergy. Allergol et Immunopathol (Mad). 2013;41(3):143–50.

[112] Vickery B, Pons L, Kulis M, Steele P. Individualized IgE-based dosing of egg oral im-munotherapy and the development of tolerance. Ann Allergy Asthma Immunol. 2010;105(6):444–50.

[113] Sudo K, Taniuchi S, Takahashi M, Soejima K, Hatano Y, Nakano K, et al. Home-based oral immunotherapy (OIT) with an intermittent loading protocol in children unlikely to outgrow egg allergy. Allergy Asthma Clin Immunol. 2014;10(1):11.

[114] Dello Iacono I, Tripodi S, Calvani M, Panetta V, Verga MC, Miceli Sopo S. Specific oral tolerance induction with raw hen's egg in children with very severe egg allergy: a randomized controlled trial. Pediatr Allergy Immunol 2013;24(1):66–74.

[115] Brożek JL, Terracciano L, Hsu J, Kreis J, Compalati E, Santesso N, et al. Oral immunotherapy for IgE-mediated cow's milk allergy: a systematic review and meta-analysis. Clin Exp Allergy. 2012;42(3):363–74.

[116] Yeung J, Kloda L, McDevitt J, Ben-Shoshan M, Alizadehfar R. Oral immunotherapy for milk allergy (Review). Cochrane Database Syst Rev. 2012;(11).

[117] Alonso-Lebrero E, Fuentes V, Zapatero L, Pérez-Bustamante S, Pineda F. Goat's milk allergies in children following specific oral tolerance induction to cow's milk. Allergol et Immunopathol (Mad). 2008;36(3):180–1.

[118] Rodríguez del Río P, Sánchez-García S, Escudero C, Pastor-Vargas C, Sánchez Hernández JJ, Pérez-Rangel I, et al. Allergy to goat's and sheep's milk in a population of cow's milk-allergic children treated with oral immunotherapy. Pediatr Allergy Immunol. 2012;23(2):128–32.

[119] Piquer Gibert M, Machinena SA, Alvaro Lozano M, Giner Muñoz MT, Domínguez Sánchez O, Lozano Blasco J, et al. Is other bovid mammals milk tolerated by children who have been submitted to cow's milk oral immunotherapy?. Clin Transl Allergy. 2014;4(Suppl 1):P28.

[120] Ruëff F, Eberlein-König B, Przybilla B. Oral hyposensitization with celery juice. Allergy. 2001;56(1):82–3.

[121] Nucera E, Aruanno A, Lombardo C, Patriarca G, Schiavino D. Apple desensitization in two patients with PR-10 proteins allergy. Allergy. 2010;65(8):1060–1.

[122] Nucera E, Pollastrini E, De Pasquale T, Buonomo A, Roncallo C, Lombardo C, et al. New protocol for desensitization to wheat allergy in a single case. Dig Dis Sci. 2005;50(9):1708–9.

[123] Pacharn P, Siripipattanamongkol N. Successful wheat-specific oral immunotherapy in highly sensitive individuals with a novel multirush/maintenance regimen. Asia Pac Allergy. 2014;4:180–3.

[124] Bégin P, Winterroth LC, Dominguez T, Wilson SP, Bacal L, Mehrotra A, et al. Safety and feasibility of oral immunotherapy to multiple allergens for food allergy. Allergy Asthma Clin Immunol. 2014;10(1):1.

[125] Bégin P, Dominguez T, Wilson SP, Bacal L, Mehrotra A, Kausch B, et al. Phase 1 results of safety and tolerability in a rush oral immunotherapy protocol to multiple foods using Omalizumab. Allergy Asthma Clin Immunol. 2014;10(1):7.

[126] Nurmatov U, Devereux G, Worth A, Healy L, Sheikh A. Effectiveness and safety of orally administered immunotherapy for food allergies: a systematic review and meta-analysis. Br J Nutr. 2014;111(1):12–22.

[127] Burks A, Jones S. Oral immunotherapy for treatment of egg allergy in children. N Engl J Med. 2012 ;367(3):233–43. http://www.nejm.org/doi/full/10.1056/NEJMoa1200435 (Accesed 02 September 2014)

[128] Hofmann AM, Scurlock AM, Jones SM, Palmer KP, Lokhnygina Y, Steele PH, et al. Safety of a peanut oral immunotherapy protocol in peanut allergic children. J Allergy Clin Immunol. 2009;124(2):286–91.

[129] Vickery BP, Scurlock AM, Steele P, Kamilaris J, Hiegel AM, Carlisle SK, et al. Early and Persistent Gastrointestinal Side Effects Predict Withdrawal from Peanut Oral Immunotherapy (OIT). J Allergy Clin Immunol. 2011;127(2):AB26[Abstract].

[130] Sánchez-García S, Rodríguez Del Río P, Escudero C, Martínez-Gómez MJ, Ibáñez MD. Possible eosinophilic esophagitis induced by milk oral immunotherapy. J Allergy Clin Immunol. 2012 ;129(4):1155–7.

[131] Varshney P, Steele P, Vickery B. Adverse reactions during peanut oral immunotherapy home dosing. J Allergy Clin Immunol. 2009;124(6):1351–2.

[132] Keet CA, Seopaul S, Knorr S, Narisety S, Skripak J, Wood RA. Long-term follow-up of oral immunotherapy for cow's milk allergy. J Allergy Clin Immunol. 2013;132(3): 737–9.

[133] Barbi E, Longo G, Berti I, Neri E, Saccari A, Rubert L, et al. Adverse effects during specific oral tolerance induction: in-hospital "rush" phase. Eur Ann Allergy Clin Immunol. 2012;44(1):18–25.

[134] Pajno GB. Oral desensitization for milk allergy in children: state of the art. Curr Opin Allergy Clin Immunol. 2011;11(6):560–4.

[135] Takahashi M, Taniuchi S, Soejima K, Sudo K, Hatano Y, Kaneko K. New efficacy of LTRAs (montelukast sodium): it possibly prevents food-induced abdominal symptoms during oral immunotherapy. Allergy Asthma Clin Immunol. 2014;10(1):3.

[136] Fisher HR, du Toit G, Lack G. Specific oral tolerance induction in food allergic children: is oral desensitisation more effective than allergen avoidance?: a meta-analysis of published RCTs. Arch Dis Child. 2011;96(3):259–64.

[137] Nurmatov U, Venderbosch I, Devereux G, Fer S, Sheikh A. Allergen-specific oral immunotherapy for peanut allergy (Review). Cochrane Database Syst Rev. 2012;(9).

[138] Vázquez-Ortiz M, Alvaro-Lozano M, Alsina L, Garcia-Paba MB, Piquer-Gibert M, Giner-Muñoz MT, et al. Safety and predictors of adverse events during oral immunotherapy for milk allergy: severity of reaction at oral challenge, specific IgE and prick test. Clin Exp Allergy. 2013 Jan ;43(1):92–102.

[139] Rolinck-Werninghaus C, Staden U, Mehl A, Hamelmann E, Beyer K, Niggemann B. Specific oral tolerance induction with food in children: transient or persistent effect on food allergy? Allergy. 2005;60(10):1320–2.

[140] Martorell AragonésA, Félix Toledo R, Cerdá Mir JC, Martorell Calatayud A. Oral rush desensitization to cow milk. Following of desensitized patients during three years. Allergol et Immunopathol (Mad). 2007;35(5):174–6.

[141] Meglio P, Giampietro PG, Gianni S, Galli E. Oral desensitization in children with immunoglobulin E-mediated cow's milk allergy--follow-up at 4 yr and 8 months. Pediatr Allergy Immunol. 2008;19(5):412–9.

[142] Meglio P, Bartone E, Plantamura M, Arabito E, Giampietro PG. A protocol for oral desensitization in children with IgE-mediated cow's milk allergy. Allergy. 2004;59:980–7.

[143] Narisety SD, Skripak JM, Steele P, Hamilton RG, Matsui EC, Burks AW, et al. Open-label maintenance after milk oral immunotherapy for IgE-mediated cow's milk allergy. J Allergy Clin Immunol. 2009;124(3):610–2.

[144] Alvaro M, Giner MT, Vázquez M, Lozano J, Domínguez O, Piquer M, et al. Specific oral desensitization in children with IgE-mediated cow's milk allergy. Evolution in one year. Eur J Pediatr. 2012;171(9):1389–95.

[145] Staden U, Rolinck-Werninghaus C, Brewe F, Wahn U, Niggemann B, Beyer K. Specific oral tolerance induction in food allergy in children: efficacy and clinical patterns of reaction. Allergy. 2007 ;62:1261–9. http://onlinelibrary.wiley.com/doi/10.1111/j.1398-9995.2007.01501.x/full (Accesed 02 September 2014)

[146] Buchanan AD, Green TD, Jones SM, Scurlock AM, Christie L, Althage K a, et al. Egg oral immunotherapy in nonanaphylactic children with egg allergy. J Allergy Clin Immunol. 2007 Jan ;119(1):199–205.

[147] Staden U, Rolinck-Werninghaus C, Brewe F, Wahn U, Niggemann B, Beyer K. Specific oral tolerance induction in food allergy in children: efficacy and clinical patterns of reaction. Allergy. 2007 ;62:1261–9. http://onlinelibrary.wiley.com/doi/10.1111/j.1398-9995.2007.01501.x/full (Accesed 02 September 2014)

[148] Vickery BP, Scurlock AM, Kulis M, Steele PH, Kamilaris J, Berglund JP, et al. Sustained unresponsiveness to peanut in subjects who have completed peanut oral immunotherapy. J Allergy Clin Immunol. 2014;133(2):468–75.

[149] Holgate ST, Djukanović R, Casale T, Bousquet J. Anti-immunoglobulin E treatment with omalizumab in allergic diseases: an update on anti-inflammatory activity and clinical efficacy. Clin Exp Allergy. 2005;35(4):408–16.

[150] Prussin C, Griffith D, Boesel K, Lin H. Omalizumab treatment downregulates dendritic cell FcεRI expression. J Allergy Clin Immunol. 2003 ;112:1147–54.

[151] MacGlashan DW, Savage J. Suppression of the basophil response to allergen during treatment with omalizumab is dependent on 2 competing factors. J Allergy Clin Immunol. 2012 ;130(5):1130–5.

[152] MacGlashan DW, Saini SS. Omalizumab increases the intrinsic sensitivity of human basophils to IgE-mediated stimulation. J Allergy Clin Immunol. 2013;132(4):906–11.

[153] Beck LA, Marcotte GV, MacGlashan D, Togias A, Saini S. Omalizumab-induced reductions in mast cell Fce psilon RI expression and function. J Allergy Clin Immunol. 2004;114(3):527–30.

[154] Eckman JA, Sterba PM, Kelly D, Alexander V, Liu MC, Bochner BS, et al. Effects of omalizumab on basophil and mast cell responses using an intranasal cat allergen challenge. J Allergy Clin Immunol. 2010;125(4):889–95.

[155] Savage J, Courneya J. Kinetics of mast cell, basophil, and oral food challenge responses in omalizumab-treated adults with peanut allergy. J Allergy Clin Immunol. 2012;130(5):1123–9.

[156] EMEA. EPAR XOLAIR (DCI) Omalizumab EMEA© 2005. EMEA/H/C/606. :1–138. http://www.ema.europa.eu/docs/en_GB/document_library/EPAR_-_Product_Information/human/000606/WC500057298.pdf (Accesed 02 September 2014)

[157] Genentech. Xolair Label. :5–24. http://www.accessdata.fda.gov/drugsatfda_docs/label/2007/103976s5102lbl.pdf (Accesed 02 September 2014)

[158] Bousquet J, Wenzel S, Holgate S. Predicting Response to Omalizumab, an Anti-IgE Antibody, in Patients With Allergic Asthma.Chest. 2004;125:1378–86.

[159] Busse WW, Morgan WJ, Gergen PJ, Mitchell HE, Gern JE, Liu AH, et al. Randomized trial of omalizumab (anti-IgE) for asthma in inner-city children. N Engl J Med. 2011;364(11):1005–15. http://www.nejm.org/doi/full/10.1056/NEJMoa1009705 (Accesed 02 September 2014)

[160] Sorkness CA, Wildfire JJ, Calatroni A, Mitchell HE, Busse WW, O'Connor GT, et al. Reassessment of omalizumab-dosing strategies and pharmacodynamics in inner-city children and adolescents. J Allergy Clin Immunol Pract. 2013;1:163–71.

[161] Eigenmann PA. Future therapeutic options in food allergy. Allergy. 2003;58:1217–23.

[162] Morjaria JB, Polosa R. Off-label use of omalizumab in non-asthma conditions: new opportunities. Expert Rev Respir Med. 2009 ;3(3):299–308.

[163] Lieberman JA, Chehade M. Use of omalizumab in the treatment of food allergy and anaphylaxis. Curr Allergy Asthma Rep. 2013 ;13(1):78–84.

[164] Leung DYM, Sampson HA, Yunginger JW, Burks AW, Schneider LC, Wortel CH, et al. Effect of anti-IgE therapy in patients with peanut allergy. N Engl J Med. 2003;348(11):986–93. http://www.nejm.org/doi/full/10.1056/NEJMoa022613 (Accesed 02 September 2014)

[165] Sampson HA, Leung DYM, Burks AW, Lack G, Bahna SL, Jones SM, et al. A phase II, randomized, double blind, parallel group, placebo controlled oral food challenge tri-

al of Xolair (omalizumab) in peanut allergy. J Allergy Clin Immunol. 2011;127(5): 1309–10.

[166] Kuehr J, Brauburger J, Zielen S, Schauer U, Kamin W, Von Berg A, et al. Efficacy of combination treatment with anti-IgE plus specific immunotherapy in polysensitized children and adolescents with seasonal allergic rhinitis. J Allergy Clin Immunol. 2002;109(2):274–80.

[167] Rolinck-Werninghaus C, Hamelmann E, Keil T, Kulig M, Koetz K, Gerstner B, et al. The co-seasonal application of anti-IgE after preseasonal specific immunotherapy decreases ocular and nasal symptom scores and rescue medication use in grass pollen allergic children. Allergy. 2004;59(9):973–9.

[168] Massanari M, Nelson H, Casale T, Busse W, Kianifard F, Geba GP, et al. Effect of pretreatment with omalizumab on the tolerability of specific immunotherapy in allergic asthma. J Allergy Clin Immunol. 2010;125(2):383–9.

[169] Casale TB, Busse WW, Kline JN, Ballas ZK, Moss MH, Townley RG, et al. Omalizumab pretreatment decreases acute reactions after rush immunotherapy for ragweed-induced seasonal allergic rhinitis. J Allergy Clin Immunol. 2006;117(1):134–40.

[170] Nadeau KC, Kohli A, Iyengar S, DeKruyff RH, Umetsu DT. Oral immunotherapy and anti-IgE antibody-adjunctive treatment for food allergy. Immunol Allergy Clin North Am. 2012;32(1):111–33.

[171] Nadeau KC, Schneider LC, Hoyte L, Borras I, Umetsu DT. Rapid oral desensitization in combination with omalizumab therapy in patients with cow's milk allergy. J Allergy Clin Immunol. 2011;127(6):1622–4.

[172] Bedoret D, Singh A, Shaw V, Hoyte EG. Changes in antigen-specific T-cell number and function during oral desensitization in cow's milk allergy enabled with omalizumab. Mucosal Immunol. 2012 ;5(3):267–76. http://www.nature.com/mi/journal/v5/n3/abs/mi20125a.html (Accesed 02 September 2014)

[173] Schneider LC, Rachid R, LeBovidge J, Blood E, Mittal M, Umetsu DT. A pilot study of omalizumab to facilitate rapid oral desensitization in high-risk peanut-allergic patients. J Allergy Clin Immunol. 2013;132(6):1368–74.

[174] Bégin P, Dominguez T, Wilson SP, Bacal L, Mehrotra A, Kausch B, et al. Phase 1 results of safety and tolerability in a rush oral immunotherapy protocol to multiple foods using Omalizumab. Allergy Asthma Clin Immunol. 2014;10(1):7.

[175] Bégin P, Winterroth LC, Dominguez T, Wilson SP, Bacal L, Mehrotra A, et al. Safety and feasibility of oral immunotherapy to multiple allergens for food allergy. Allergy Asthma Clin Immunol. 2014;10(1):1.

[176] Cox L, Platts-Mills T a E, Finegold I, Schwartz LB, Simons FER, Wallace D V. American Academy of Allergy, Asthma & Immunology/American College of Allergy, Asth-

ma and Immunology Joint Task Force Report on omalizumab-associated anaphylaxis. J Allergy Clin Immunol. 2007;120(6):1373–7.

[177] Cox L, Lieberman P, Wallace D. American Academy of Allergy, Asthma & Immunology/American College of Allergy, Asthma & Immunology Omalizumab-Associated Anaphylaxis Joint Task Force Follow. J Allergy Clin Immunol. 2011;128(1):210–2.

[178] Long A, Rahmaoui A, Rothman KJ, Guinan E, Eisner M, Bradley MS, et al. Incidence of malignancy in patients with moderate-to-severe asthma treated with or without omalizumab. J Allergy Clin Immunol. 2014;(June 2004):In press.

[179] Noh G, Jang EH. Dual specific oral tolerance induction using interferon gamma for IgE-mediated anaphylactic food allergy and the dissociation of local skin allergy and systemic oral allergy: tolerance or desensitization? J Investig Allergol Clin Immunol. 2014;24(2):87–97.

[180] Pajno GB, Cox L, Caminiti L, Ramistella V, Crisafulli G. Oral Immunotherapy for Treatment of Immunoglobulin E-Mediated Food Allergy: The Transition to Clinical Practice. Pediatr Allergy Immunol Pulmonol. 2014;27(2):42-50.

Permissions

The contributors of this book come from diverse backgrounds, making this book a truly international effort. This book will bring forth new frontiers with its revolutionizing research information and detailed analysis of the nascent developments around the world.

We would like to thank all the contributing authors for lending their expertise to make the book truly unique. They have played a crucial role in the development of this book. Without their invaluable contributions this book wouldn't have been possible. They have made vital efforts to compile up to date information on the varied aspects of this subject to make this book a valuable addition to the collection of many professionals and students.

This book was conceptualized with the vision of imparting up-to-date information and advanced data in this field. To ensure the same, a matchless editorial board was set up. Every individual on the board went through rigorous rounds of assessment to prove their worth. After which they invested a large part of their time researching and compiling the most relevant data for our readers.

The editorial board has been involved in producing this book since its inception. They have spent rigorous hours researching and exploring the diverse topics which have resulted in the successful publishing of this book. They have passed on their knowledge of decades through this book. To expedite this challenging task, the publisher supported the team at every step. A small team of assistant editors was also appointed to further simplify the editing procedure and attain best results for the readers.

Apart from the editorial board, the designing team has also invested a significant amount of their time in understanding the subject and creating the most relevant covers. They scrutinized every image to scout for the most suitable representation of the subject and create an appropriate cover for the book.

The publishing team has been an ardent support to the editorial, designing and production team. Their endless efforts to recruit the best for this project, has resulted in the accomplishment of this book. They are a veteran in the field of academics and their pool of knowledge is as vast as their experience in printing. Their expertise and guidance has proved useful at every step. Their uncompromising quality standards have made this book an exceptional effort. Their encouragement from time to time has been an inspiration for everyone.

The publisher and the editorial board hope that this book will prove to be a valuable piece of knowledge for researchers, students, practitioners and scholars across the globe.

List of Contributors

Celso Pereira, Frederico S. Regateiro, Graça Loureiro, Beatriz Tavares and António Martinho
Clinic Immunology, Medicine Faculty, Coimbra University. Immunoallergology Department, Coimbra University Center Hospital. Blood and Transplantation Center of Coimbra / Portuguese Institute of Blood and Transplantation., Portugal

Rebecca Scherr
Division of Gastroenterology, Hepatology, and Nutrition, University of Nevada School of Medicine, Department of Pediatrics, USA

Mary Beth Hogan
Division of Allergy and Immunology, University of Nevada School of Medicine, Department of Pediatrics, USA

Abdulghani Mohamed Alsamarai, Mohamed Abdulsatar Hamid and Amina Hamed Ahmed Alobaidi
Tikrit University College of Medicine, Tikrit, Iraq

Elodie Neau, Marie-José Butel and Anne-Judith Waligora-Dupriet
EA 4065, DHU Risques et Grossesse, Faculté des Sciences Pharmaceutiques et Biologiques, Université Paris Descartes, Sorbonne Paris-Cité, France

Evgenia Bogomolova
Komarov Botanical Institute of the Russian Academy of Sciences, St. Petersburg, Russia

Olga Ukhanova
Department of Allergology-Immunology, Ministry of Medical Care of the Stavropol Territory, Stavropol, Russia

Ramla Hamed Ahmed Alobaidi
Al Mansour Constructive Company, Kirkuk, Iraq

Amina Hamed Ahmed Alobaidi
Tikrit University College of Medicine, Tikrit, Iraq

Abdulghani M. Alsamarai
Tikrit Teaching Hospital, Tikrit, Iraq

Lauren Folgosa Cooley
Center for Clinical and Translational Research (CCTR), Virginia Commonwealth University, Richmond, VA, USA
Department of Microbiology and Immunology, Virginia Commonwealth University, Richmond, VA, USA
Lauren Folgosa Cooley and Rebecca K. Martin equally contributed to the writing of this review

Daniel H. Conrad
Department of Microbiology and Immunology, Virginia Commonwealth University, Richmond, VA, USA

Rebecca K. Martin
Department of Microbiology and Immunology, Virginia Commonwealth University, Richmond, VA, USA
Lauren Folgosa Cooley and Rebecca K. Martin equally contributed to the writing of this review

José Manuel Lucas, Ana Moreno-Salvador and Luis García-Marcos
Pediatric Clinical Immunology and Allergy Unit, "Virgen de la Arrixaca" University Children's Hospital, University of Murcia, Murcia, Spain

Index